Elizabethan Dyetary of Health

Jane O'Hara-May

C/P

CORONADO PRESS   1977

ISBN 87291 074 1

Set in ten on twelve point Press Roman
Published by
Coronado Press
Box 3232
Lawrence, Kansas 66044

Manufactured in the USA

CONTENTS

*THE ELIZABETHAN
DYETARY OF HEALTH*

PREFACE

THERE ARE FEW aspects of Elizabethan life which have not been scrutinized during the progressive expansion of Elizabethan studies over the last twenty-five years. One field of study which has received little attention is that of medicine and within this area one aspect which has been overlooked is the mass of advice on the preservation of health, presented to the public in the vernacular printed books of the period. This material provides side lights on medical theory and social conditions and illuminates many attitudes of mind of the educated layman.

The Elizabethan Dyetary of Health is intended as an introduction to Elizabethan ideas about the preservation of health and as an introduction to this wide subject inevitably raises a number of points which need to be studied in greater depth. Probably the most important aspect which requires investigation is the English sixteenth century view of heat, while at the other end of the scale one might ask somewhat frivolously whether the Elizabethans really took cold baths?

The advice given by contemporary writers is not original but is derived from ancient teachings. The temptation to look backward from the sixteenth century has been resisted as far as possible. Expressions such as "The Elizabethans believed. . ." are used frequently in the text of this book but, in this context, do not imply that they were the first to hold the beliefs described.

The whole subject of the Elizabethan "Preservation of Health" with its particular emphasis on "Meats and Drinks," would today be covered by the combined disciplines of Nutrition and Hygiene. Much of the material in this study was submitted in a Ph.D. Thesis in the University of London and was intended as a starting point in a study of the history of nutrition. It is a pleasure to acknowledge the debt owed to Professor J. S. Wilkie of London University for his advice and interest in this work. I am much indebted to Dr. Edwin Clarke for his teaching on the development of medical theories and the benefits I have derived from association with the Sub-Department of the History of Medicine, University College, London. An invaluable guide to the general background of this study, including the work of Arabic writers, medieval ideas and sources, and a general historical perspective to Elizabethan thought, was provided by informal conversations with friends. My thanks go to Dr. Jean Cadden, Dr. A. Z. Iskandar, Dr. S. H. Mauskopf, Dr. Walter Pagel, Dr. C. H. Talbot and Miss Marianne Winder. Professor Jerry Stannard and Mrs. Antonia McLean have made helpful comments on sections of the text.

It is common practice to acknowledge the help received from libraries. In this case my recorded acknowledgements are certainly far from perfunctory. The Book List of primary sources indicates the debt I owe to the Superintendent and Staff of the British Museum, North Library for their courtesy and help. For the excellent facilities and help provided by the Wellcome Institute for the History of Medicine I am extremely grateful to the former Director and Librarian, Dr. F. N. L. Poynter and Mr. E. Gaskell. I thank most sincerely all the Staff of the Library for their enduring interest in this book and am particularly grateful to Mr. E. J. Freeman, Librarian, whose wide knowledge of late medieval medical manuscripts and sixteenth century printed books and orthography has been invaluable. For clarifying and cross referencing the Book List I am indebted to Mrs. H. J. M. Symons. Miss C. Tonson Rye kindly took care of the mechanics of revision. My final acknowledgement is one that any student of this period makes with very great gratitude; it is to Pollard and Redgrave, compilers of the *Short Title Catalogue of English Printed Books 1475-1640* and to all who compiled the *Oxford English Dictionary*.

QUOTATIONS AND REFERENCES

IN QUOTATIONS the spelling of the original text has been preserved but obsolete orthographic symbols have been modernized. The use of sixteenth century spelling has been retained in the modern text where the old meaning has a particular significance, e.g. physick. The use of "sic" has been avoided unless its omission would cause confusion.

Books referred to infrequently will be given in full at the first mention in each chapter; thereafter they will be indicated by the author's name plus (if necessary) an abbreviated title. Where translations, facsimiles or modern reprints are used the name of the original author is given as reference when his material is quoted. The editor's name is given when a comment on the work is referred to. The exception to this is the use of the reference "Batman" for the translation of and additions to the work of Bartholomaeus Anglicus.

Books referred to repeatedly can be identified by the following key:—

Aristotle:	W. D. Ross (ed.), *The Works of Aristotle* (Vols. I-XI), Oxford, 1908-1931.
Batman:	S. Batman, *Batman uppon Bartholome, his book de proprietatibus rerum,* London, 1582.
Boorde:	F. J. Furnivall (ed.), *The Fyrste Boke of the Introduction of Knowledge made by Andrew Borde,* London, 1870. (E.E.T.S. Extra Series No. X).
Bullein:	W. Bullein, *The Government of Health,* London, 1595.
Celsus:	W. G. Spencer, *Celsus de medicina* (Vol. I), London, 1935.
Cogan:	T. Cogan, *The Haven of Health,* London 1589.
DNB:	L. Stephen, *Dictionary of National Biography,* London, 1885.
Elyot:	T. Elyot, *The Castel of Helth* corrected, London, 1541. (British Museum shelf mark C112-b-23).
Emmison:	F. G. Emmison, *Tudor Secretary,* London, 1961.
Galen:	A. J. Brock, *Galen on the Natural Faculties,* London, 1916.

Galen (Daremberg):	C. H. Daremberg, *Oeuvres anatomique physiologiques et médicales de Galien,* Paris, 1854-56.
Galen (Kühn):	C. G. Kühn, *Opera Omnia Galeni,* Leipzig, 1821-33.
Galen (MTM):	M. T. May, *Galen on the usefulness of the parts of the body,* Ithaca, N.Y., 1968.
Gratarolus:	G. Gratarolus (trans. T. Newton), *A direction for the health of magistrates and students,* London, 1574.
GHH:	Anon, *The good Huswives handmaid,* n.p., n.d. (British Museum shelf mark 1037-e-1).
GHJ:	Thomas Dawson, *the good huswifes jewell,* London, 1596.
Harrison:	J. Furnivall (ed.), *Harrison's Description of England in Shakespeare's Youth,* London, 1877-1909.
Hippocrates:	W. H. S. Jones, *Hippocrates* (Vols. I and IV), London, 1923 and 1931.
Hippocrates (Littré):	E. Littré, *Oeuvres complètes d'Hippocrate* (Vols. I-X), Paris, 1839-1861.
Jones, *Bathes Ayde:*	J. Jones, *The Bathes of Bathes Ayde,* London, 1572.
Jones, *Body and Soul:*	J. Jones, *The Arte and Science of preserving Bodie and Soule,* London, 1579.
Jones, *Bucks baths:*	J. Jones, *The Benefit of the ancient Bathes of Buckstones,* London, 1572.
Jones, *Galen's Elements:*	J. Jones, *Galens Bookes of Elements,* London, 1574.
Jones, *Growing and Living:*	J. Jones, *A Briefe Excellent, and profitable Discourse, of the naturall beginning of all growing and living things. . .,* London, 1574.
Langton:	C. Langton, *An introduction into phisycke with an universal dyet,* London, 1550.
Langton, *Prin. parts:*	C. Langton, *A very briefe treatise ordrely declaring the principal parts of phisick,* London, 1547.
NHB:	T. Percy, *The Northumberland Household Book,* London, 1770.
OED:	*Oxford English Dictionary*
Regimen Sanitatis:	T. Paynell, *Regimen Sanitatis Salerni,* London, 1528.
WT	Anon., *The Widdowes Treasure,* London, 1595.

The choice of edition used depended upon the availability and condition of the book as well as its contents. Wherever possible the edition chosen was one that had appeared within the lifetime of the author.

Where Latin names have been assigned to plants according to the modern binominal system the information is from William Turner,

Libellus de Re Herbaria etc., Ray Society Facsimile edition, London, 1965.

Wherever possible and reasonable, reference has been made to English translations of ancient texts on the assumption that a number of modern readers, like their Elizabethan counterparts, are, in Cogan's words, "no good Latinistes."

PART I

CHAPTER I
INTRODUCTION

The excellence of the body is health; that is, a condition which allows us, while keeping free from disease, to have the use of our bodies for many people are 'healthy' as we are told Herodicus was; and these no one can congratulate on their 'health', for they have to abstain from everything or nearly everything that men do.

Aristotle *(Rhetorica)*

Health is the most beautiefull and rich present that Nature can bestow upon us, and above all other things to be preferred, not only Science, Nobility, Riches, but Wisdome it selfe, which the austerest amongst the wise doe affirme. It is the only thing that deserveth our whole imploiment, yea our life it selfe to attaine unto it; for without it life is no life, but a death.

P. Charron (trans. Lennard, 1606)

MAN'S CONCERN with his own health has never been confined to any particular place or period. The fact that there are extant today at least twenty different sixteenth century English books which contain the word "health" in their title, apart from many others on diet, is surely an indication that the literate Elizabethan's preoccupation with his health was probably as great as is our own.

In the sixteenth century it was considered that the physician had three instruments in physick. They were: Diet, Medicine, Surgery, and the most important of these was diet. This did not merely refer to food and drink but to the whole regimen or way of life of the individual: the air he breathed, the food he ate, his activities and emotions.

English medical theory at this time was firmly based on ancient teachings. Such was the attachment of the College of Physicians to Galenic writings that John Geynes was disciplined as late as 1560 for stating that "Galen had committed errors."[1] Errors of Galenism had already been accepted on the Continent but the ideas of Paracelsus came late to England. These new theories introduced the extra principals of sulphur,

N.B. Footnotes to this chapter appear on pages 299-300.

mercury and salt to the four Aristotelian elements. They also united more strongly than before neo-platonic cosmology (including its astrology) with alchemy. The overall philosophical effects of Paracelsian theories have been dealt with recently by Pagel, Wightman and Debus.[2] England did not feel the full impact of iatrochemical ideas until the seventeenth century, though Paracelsian doctrines in their practical application exaggerated factors which were already present in sixteenth century writings and did not introduce them as completely new factors. Alchemy had always had the search for health as one of its avowed aims.[3]

Today our concepts are biochemical, having been developed from basically new ideas postulated in the late eighteenth and early nineteenth centuries. We now recognise that energy is essential for life and that the warmth and movement of the body are manifestations of it. The bodily changes which produce the effects required for living are accepted as being physico-chemical changes. On the whole we take an optimistic view of evolutionary changes, believing that they lead toward improvements and we expect that the application of good dietary practices (by which we mean good eating habits) will help to extend man's expectation of life. The twentieth century scientific attitude demands a continuous re-evaluation of our theories and their application.

The Elizabethans differed from us in all these points. Unlike our continuous attempts to find the true answer Elizabethan physicians, with few exceptions, clung to the traditional concepts of ancient teachers. The general belief was that the truth, in so far as it was a proper subject for man to be concerned with, had already been ascertained and written down in the Scriptures and writings of ancient thinkers. This respect for ancient thought is related in part to the persistent belief, derived from Medieval times, that the world and man had been created perfect, had declined to a less perfect state and were slowly degenerating. The ancients were considered superior mentally and physically and because they were nearer to the original perfection, were better able to perceive the truth. Sixteenth century writers rarely felt at ease without the support of the authority provided by references to respected writers of the past.

The "grave menace" of astrology to religion as seen by Elizabethan clergy has been discussed by Kocher. Here the danger was seen to lie in the increase in Judicial Astrology.[4] Previously public forecasts according to the stars had been acceptable but the change taking place was towards private, individual forecasts which, as they became "more specific [were] more presumptious against mans free will and gods Providence."[5] Philosophically it was considered that the effect of the increased attention to astrology was an attack upon religion and the counter attack was naturally based on religious tenets.

The influence of the astrological herbalists was not great in the late sixteenth century and no significant reference to astrology in relation to diet has been found in the works studied. Arber has shown that the idea of astrological influences in relation to plants reached its height in England in the seventeenth century.[6]

The Elizabethan period is significant for medicine because it falls at the threshold of a time of great changes. Soon English medicine was to feel the real impact of Paracelsian theory and then of Harvey's revolutionary discovery — ideas which would eventually lead towards modern medicine. The place is significant because the new ideas did not have their full impact until after a sharp increase in the number of books printed in the vernacular. This has provided a large body of material in English based predominantly on ancient theories.

Christopher Langton, writing in the middle of the sixteenth century, makes it quite clear that he follows the Galenist school of thought, but divides physicians into three sects, namely:

(i) Empiricists. This sect included Thessalus and Cornelius Celsus.

(ii) Methodists. This sect included Erasistratus and Asclepiades.

(iii) Dogmatists. This sect included Hippocrates and Galen.[7]

These divisions are the traditional grouping, but Langton's general classification of individuals into these three sects does not always agree with the named individual's own view, or with that of modern commentators. Spencer[8] puts Cornelius Celsus between the Dogmatic and the Empiric schools: modern writers see a much more tenuous link between Erasistratus and the Methodists. Galen himself, in his *De sectis medicorum,*[9] criticizes all three sects and considers himself to be an Eclectic, though in most general terms of the three schools listed above he is nearest to the Dogmatists.

Langton describes the characteristics of the three schools of physick. These, in general terms, agree with Galen's views, and no attempt has been made here to present any detailed comparison. According to Langton:[10]

(i) *Empiricists* used experiments and abolished reason. They disregarded the importance of the time of year, climate, powers of the patient, age of the patient, characteristics of being weak or strong, hot or cold, dry or moist, "but thoughte that they might safelye venture that upon one, wyth the whych they had healed another in lyke disease."[11] That is, if they cured a disease in one patient by a certain method, they assumed the same treatment would suit another patient with the same symptoms.

(ii) *Methodists* disregarded the "place" (i.e. part of the body) affected, the cause of illness, age of the patient, time of year, climate, habit and the kind of life formerly led by the patient. They assumed that there were only two kinds of diseases, the one due to the stopping of the pores, the other caused by too much opening of the same.

This group condemned Hippocrates because he said that "physike was a longe arte and that mans lyfe was very short."[12] They believed the opposite and said that if the "superfluities" were removed, physick could be learnt in six months. This school of thought rejected the ideas of the Empiricists and believed that there was no profit to be gained from experience until the virtues and effects of medicines and remedies were known directly and *per se*. Their knowledge of remedies was based on information obtained through their senses. Langton says that the Empiricists believed that "it is not possible to fynde any remedye or medicyne, by diligent markynge, seing that all remedyes, be gathered of suche thinges as be evident to the sense."[13]

(iii) *Dogmatists*, to which group Langton and most sixteenth century physicians belonged, are said by Langton to join experience to reason. They considered very carefully both the obvious and the obscure courses of disease. They thought the condition of the air, water and region where the patient lived was important.[14] They considered the accustomed diet (in its fullest sense) of the patient and compared past and present conditions and habits. The Dogmatists believed they must know the powers and virtues of the medicines they used, believing that these powers could be "proved and improved" if the physician was properly trained. To be properly trained a physician must know anatomy and have practical experience in dissection besides acquiring a knowledge of logic, philosophy, astronomy, mathematics and arithmetic. Langton particularly stresses that diagnosis must not be made from an examination of urine alone without an examination of the patient, as it appears some were wont to do.[15]

Writing on nutrition from Classical Antiquity to the Baroque, Temkin starts his paper with the words "Nutrition and medical ideas on nutrition cannot be independent of the style of living."[16] Similarly the conditions in sixteenth century England influenced the theoretical advice given on the preservation of health and, of course, the application of these theories. English records of the sixteenth century give a wealth of information about the nobility, the well-to-do and their employees. Information about groups of the poor is harder to find. These groups will have been very much affected by changes in harvests and the economic situation. Modern historians of Agriculture have shown that there was a general improvement in the economic conditions for farming in the latter part of the century.[17] However, in terms of what was available for the people, this must have been counterbalanced by the sequence of dearths which occurred in the 1590s.

Jordan, discussing the problem of poverty in that period, refers to the previous critical state of want and starvation in England in 1480, but is confident that there was "no real increase in poverty in England during the sixteenth century. He suggests that the illusion of the increase in poverty, at this time, was fostered by men addressing themselves "with such persistence, such eloquence, and on occasion with such exaggeration to a great social problem,"[18] and that the cure itself was close at hand. The shaping of society was being taken into men's own hands and they were beginning to build it to a pattern supplied by their own aspirations. That the Authorities attempted to alleviate the conditions of the poorer sections of society is obvious from the many regulations which were intended to deal with the social problems of the poor. These ranged from the new Poor Law Statutes and the Statute of Artificers, to the attempted control of prices in London markets. The recognition that the community is responsible for its weaker members in time of stress is illustrated by the regulations provided in time of pestilence.*

The imagination and initiative, for which the Elizabethans are famous in many spheres is singularly lacking in works of medicine and allied fields. As will be seen, advice on the preservation of health followed the Galenic texts very closely, this information being reconciled wherever possible with Biblical texts. The summary of Elizabethan advice, presented here, does not convey adequately the sense of the all pervading will of God in men's lives which is apparent in the Elizabethan texts.

Galen's physiology, which played such a large part in sixteenth century thought, was rooted in philosophical concepts.[19] He accepted the Empedoclean doctrine of the four elements (air, fire, water and earth) but depended, for his interpretation of this doctrine, on the writings of Hippocrates and Aristotle. The four elements embodied the four quali-

---

*See Chapter VII.

ties of hot, cold, moist and dry. Everything contained a proportion of each element, and therefore each quality, but was characterized by the predominance of certain qualities. Corresponding to these elements and qualities were four essential humours of the body namely, blood, yellow bile, black bile and phlegm. Galen believed that the bodily parts and their actions resulted from various combinations of these four elements or qualities or humours. The precise proportions in which the qualities were combined was very important and a proper *crasis,* or blending of temperament, produced health; an improper blending caused ill-health. Galen attributed the varying characteristics of individuals to various admixtures of the four qualities. The present interpretation of the names sanguine, choleric, melancholy and phlegmatic are Arabic rather than Galenic.

Linked to these ideas was Galen's fundamental acceptance of the Platonic idea of three souls ruling yet serving the body. These souls were placed in the brain, heart and liver; reasoning thought, sensation and motion were controlled by the *rational soul,* in the brain; the passions by the *vital soul,* in the heart; what is now called nutrition and metabolism, by the *vegetative soul* in the liver. These three souls were regarded as different phases or divisions of one soul which inhabited the body. Serving the soul are *pneumas*[20] or spirits, the source of which is inspired air. This is a complex concept inherited and altered by Galen, who stressed two pneumas, though some later Galenists accepted the third "natural pneuma" or spirit.

Each division of the soul is endowed with a special power (which is sometimes termed a faculty). Besides these faculties each part of the body had the ability to attract, hold or expel nutriment appropriate to them, through the attractive, retentive, and expulsive faculties respectively. Galen himself was aware of the multiplication of faculties and said "so long as we are ignorant of the true essence of the cause which is operating we call it a faculty . . ."[21]

The preservation of life depended upon an adequate amount of innate heat, the loss of which led to death. Galen believed that the heat of the living body was not acquired after generation but was "primegenial and innate,"[22] and was, to say the least, the first instrument of the soul. Galen was not able to explain, or give an adequate description of this heat, but believed that it was found in its most intense and pure form in the heart and that it gave support and protection to the whole body.

Heat also played an important part in digestion and concoction. In his description of the changes food underwent before it could provide nourishment for the body, Galen used two illuminating analogies. The first was the preparation of wheat for and by the public baker, the second was the fermentation of wine. The changes in foods took place through a series of concoctions. The first occurred in the stomach; here unwanted parts of the food were thrust on by the stomach, just as in the case of wheat being cleaned and the earth and stones removed. The remaining material in the stomach was "improved" and turned into chyle. Just as cleaned wheat then went to a public baker, so the chyle went to be further concocted in the liver for the benefit of the whole body.

In the liver the chyle became blood, but still required further cleansing from impurities. The fine thin residue, like the "flower" on the top of light wines, went to the gall-bladder. The heavier residue, like the dregs of wine, went to the spleen. The remaining blood in the liver still contained a watery fluid called by Hippocrates "the vehicle of nutrition."[23] This fluid was drawn through the veins to all parts of the body by the attractive faculty. It was retained and altered into the part, as appropriate, or passed on. When this work was completed the thin fluid was expelled through the kidneys by the expulsive faculty.

In describing the use of the intestines Galen explained that when chyle from the stomach escaped into the intestines *anadosis*[24] takes place with the result that material passed into the veins, and "No juice useful for nourishment escapes and passes out of the animal."[25] The idea of the movement of residues back to the stomach from the liver is referred to by sixteenth century writers. May comments on the basis of this idea in her lengthy discussion of the washing back and forth of the blood.[26]

Galen believed that the foetus was formed from a mixture of male semen, female semen[27] and blood furnished by the mother. Both semina had the material and efficient faculties. The liver was formed from the thickest venous blood, the heart was formed around the arteries, and the brain from the semen. Galen contradicts himself in different works in describing the order in which these organs were formed, but in *De foetuum formation*[28] gave the order as liver, heart, and then brain. This disagrees with the Aristotelian view.[29] The chief actions of the foetus, according to Galen, were generation, growth and nutrition presided over by the generative, augmentative and nutritive faculties. The nutritive faculty itself was comprised of the faculties of attraction, retention, concoction and expulsion.[30] Galen considered *genesis* to be the result of alteration together with shaping. Growth and the nutritive faculty were present *in utero* but these two faculties were considered to be like "handmaidens" to genesis. After the animal was completely formed and during the period following its birth until the acme of growth was reached, the faculty of growth predominated and the alterative and nutritive faculties were accessory. Galen recognized that growth could not occur "without the nutriment which flows into the part and is worked up into it."[31] Nutrition, caused by the nutritive faculty, was a form of alteration. This was a different alteration from that of genesis. In nutrition the "inflowing material becomes assimilated to that which has already come into existence" and so the alteration due to nutrition was called assimilation.[32]

The importance of food in Galen's regimen for health, either as "meat" or medicine, cannot be over-emphasized. Not only does he describe the attributes of different foods at length in *De alimentorum facultatibus*[33] but references to the value of foods to be taken under different circumstances are found throughout his medical works, as in, for example, *De simplicium medicamentorum temperamentis et facultatibus.*[34]

In estimating the value of food, two objectives of healthy living were, the proper replacement of waste and the elimination of excrements. Galen not only considered the proportion of primary qualities (hot, cold, moist, dry) present in foods but also such characteristics as colour, taste, hardness, softness, density, their ease of digestion, tendency to putrification, the natural waste material present in the food and the purging or oppilative effects on the body.

In recommending foods for individuals, all these characteristics had to be considered in relation to the condition of the individual for whom they were to be prescribed, all this within a framework of what the Elizabethans called the "things non-natural."*

---

*See Chapter V.

CHAPTER II
CHANNELS OF INFORMATION

For dyvers pregnaunt wytts be in this lande
As well of noble men as of meane estate whiche
          nothynge but englyshe can understande
Than yf connynge laten bokys were translate
In to englyshe wel correct and approbate
All subtell sciens in englysh myght be lernyd.

Rastell (c. 1520)

. . . for I confesse that I have taken *Verbatim* out of others where it served my purpose, and especially out of *Sch. Salerni*: but I have so interlaced it with mine owne, that (as I thinke) it may be better perceived.

Thomas Cogan (1584)

THE PRODUCTION of popular treatises in the vernacular was not new. Alfred the Great had encouraged the translation of theological, historical and physiological works into Anglo-Saxon, and a large portion of the translations of classical medical texts, by unknown hands, had been incorporated into the Leech books.[1] The use of the material in the vernacular continued until the coming of William the Conqueror. Being in positions of authority and knowing only their own language and Latin, the Normans arrested the continuation of translations into Anglo-Saxon, and even reversed the process by having some manuscripts in the vernacular translated into Latin.[2] Documents for instruction of those unacquainted with Latin were available from an early period in English history. T. Wright points out that ". . . science was not concealed from the unlearned. . . . Our forefathers at all times published treatises for the uninitiated."[3] These works, he says, show both the methods of popularizing instruction and the quantity of information thought necessary. He gives as examples a tenth century work on Astronomy (in Anglo-Saxon), a twelfth century Bestiary (Anglo-French), and a *Lives of the Saints,* including a section on physiology, written in English

---

N.B. Footnotes to this chapter appear on pages 300-305.

during the reign of Edward I (1272-1307). A more recent description of
this type of literature is given in the *Cambridge Bibliography of English
Literature,* which illustrates the continual growth in the quantity of
vernacular material.

The marked increase in the use of the English language for all literary
purposes (including instructional and scientific), in the second half of
the fourteenth century, can be seen from collections such as the Sloane
Manuscript Collection in the British Museum. O'Malley has shown that
the sixteenth century texts of Thomas Geminus' "Compendius Anatomy" and Vicary's *Treatise of the Anatomie of Man's Bodie,*[4] are related
to a late fourteenth century English manuscript on anatomy based on
the works of Lanfranc and Henri de Mondeville.[5] Besides these a number of alchemical and plague texts written before the sixteenth century
– in Latin and the vernacular – have been catalogued by Dorothy
Singer.[6]

A large proportion of the books printed in English in the sixteenth
century were concerned with religion, but the number on "science" was
growing. In the second half of the century the production of medical
and allied books increased greatly when compared with the first half.[7]
By this time experience had shown the book trade that there was a
steady demand for English books setting out the basic rules of hygiene
and the dietary, or making observations and providing precepts necessary to the prolonging of life. The public wanted books of reasonable
size which they could understand and turn to in time of trouble.

It is impossible to determine the number of books actually printed
and sold. Though legal limits in the form of licences had been set for
the numbers of books permitted to be printed for each edition,[8] these
limits were certainly exceeded. Some indication is given by booksellers
complaining that their patents to print a given title had been infringed.
John Day complained to the Star Chamber in 1582, saying that this
patents had been infringed and ten thousand copies of the *ABC with a
little Catechism* had been printed by Roger Ward, who admitted the
offence.[9] This work was one of the most popular and numbers would
be greater than for other types of books but the quantity of books
involved does indicate that printings were not small.

Readership of the books

There is no reliable information as to what proportion of the population could read in sixteenth century England. There is abundant
evidence that in the fifteenth century the ability to read and write was

no longer confined to the clerical class. The wives and sisters of country gentlemen could commonly read and write as well as the male members of the family.[10] Frequently servants were required to keep accounts, and merchants and their employees needed at least to be able to read in order to transact their business.[11]

The Act of 1543 "For the advancement of true religion and the abolition to the contrarie" forbade the reading of the Bible in English by various groups. These included: women (excluding noble and gentlewomen), artificers, apprentices, journeymen, serving men (of the rank of yeoman and under), husbandmen and labourers. The range of people listed in this Act indicates that the authorities recognized that the ability to read was widespread. The Act also forbade the reading aloud of the Bible in English by certain people to various groups; only noblemen, gentlemen and merchants might read it to their families.[12]

In his study of Elizabethan middle-class culture, Louis B. Wright points out that from the middle of the sixteenth century the ordinary citizen was showing an increasing interest in school learning. This tendency was encouraged by the increased movement towards secular responsibility for education.[13] Adamson concludes that English society of the sixteenth century was by no means illiterate and that facilities for rudimentary instruction, at least, were so distributed as to reach even small towns and villages.[14]

The position regarding literacy in other languages was naturally different. In the sixteenth century Latin was a language of the educated and was taught in the grammar schools. However, lack of use produced many a "poor Latinist" as can be seen from certain alterations Cogan made in the third issue of his *Haven of Health* of 1589 (1st edition 1584). He explains "To the Reader" that he has altered the first edition as a result of "the request of divers of my friendes, which being no good Latinists could not well wade in the reading of my booke by reason of much Latin."[15] In fact, this refers mainly to a number of Latin quotations of which he left only a few Latin verses for "them that be Latinists." Greek was also taught in some schools, and French was known to the nobility and many of the merchant class. Erondell's French language handbook, published in 1605, is a remarkable source of information about contemporary everyday behaviour. There was some knowledge of Italian, a printed Italian grammar appearing in 1550.

Type of books available

Some idea of the range of vernacular books related to the dietary can be seen from the titles listed in the Book List of Primary Sources. Only a brief comment is given here. Regardless of source, works related to advice on the diet can be grouped in a very general way as follows:

(a) *Books on the preservation and restoration of health.* Comprehensive books on the diet or regimen for preserving health contained sections on (i) the theory required by an individual to enable him to understand his needs related to his particular physical characteristics e.g. to his complexion, age, occupation and habits, and (ii) information about external influences, particiularly in relation to the "non-naturals" with emphasis on the value of different foods and drinks.

Elyot's *Castel of Helth* and G. Gratarolus' work translated by T. Newton are examples which cover the whole range of information.[16] Some authors like Langton put emphasis on theory with little information about foods,[17] while Buttes gives information about foods with no "theory."[18] Most books on diet fall somewhere between these two extremes.

Books dealing with the restoration of health or the regimen in sickness contained mainly descriptions of conditions and recipes or prescriptions for their treatment. Sometimes a book on health and a book on treatment were written to be supplementary to one another, as in the case of Andrew Boorde's *A compendyous regyment or a dyetary of helth* (London, 1542) and his *The breviary of Helthe* (London, 1547). Here the author includes a number of cross references from one book to the other.

(b) *Books on husbandry, cookery and advice to housewives or householders.* A wide variety of types of books come under this heading. Most do not give direct advice on the choice of diet or regimen, but refer to it indirectly. These books lack theoretical information but give practical advice about husbandry and the use of foods and the ordering of the household. An early cookery book, called *A Proper Newe Booke of Cokerye*[19] (the title is open to a number of different spellings) contains only recipes and menus. *The householders philosophie*[20] gives advice on the ordering of the household, and *The treasurie of commodius conceites and hidden secrets*[21] gives snippets of information on a large range of subjects connected with the family and the running of the home. This sort of book can be traced in a direct line to the "Domestic Medicine" and "Home Encyclopaedias" of today.

Bennett estimates that many books published in the first half of the sixteenth century were constantly in demand in the second half and made up about one third of the total output at that time. Elyot's *Castel of Helth,* first printed in the fifteen-thirties, had gone through twelve editions by 1595. Books were often reprinted when more than sixteen years old; they survived not because of amendments, but because they contained what the public needed in a form that could be understood.

It is reasonable to assume that it was possible, in the last half of the sixteenth century, for some knowledge of dietary ideas to reach a comparatively large number of people. This assumption is based on the range and increasing number of books in the vernacular, the variety of people able to read them, the possible dissemination of information through such channels as the Housewife reading to her household, the Merchant to his apprentices and the ever present curiosity of people to hear things which might be to their advantage. This is supported by the wide interest and knowledge shown by poets and dramatists in dietaries.[22] It follows that this interest and some knowledge of diet must also have been held by their audiences.

Authors of works in English

The impression has sometimes been given that "good doctors" only wrote in Latin, never in the vernacular. This is certainly not the case. In the sixteenth century the great John Caius had translated a number of theological works into English before he decided, for reasons given below, not to use English for learned works again. He broke this rule with an English and a Latin work on the sweating sickness *(sudor anglicus)* only because the subject was particularly relevant to English people.[23] The reasons Caius gave for neglecting the vernacular were:

Firstly, the readership of the book would be restricted to England.

Secondly, the effort put into the work would be only half appreciated by "them whiche sette not by learnyng."

Thirdly, a learned man is often forced to disagree with the popular view, and it was better to avoid "the judgement of the multitude."

Fourthly, because of the foolish things printed in English, learned material in the vernacular would be debased.

Lastly, he did not wish to set his countrymen an example by writing in the vernacular because they needed a knowledge of other languages to maintain their standard of learning.[24]

These are Caius' personal views. Others felt more strongly about the matter, and untold dangers were forecast if learned works were put, through translation, into the hands of ordinary people. Opposition came from what might be called "scholarly circles." The basis of antagonism seems to have been the danger of professional secrets getting into the wrong hands and the belief that the status of both author and works would be lowered. Robert Burton complained in the introduction to *Anatomy of Melancholy*, that it had not been his intention "to prostitute my muse in English" and after having his Latin rejected, added rather peevishly, "Any scurrile pamphlet is welcome in English."[25] Much of the dislike of the vernacular was based on its supposed crudeness and on the belief that aesthetically Latin was superior to English. The need of an explanation and justification for the use of the vernacular was felt well into the seventeenth century.

The main argument for the use of English was that the ancients had written in *their* own tongue, e.g. Greek or Arabic, and therefore English for the English was acceptable. Besides, others in France and Italy wrote in their own language.[26] William Turner actively supported the use of the vernacular, dismissing the supposed dangers in these terms:

> ... if they [foreign authors] writing in their own tongue gave no occasyon unto every old wyfe to practise physicke than I give none. If they give no occasyon of murther then I gyve none.[27]

On the other side of the coin we find Langton complaining, quite irritably, at the slackness of English doctors in not finding an English word to use instead of cerebellum![28]

Turner was not the only man of repute who advocated the use of English. Thomas Newton in his translation, *The Olde man's Dietarie* (1586), discussed other works he had translated out of Latin, argued for the English language for the English, and acknowledged

> The great benefit and furtheraunce that wee still enjoye by the painfull pennes and English treatises of many our owne Countrymen, as well in Phisicke as Chyrurgerie.

He lists the following names, adding thereafter, "and some others, whose works I either have not yet seene, or at this present come not to remembrance."[29]

Knight Sir Thomas Eliot*	Master Lyte
Master Doctor Turner	Master Carye
Master Doctor Record	Master Coxe
Master Doctor Phaer	Master Hill
Master Doctor Cunningham	Master Gale

---

*English works by these authors are given in the Book List of Primary Sources. Hill is not definitely identified.

Master Doctor Bulleyn	Master Baker
Master Doctor Caldwell	Master Banister
Master Doctor Johnson	Master Hall
Master Doctor Jones	Master Clowes
Master Doctor Boord	Master Moore
Master Traheron	Master Paynell
Master Bright	Master Vicars [Vicary]
Master Barowe	Master Hester
Master Securis	Master B[r]asebridge

This is an impressive list of well respected men of the period up to 1586. Even so it is incomplete, omitting such well known physicians as Thomas Cogan and Christopher Langton.

An idea of the background of the writers and the level of their work can be obtained from an examination of some of the reasons given for the preparation of these books.

Sir Thomas Elyot's *Castel of Helth* was intended as an aid for the layman to understand his condition and so indirectly to help physicians in their diagnosis. Sir Thomas was not himself a qualified physician and, he tells his readers in later editions, the work was not too well received by the medical profession though otherwise it was very popular and frequently imitated.

Andrew Boorde claimed that he wanted to reach the unlearned with his *Breviary of Helth.* Here the word unlearned means not learned, deeply read or erudite and not "without learning." Other authors such as Newton in his translation (from Gratarolus) of *A Direction for the Health of Magistrates and Studentes* clearly aimed at a lay readership, though from the content of the book the reader was expected to be a person of intelligence and education.

Timothy Bright, in his *A Treatise wherein is declared the sufficiency of English medicines*, expressed his object in the title, while his *Treatise of Melancholie containing the causes thereof* was written to comfort and reassure a friend suffering from the condition. Besides trying to raise the standard of practitioners in physick Henry VIII had also encouraged the Barber-Surgeons to improve their situation. The four surgeons — Banister, Clowes, Gale, and Vicary — all had this object in view with their vernacular publications. Richard Caldwell had his translation of Morus' surgical work printed with the Latin and English texts opposite one another. Gale had found his Latin inadequate for the preparation of *Certain works of Chirurgerie* and the translation from the Latin of Vigo was undertaken by his friend Dr. Cunningham. Physicians, as might be expected, were on the whole better at Latin than the surgeons, Dr. Christopher Johnson being "reckoned as the most elegant Latin poet of his time,"[30] though he of course was exceptional.

John Securis, following the trend of his time, laid down rules for the education and conduct of physicians, surgeons and apothecaries in his *Detection of abuses committed in physick* in an attempt to improve the standard of medical men.

Henry Lyte, the botanist, translated the *Newe Herball or Historie of Plantes* from the French version of Rembert Dodoen's original Dutch work. Lyte explained in the introduction that he undertook the translation because he believed "Bonum quo communius, eo melius et praestantius: a good thing the more common it is the better it is." Also he wished to put the information at the disposal of the lowliest of his countrymen. However, according to William Ram this big book became too costly for poor people and, what was claimed to be a shortened version was published in 1606, under the title *Ram's little Dodoen.*[31] Barlow, however, dismisses this later book as nothing more than a book of recipes, unworthy of being associated with the name of Dodoens who was a leading authority on plants.[32]

Philip Moore, who practised physick and surgery in Suffolk also wished to disseminate a knowledge of medicinal herbs among the poor through his *The Hope of Health.* George Baker had published the *Oleum Magistrale* in 1574; this contained Galen's book on the "curing of pricks and wounds of Sinowes," one of a number of translations made of Galen's works. Two years later Baker published his translation of Gesner's work as *The Newe Jewell of Health,* the most advanced treatise on the chemical preparation of medicines printed in English up to that time. Baker explained that it was for the good of the nation as a whole that knowledge should be widely spread and that information on distilled medicines could be of benefit to individuals. He clearly states that in order to understand his book the reader required a knowledge of the works of Hippocrates and Galen, not then readily available in English. In this book Baker recommended three skilful apothecaries – Kemech, Geffroy and John Hester. Recently Kocher has described Hester's lone defense of Paracelsian ideas in England. Though much of Hester's translations from other languages were of practical advice, Kocher points out that,

by translating from *Centum quindecim curationes* the anti-Galenic polemical prefaces of Bernardus Georgius Penotus, the French Paracelsian, Hester gave to English readers their first large dose of Paracelsian theory.[33]

It is clear that not all books were prepared on a comparatively simple level as can be seen from the fact that Paracelsian theory can hardly be called simple in any language; the translations of Galen's works included the "theoretical" *Methodus Medendi*[34] and the availability of works of the calibre of Blundeville's *The Arte of Logicke plainly taught according to the doctrine of Aristotle.*[35] This despite John Caius' comments in his books on the sweating sickness, where he said that he "finished one boke in Englishe, onely for Englishe men not learned, one then in latine for men of learninge more at large."[36]

Background sources for English writers

It can be seen that most of the authors consulted would have had the usual education of their time, enlarged perhaps by the fashion of travelling on the Continent. Whatever the background of author or translator the basic sources of information related to diet and health were the same for all Renaissance Europe and were derived from ancient texts. Talbot has described the way in which the works of important scientific writers of antiquity became available to scholars in western Europe.[37] This was through a number of translations, first into Syriac and then into Arabic, under the guidance of Hunaim ibn Ishaq* and his disciples. These texts with additional material from leading Arab physicians, such as Avicenna, were then translated into Latin in the eleventh and twelfth centuries through the efforts of scholars such as Constantine the African and Gerard of Cremona. The ideas contained in these writings were spread through the wide influence of the schools of Salerno and Montpellier[38] and in the sixteenth century many of these works were retranslated from manuscripts in the original Greek,[39] thus giving more precise versions.

Below are suggested the main channels and basic sources of information for English writers on health.

1. The Bible. Very great use was made of the Old Testament. The English printed translation became available generally in 1539.[40] The restrictions on its use were not likely to affect the authors under consideration.

---

*(809-873 A.D.). The Westernized version is Honain ben Isaac, the Latinized form being Joanittius.

2. The works of Hippocrates, Galen, and Aristotle. Some of the works
of the Hippocratic school had long been available in garbled Latin translations. The finding of a manuscript of Celsus' *De Medicina* in 1443
provided an opportunity of studying the best side of Hippocratic medicine from a more authoritative source. The work of Thomas Linacre in
the period 1517-1524 provided a direct translation from Greek to Latin
of some of Galen's works. This material was used by Elyot. That a large
number of translations of Galen's works were undertaken at that period
can be seen from Durling's "Chronological census of Renaissance editions and translations of Galen."[41]

Another influential work reflecting much of Galen's works is *De
Natura Hominis Liber,* said to be written by the Bishop of Emesa
(c.A.D. 400).   The material is not purely medical or ethical but religious and spiritual. It combines philosophy about the interaction of the
body and soul with some description of medical theory. Originally written in Greek, it was printed in Latin by Plantin at Antwerp in 1564. It
was not available in an English edition until it was translated by George
Withers in 1636.[43]

In the sixteenth century English translators were attracted to Aristotle's writings on Logic more than to any other branch of his work.[44]
Thorndike has commented on the pseudo-Aristotelian books printed at
that time.[45] A common example was *Secreta Secretorum,* which was
reprinted through later centuries, the material and illustrations being
adapted to the period. A seventeenth century version includes a charming frontispiece of Aristotle in the dress of an Elizabethan cleric.

3. The works of Arab and Jewish authorities. Reference has been
made to the translations of the eleventh and twelfth centuries. English
writers on diet in the sixteenth century referred frequently to the Latin
translations from Rhazes, Avicenna and Averroes. Constantine the
African's translations of works on diet by Isaac Judaeus were available
in printed books, and a Latin version of Avicenna's *Canon of Medicine*
was published in Venice in 1524. Much material from these sources was
incorporated into the *Articella.*

4. The Articella. This work was a basic part of the medical curriculum
from medieval times, and it continued to be used well into the seventeenth century. Talbot has shown that in the middle of the twelfth
century there was a discernible change in the character of the writings
from the School of Salerno. This was probably brought about by the

production of works for teaching purposes with a movement from practical manuals toward theoretical treatises intended for the instruction of students. A manuscript of the time shows that the teaching texts contained a set of commentaries which later came to be called the *Articella*.[46] The main items usually included in medieval manuscripts of the *Articella* were:

Johannitius	*Isagog e ad Tegni Galeni*
Philaretus	*De pulsibus*
Hippocrates	*Prognostica*
	Liber de regimine actuorum
Theophilus Protcspartharius	*De urinis*
Galen	- *Ars parva*

Many variations of contents can be found, and possibly some additions included the pseudo-Aristotelian work *Secreta Secretorum* and the *Antidotarium* of Rhazes. These are present in a number of fourteenth century manuscripts. In addition to the basic works referred to above, printed editions of the sixteenth century included extracts from Celsus, Avicenna, Mesuë the Elder (d. 857) and Arnald of Villanova.* The manuscript Latin text was freely available in England, and a number of copies were printed in the late fifteenth century. The first printed edition was by N. Petri in Padua about 1476. In the sixteenth century the printing of the *Articella* spread to many parts of Europe.

5. Regimen Sanitatis Salernitanum. This Latin poem is usually called "Regimen Sanitatis Salernitanum," but there are a number of variations, e.g. "Schola Salernitana" or "De Conservanda Valetudine" or "Flos Medicinae." It is believed that the text was originally limited to the subject of dietetics.[48] It is said to have been written for "The king of the English," Robert II, son of William the Conqueror, which would place the date of its composition around the end of the eleventh century.

The author[49] is traditionally John of Milan, who is supposed to have been head of the faculty of medicine at Salerno when the poem was written. The original text is said to have contained some 362 lines. Sir Norman Moore refers to a number of manuscript copies in England, one

---

*The list of the contents printed by J. Myt for C. Fradin in Lyons in 1519 is given at the end of this chapter.

containing about 1,400 lines.[50] The number of manuscript copies made
of the original and of the variations was enormous. Moore concludes
that by the reign of Henry III (1216-1272) it must have been familiar
to any educated person interested in health.

The most important early commentator on the poem was Arnald of
Villanova who was familiar with the original poem and indicated in his
commentary any additions he had made. The first printing was at Montpellier in 1480[51] and the first printed translation into English (by
Thomas Paynell) appeared in 1528.[52] Paynell retained the poem in
Latin but translated the commentary into English. This version went
through a number of editions, the last with Paynell's name being in
1597. Thomas Phayer translated the French version of J. Goevrot into
English in 1544.[53] William Withye made a translation into English verse
in 1575.[54] Both the poem and commentary were translated into English
by Philemon Holland in 1617.[55] Sir John Harrington's well known ren-
dering without commentary appeared in 1607.[56]

Elyot cites the dedication as being proof that medicine was well
respected in England. He says:

> It semith that physicke in this realme hath ben well estemid . . . sens
> the hole studye of Salerne [was prepared] at the request of a Kynge
> of England.[57]

This seems a somewhat grandiose claim when the comments of later
writers are considered. Packard, after a study of previous authorities,
describes the "Regimen — as a handbook of domestic medicine. It was
not intended for the medical profession, but for the guidance of lay-
men. . ."[58] Its merits were such that it was copied many times and
translated into many languages. All translations bear the same characteristics as the English version, namely that of a series of wise maxims,
written in plain language, on the care of the health. The number and
variety of translations indicate that the work was of practical value. A
manuscript of a Gaelic version dated as early sixteenth century or before is believed to have belonged to John McBeath, one of the family of
hereditary physicians to the Lords of the Isles and Kings of Scotland.[59]

Another link with Salerno, which illustrates the continuity of thought
between the Middle Ages and the Renaissance, is discussed in Brian
Lawn's *The Salernitan Questions* (1963). He contends that the use of
questions for conveying information was of pre-Salernitan origin and
that the influence of this type of question was particularly strong in
England. The range of questions listed is wide. Examples related to diet

are: What makes the East wind warm and the West increasingly cold? How is it that milk or fish is changed into nourishment? Why is it that pepper and mustard applied externally hurt the skin but are harmless if swallowed?[60] The question-answer approach is not used in the *Regimen Sanitatis* itself though a number of sixteenth century vernacular books on health use the dialogue form to instruct their readers.[61]

6. **Encyclopaedias.** With a growth in literacy the demands for information increased. Information was wanted on practical everyday matters. The manuscript writers had begun long before to gather storehouses of information, in forms we might call encyclopaedias, and the printers continued this task of producing anything from large folio encyclopaedias to small pamphlets.

An outstanding work of this nature was *De Proprietatibus Rerum* by Bartholomaeus Anglicus. This work includes material as varied as that dealing with the nature of God, the properties of the soul, infirmities, animals, herbs, plants and foods.

Bartholomaeus Anglicus, author of the original work, was a thirteenth century Franciscan friar. The earliest known manuscript in England is dated 1296. The work became widely known and popular, because it was carried about by the friars. Steele gives a long list of printed Latin editions ranging from 1480 to 1609.[62] It was also translated into Dutch, French and Spanish. The first English translation was made by John Trevisa in 1397 and printed by Wynkyn de Worde in 1491. In 1535 Trevisa's translation was reprinted by Bertholet and later revised by Dr. Stephen Batman in 1582.[63] Batman acknowledges the "Authors of this Booke." These include the expected familiar names of Greek, Roman and Arab physicians, historians and philosophers and also some contemporary European writers. The work is a popular one and follows the conventional ideas of the period in diet and health. Useful information on herbs and foods is given, and authors continued to make use of this material in the seventeenth century.[64] This kind of book was a source of advice to the layman. Batman's additions provided new material in some fields, but reproduced knowledge on diet and health that had been current for centuries.

7. **Herbals and books on husbandry and gardening.** A herbal has been defined as a book containing the names and descriptions of herbs or plants in general, with their properties and virtues. During the most active period of the printed herbal, that is from the first quarter of the

sixteenth century until about 1670,[65] the term herbal also covered books which included information on animal and mineral material and some could be described as illustrated medicinal recipes. These herbals formed the materia medica of the sixteenth century and were derived for the most part from *De Materia Medica libri quinque* of Dioscorides, prepared in the first century of the Christian Era. From its beginning this work exerted a strong influence which increased during the Renaissance with the realization that Dioscorides represented "not only classical materia medica in its fullest form, but Greek materia medica unspotted by the taint of arabism."[66]

The herbal medicine of southern Europe was probably brought to England through the *Herbarium Apuleii Platonici*, of which a number of manuscripts of Anglo-Saxon translations still survive.[67] The earliest printed herbal information in English is in the encyclopaedia of Bartholomaeus Anglicus, where one section consists of an account of a large number of trees and herbs arranged in alphabetical order with a description of their medicinal properties. Some theoretical consideration was also given to plants, along Aristotelian lines.

Strictly speaking, the first printed English herbal was a small quarto volume in black letter, without illustration, prepared anonymously and printed by Richard Bankes in 1525. This came to be called *Bankes Herbal* and was the first of a series of similar works which appeared in the next thirty years and which included *Macer's Herbal* and *Askam's Herbal*.[68] Of a different style was the English translation of *Le Grant Herbier*, published in 1526.[69] This was the first example of a number of large illustrated books based chiefly on Continental works. This series included Lyte's *Historie of Plantes* and the famous *Gerard's Herbal* of 1596.[70] The preparation of the latter involved controversy and some acrimony between Gerard and the Flemish botanist Matthias de l'Obel.[71] Despite this, Gerard's arrangement of the herbs was altered from that of Dodoens to the method de l'Obel had used.[72] Though de l'Obel spent a great part of his life in England he did not publish any works in English.

The greatest English authority on herbals in that period was William Turner. His book, *The names of herbes in Greke, Latin, Englishe, Duche and Frenche Wyth the commune names that Herbaries and Apothecaries use*, was published in 1548, ten years after his Latin version. Turner was the first Englishman to study plants scientifically and his herbal marked the beginning of the science of botany in England. He included little folklore and qualified it with expressions such as "some do say."[73] Though many authorities had accepted, uncritically, information about plants indigenous to southern Europe, Turner carefully included plants particular to England, a practice followed by Bright and Gerard.

Another new influence at this time was the information on plants coming from the Americas, of the sort presented in John Frampton's *Joyfull Newes from out of the newe founde worlde,* translated from the original of Nicholas Monardes.[74]

The foundation of nearly all English writings on husbandry and gardening was *De Re Rustica* of Palladius,[75] written in the fifth century A.D. This work in turn was based on the works of Hesiod, Cato, Varro, Virgil, Columella and Pliny,[76] and was translated into English around 1420. Other important manuscripts from the twelfth and fourteenth century were Walter of Henley's *Treatise on Husbandry,* a survey of management, of men and animals; the anonymous *Husbandry,* which was concerned with estate accounts; *Senescalcia,* which dealt with the division of labour, and *Bishop Grosstestes Rules*, with instructions on the production and consumption of crops and the management of the household. All were in Anglo-Norman.[77]

The first printed book on agriculture was the *Liber ruralium commodorum* of Petrus Crescentius, printed in Augsburg in 1471. The first printed book on farming in English was Fitzherbert's *The Boke of Husbandrye* of 1523.[78] Though there are a number of extant English manuscripts on gardening, including John Gardener's poem, the *Feate of Gardeninge,*[79] the first printed book on the subject was Thomas Hill's *A most briefe and pleasaunt treatyse, teachynge howe to dress, sowe and set a garden* (with acknowledgements to Palladius) of 1563.[80] Towards the end of the century, with the increased interest in agricultural improvement, more works appeared in the vernacular, as illustrated by the following examples (references to purely veterinary works[81] and surveying are omitted): Tusser wrote on husbandry and housewiferie; Reynolde Scot on hops; Mascall on cattle, poultry and orchards; Hugh Platt advised on proper manuring; Taverner wrote on experiments concerning fish and fruits; Googe translated Herebachius; "R.E." translated Le Choyselat on poultry, and Surphlet translated the all-embracing *d'Agriculture et Maison Rustique* of Etienne and Liebault.[82] All these books contain material relevant to the place of foods in the diet.

8. Cookery Books. The many extant early English cookery manuscripts demonstrate that the instructions they contain are derived basically from Roman recipes of the form found in Apicius' *De re coquinaria*.[83] The first English cookery book is believed to be that of Neckam in the twelfth century, but the oldest and best known practical work is the *Forme of Cury* compiled by the Chief Master Cook of King Richard II around 1390. A version of this was published by Samuel Pegge in the eighteenth century and gives some 196 recipes.[84] Recipes of the same general type are found in Austin's *Two Fifteenth-Century Cookery-Books*, which are derived mainly from two Harleian manuscripts. The Harleian MS 279, dated about 1430, deals with soups (153 recipes), "leche metys" or sliced meats (64 recipes) and "baked metis" (41 recipes).[85]

The first printed cookery book was *De Honesta Voluptate* (Venice, 1475) by Platina — that is, Bartholomeo Sacchi (1421-81), an Italian historian and Vatican Librarian. This work, which was part cookery book and partly a philosophical guide to good health, went through many editions in the sixteenth century, and though referred to by English authors was not translated into English.

One of the first English printed cookery books is said to be *This is the Boke of Cokerye* of [1500] described as "Here beginneth a noble boke of festes royalle and Cokery a boke for a pryncis householde or any other estates. . . ."[86] A later work, *A proper newe Booke of Cokerye,* first edition about 1525, went through a number of editions with variations of title but with comparatively little alteration in content. In general, sixteenth century printed cookery books are very similar in content; in any case they would have been supplemented by family recipes written down or remembered. At Court and in noble houses, where the serving of meals followed a definite ritual, the appropriate "bouche of court" and diet book of the establishment would also have been consulted.

Duffy has suggested that recipe books had their greatest vogue in the sixteenth century between 1535 and 1550, and were not frequently printed after that date.[87] Here Duffy must perhaps refer to books containing only recipes, with lists of ingredients and menus. Books including recipes, menus and advice are shown by A. W. Oxford's bibliography to have increased towards the end of the century.[88] The "readership" towards which the books were directed had changed subtly. No longer were the directions intended for princely or noble establishments, but they were more and more directed toward the mistress of a good sized household and often contained "Housewife" in the title. There still had been no great revolution in recipes, however, for in the

Good Hous-Wives Treasurie of 1588[89] medieval and early Roman overtones can still be seen in some recipes.

A change in form and content of cookery books became apparent in
the middle and later part of the next century. Austin says that the earliest books that can be called English date from this time.[90] Unhappily,
few studies have been made of the early development of "English"
cookery, though recent practical approaches are P. Pullar's and R. Barber's attempts to trace the development of English recipes from Roman
techniques by a comparison of actual recipes, given in a modernized
form.[91]

Many factors must have contributed to the changes in English cookery practice, not least the influences from the Continent. Catherine de'
Medici had brought Italian ideas on the use of food to the French Court
and English nobility, according to Harrison, for the most part employed
"musicall-headed" Frenchmen as their cooks.[92] The controversy over
benefits from French influences on English cookery reappears at regular
intervals. The famous Mrs. Glasse, in the eighteenth century, had strong
views on the subject.[93]

New ideas are worthless without the proper materials to put them
into practice. Fortunately these became increasingly available with improved agricultural techniques and the increased import of new foods
and spices from distant countries. Proud as the English were of their
own country's produce, writers on food and diet frequently reminded
them of the old proverb, "God may sende a man good meate, but the
devyll may sende an evyll coke to dystrue it."

The reliance placed on ancient advice in sixteenth century English
works is obvious both from the many references given and from the
marked similarity of the advice provided to that found in modern translations of Greek and Latin texts. Langton, for example, uses Galenic
analogies in his physiological information, frequently with a wording
identical to the modern translation of the Galenic texts.[94] This uncrit-
ical repetition of material is, of course, not only characteristic of Elizabethan dietaries of health but can also be found in some modern text-
books. Fortunately, few examples are carried to the extreme length
found in Lupton's *One thousand notable things,* which despite changes
in "author" through over twenty editions has two items, both related
to diet, which are repeated word for word over two and a quarter centuries.[95]

The repetition of old material does indicate a lack of original thought,
which was the case in sixteenth century English medicine. However,

even in situations when there is vigorous original thought and new concepts are being introduced and accepted, they exist concurrently with a
mass of material based on the traditional ideas at a different but possibly wider level — a level which though it is not likely to be of direct
influence in the development of man's thought will certainly affect his
way of life.

Despite the marked changes in thought that took place in the seventeenth century and the gradual rejection of Galenic medicine in terms
of practical advice, many books, such as those of Gervase Markham, are
taken directly from earlier works.[96] Writers in the nineteenth century
were aware of ancient teaching, and many of the terms used remained
unchanged through the centuries, but with an altered connotation suited to the new concepts. For example, in Day's translation of Simon's
Animal Chemistry (1846), in the section on urine the explanation of a
certain result is given as being due to the individual's ". . . taking only a
very little drink as is the usual habit of the sanguineo-bilius temperament."[97]

CHAPTER III
THE REGIMEN OR DYETARY

To the conservation of the body of mankynde within the lymita-
tion of helthe (whiche as Galene saythe) is the state of the body,
wherein we be neyther greved with peyne, nor lette from doing our
necessary busynesse.

T. Elyot (1541)

A MODERN DEFINITION of the word diet, in general use today, is a
way of feeding: prescribed courses of food, or regimen. The word diet
is derived through the Latin *diaeta* from the Greek word διατα, which
means a way of life. To the Elizabethans the dietary, or regimen, to be
followed for health included consideration of every aspect of a man's
life: his physical and mental condition, age, habits, and all the circumstances of his surroundings. These many factors were considered under
the three main headings of things natural, things not-natural, and those
things against nature. The last group was concerned with disease, and so
is not dealth with further. The first two groups are the basis for all
advice on health and form the foundation of this study.

The object of books on dietary advice (as opposed to those on medicine) was to help both in the preservation of health and the lengthening
of the individual's span of life. The expected span of life for man is
discussed in *Regimen Sanitatis*. It is asked why people like Adam lived
930 years, King Arganton of the Tartars 97 years, and Galen 140 years,
whereas in contemporary times "if a man may approche to xl or lx
yeres men repute him happy and fortunate."[1] The cause of "this
sodeyne and strange alteracion" is sought, and it is concluded that the
reasons are twofold. One is "because we fulfyll not the commande-
ments of almighty god," and secondly "that is chaunceth by our
mysdiete and to moche surfettyng." It can be concluded from this that
a short life was thought to be due to sin or to "mys-diete." It is not
specifically stated, but it is implied, that the effects of an otherwise
good diet can be negated by sinful behaviour, although a good regimen
of life and righteousness cannot be considered identical.

N.B. Footnotes to this chapter appear on page 305.

Andrew Boorde puts the matter somewhat differently in his *Breviary of Helthe*. He explains that God has "pyt a tyme to everyman, over which tyme no man by no arte nor science can not prolong." God knows the length of a man's life. However, man is able to alter this in one direction. "God hath given man in this lyfe fre wyl"; this enables him to "abreviate" (but not extend) his life by his own behaviour. Boorde lists such things as surfeiting, drunkenness, worry, infectious sickness and "going against Gods will" as those items which will shorten life. He does make it quite clear that provided man avoids all these pitfalls the number of his days is set and will not be arbitrarily cut short by God.[2] This attitude gives the modern reader a feeling of greater flexibility than the approach in *Regimen Sanitatis*, but it still remained that sinning against God was considered as potent a shortener of life as bad diet.

Alexis of Piemont took another view.[3] He starts by speaking with scorn about "those Christians" who despise medicines and who say that if a sick man has been appointed by God to die, all the medicines in the world cannot save him. Alexis himself disagrees with this idea and argues that God has created things to give man "ease and remedy." He does not believe that every man that is vexed with disease is appointed to die of the same but that the infirmity is sent to him as a punishment for his offences. The influence of the will of God in man's life and health is apparent throughout the Elizabethan texts.[4]

Basically the advice on the preservation of health revolves round the maintenance of the proper level of vital or innate heat and radical moisture in the body. This heat, which is recognized as being essential for life, is nourished by the appropriate balance of humours. By the humours "are nourished the entyer parts of all Creatures and for this cause, so long as a man lyveth, he can never want these without great detriment and daunger to his health."[5] The humours, in turn, receive their nourishment from "outward sustenance" — that is, air, food, or drink. Thus indirectly the vital heat of the body is maintained by the food eaten though Elizabethan writers do not seem to make the direct connection but habitually link the two through the humours and qualities. Cogan says,

For such is a state of man and beast touching the bodie that the spirites humours yea the sounde substance of all parts doe continually wast and weare away. So that unless nourishment other like be restored of necessitie the whole must shortly be consumed.[6]

Great trouble was taken in the sixteenth and seventeenth centuries to investigate or refute situations where life and reasonably good health were maintained during long periods without food. These investigations did not include the behaviour of holy persons whose miraculous action would be acceptable. A well known example, translated into many languages, is that of a young girl who was said "not to have eaten, dronke, or voided anie thing out of her body for these seaven yeeres." Her name was Katerin of Schmidweiler. On the instructions of the noble Prince, "Lord Duke John Casimire, Countie Palatin of Rhin," the girl's case was investigated in 1584. The examiners included two doctors, a magistrate and respected local citizens. Despite the supervision of the girl by four "honourable women" for two weeks, the Commissioners were non-committal in their verdict. The report of the incident ends by saying that Katerin had now completed nine years without food, drink or sleep and yet she "miraculouslie liveth through the singular pure and incomprehensible grace of almighty God."[7] When faced with specific cases of individuals who could live in health without food, drink or sleep, scepticism was overruled (in part anyhow) by the recognition of God's mysterious ways with the humble individual as well as with the holy man.

The place of food in the regimen of health was clearly recognized by the Hippocratic school. It is referred to in *Regimen of Health, Nutriment,* and particularly in *Regimen I* and *Regimen II*, where the effect of food on the body is considered: "[the] author must know and further the power possessed severally by all the foods and drinks of our regimen including the power by nature and the power by contrast of human art."[8] In *Regimen II* the powers of various foods are considered along with the effects of cooking methods on these powers.[9]

The effect of cooking on foods was also considered carefully in the sixteenth century. Boorde says,

For a good coke is halfe a physycyon. For the chefe physycke (the counceyll of a physycon excepte) dothe come from the kytchyn; wherfore the physycyon and the coke for sycke men must consult togyther for the preparacion of meate for sycke men.[10]

Sixteenth century theories of diet and metabolism are formal and elaborate but lack the precision which comes with the modern concepts of chemical formulae and the recognition that heat can be measured in terms of energy and intensity. The interrelationships between the basic factors of the theories were complex and had to be considered within the framework of their philosophical background and the Elizabethan habit of describing material things by the use of metaphors as well as being considered in practical terms.

The factors relevant to this study are summarized below and elaborated in subsequent chapters.

1. In relation to MAN—

Four elements: fire, air, water, earth.

Four qualities: hot, cold, moist, dry. These can produce different effects in different circumstances. The qualities are active both in the organs and the faculties of the body.

Three spirits: vital, animal, natural.

Three powers: spiritual, animal, natural with subservient powers or faculties.

Seven faculties: generation, auction, nutrition, attraction, concoction, retention, expulsion. These are the main faculties; there are others.

Four natural humours: blood, phlegm, yellow bile (choler), black bile (melancholy).

Eleven unnatural humours: blood (two), phlegm (four), choler (four), melancholy (one). Writers vary; some refer only to four natural and four unnatural humours.

One complexion: applicable to the individual, this may be sanguine, phlegmatic, choleric or melancholy and will gradually change with ageing.

Fourteen members: the parts referred to particularly by writers on diet are: the brain, heart, liver, testicles, nerves, arteries, veins, spermatic vessels, bones, gristle, membranes, muscles, fat and flesh.

Also to be considered are the age, activity, emotional condition and habits of the individual.

2. In relation to FOODS—

Four elemental qualities: hot, cold, moist, dry.

Four degrees of qualities: each degree may be subdivided into three parts — the beginning, the middle, and the end.

Eight tastes: tastes are linked to qualities, four being hot, three cold and the eighth without predominant qualities.

Smell: generally divided into pleasant (or fragrant) and unpleasant (or rotten).

Substance: the generalized division is "gross" and "fine."
Production of "juice:" which can be good, ill, thick.

Foods also have some generalized characteristics. These include digestibility, being costive or laxative, putrefying effects, causing oppilations, causing sweating, diuretic, aphrodisiacal, flatulent, containing superfluities, or nourishing — plus a number of vague terms.

It is the "matter" of foods which causes effects, not the foods themselves, any more than "an Oake [is] a Table or Ship, or a quarrie of stones an house."[11] The value of this matter is related to the individual (country of residence, age, sex, time of year and custom) and will be needed differently by people in different circumstances.

CHAPTER IV
THINGS NATURAL

> For no man can do any good with a medicine; whiche is ignorant in the constitution of mannes bodie, therefore the thinges naturall wherof mannes bodye is compact and made, be seven in number.
>
> C. Langton (1547)

IMPORTANT AS a knowledge of the seven things natural was for the physician, this did not apply to the same extent to the reader seeking advice on the preservation of his health. The seven innate factors of the body — namely elements, humours, complexions, members, powers, operations and spirits — are all introduced but they are not usually described in detail. Most attention is given to the elements (and their qualities), the humours, complexions and spirits. These are the things most obviously and frequently affected by the things non-natural and it is on this relationship that advice about health is based. Vernacular books cannot be classed precisely according to the detail with which they do or do not cover the things natural, though in general those which provide detailed information about foods tend to give less on physiology. The attitude of the author towards providing definitions also has some influence. Some writers, like Langton, try to be precise, explaining:

> Tully that eloquent Romain, counselleth very wel every man, first of all and before he make any far procedynge to defyne the thing which he pourposeth to entreat.[1]

Others are more diffuse in their explanations. Because of Langton's attempts to give definitions and the simplicity of his style, much of the material in this chapter is taken from his two books on physick and on diet.

Elements and their qualities

Sixteenth century English writers accepted the basic elements of fire, air, water and earth. Their descriptions are based on, but not always

---

N.B. Footnotes to this chapter appear on pages 305-311.

identical with the Aristotelian view, which implies a common substratum or prime matter for the elements. This has no separate existence; it exists only as qualified by certain contrary qualities, which in turn exist only in this substratum. Contraries and substratum are logically distinguishable but inseparable basic parts in fire, air, water and earth which, as Ross says, "though not strictly elements since they are logically analysable, are the simplest of sensible bodies."[2]

None of the four elements is primary, underivative or unchangeable: all alike pass into one another in a cycle. The quickest transformation is that of an element into the one which stands next to it in the series of fire, air, water and earth.[3]

Langton goes to considerable lengths to try and define and clarify the meaning of elements for his readers.[4] He begins by explaining that the word "Elementum" means "a begynnynge of anythynge" and is used to refer to such things as letters of the alphabet. Similarly the "principles also of every arte be called Elementes, bycause they are the begynners of the same." A pure element "is the last part of that thynge of which it is an element," but this sort of "fyre ayre water and earth (of which all thynges under the moone be made) can not be perceyved by any sence." Also the pure element is without generation or corruption.

> Howe be it of fyre made thycke, commeth ayer: and of ayer made thycke, commeth water: and of water made thycke, commeth earth. And yet here is neyther corruption nor yet generation of the whole, for this is a mutation of the partes only.

Langton realizes that not all his readers will be familiar with this concept of the Aristotelian elements, and some may say "that there is no man so madde [as] to saye that the fyre, ayre, erth and water can not be felt." He tries to explain these elements, which cannot be recognized by the senses, by reiterating that as "Elementum"[5] means the beginning of anything, then naturally the very beginnings of a man's body cannot yet be sensitive, therefore the elements of which this beginning is made cannot be sensed. Answering the question "How many Elements are there?" the surgeon, Peter Lowe, says, "Two according to the contemplation of Chyrurgery viz. simples or intelligibles and composed or sensibles."[6] The "simples" or "intelligibles" are the simple pure elements comprehensible only through the intellect,[7] the composed or sensible elements are the fire, air, water and earth seen in nature. These are impure or exaggerated forms of the simple elements and it is of these sensible elements that the body is formed. In fact "the parts of the bodi do represent the elements."[8]

The heat in living bodies can be compared to fire, the breath to air, the hard parts to earth, and the moist parts to water. An altogether simpler approach is used by some authors. Elyot describes the elements as being "those original things unmixed and uncompounded," and recognizes that all corporate things are made of the temperance and mixture of elements.[9]

Aristotle assigns the qualities to elements in four combinations as follows:

hot and dry to fire	cold and fluid to water
hot and fluid to air	cold and dry to earth

These qualities apply to the simple or pure elements, in each of which one quality predominates: heat in fire, moisture in air, cold in water, and dryness in earth. However, some writers — Timothy Bright for example — maintained that "these [elements] have each of them but one quality: fire hote, ayer moist, earth dry and water cold." His argument is that if the elements had two qualities, their relation to each other would be such (i.e. in *entercommunication*) that they would no longer be elements. The answer to the question "is not the element of fire dry?" is that fire is dry, but not of its own nature "but that which is in fire beside heate, is only an absence of moistnes" as in earth, coldness is an absence of heat. However, he continues, in the body and in foods or medicines required to preserve health, the elements are not pure and it is the presence of more than one quality that gives a substance its characteristics. Giving pepper as an example, Bright explains that "The heate of pepper riseth of the fiery element; the dryness and solidity of substaunce which it hath of the earthie."[10]

An element was an essential vehicle for a quality because a quality cannot exist alone, "seeing [that] no qualitie can be founde aparte from substaunces, wee are compelled to receyve them together with the substaunces."[11] Although the lack of any one element would cause an extreme imbalance and lead to death, it is in terms of the qualities of the elements that health and disease are considered.

The "foure qualities Elementarie" are described as:

Heate, cold, drie and moist: they be the first qualities, because they slide first from the Elements. They be also called the principall qualities: for of them come all the secundarie effects.[12]

Each sensible element was considered to contain all four qualities with a preponderance of two. The two dominant qualities could never be those directly contrary to each other, i.e. heat and cold or moist and dry. Each quality has four degrees,* though moisture is not given by Newton beyond the third degree because all things are hot or cold and both can destroy moisture.[13] Heat dries it and cold congeals it, thus preventing moisture being dominant in the fourth degree. Of the four qualities, hot and cold are "able to work," i.e. are active and dominant; dry and moist are "able to suffer," or passive. Nevertheless all qualities work together "for there is none idle qualitye in the bodie."[14] Hot is the most powerful of all, but in living things is always linked in importance with the passive quality moist. Wyngfield explains:

> That same quicke and lyvelye power in our bodyes which is called lyfe, supported by naturall heat and moisture, liveth and dwelleth in the body, whiche two so together are conglutinate or knyt, that the one cannot be separate from the other, and the humiditie or moystness is a very noryce [nourisher], to this naturall heat, . . . These two qualities be the materiall causes of our livinge.[15]

Heat and moisture must be maintained in the proper proportion. Too much or too little moisture can cause death, just as with an oil lamp too much oil drowns the flame "or else if by negligence they forget to putte any oyle in, for lack of humiditie the lyght is extinguished and goth forth." Of all qualities it is the active quality hot which provokes the most discussion. This is elaborated at the end of this chapter.

Humours and complexions

The relationship between elements, qualities, humours and complexions is sometimes tabulated in this way:

Elements	Qualities	Humours	Complexions†
AIR is more light and subtle than water	hot:moist	Blood	Sanguine
WATER is more light and subtle than earth	cold:moist	Phlegm	Phlegmatic
FIRE is absolutely light and clear and is the clarifier of other elements	hot:dry	Choler or yellow bile	Choleric

*Degrees are dealt with in more detail in relation to the value of foods (Chapter VI).
† Complexions are referred to again in Chapter VIII, Section I.

| EARTH is the | cold:dry | Melancholy or | Melancholic |
| most gross | | black bile | |

The order of complexions is that used generally by sixteenth century writers. It is different from the sequence related to the elements given earlier.

The implication sometimes drawn is that the humours are derived from the elemental qualities and that the humour determines the complexion. According to sixteenth century theory both the humours and the complexions are derived directly from the qualities. This is not always made clear due to the way that contemporary vernacular authors use the words humours and complexions (see also Chapter VIII).

The difficulty of defining the humours really arises from the origin of the doctrine of the humours which, basically, was an attempt to reconcile empirical medical evidence with speculative ideas of natural philosophy. The evolution of the ideas about humours has been described by Klibansky, Saxl and Panofsky.[16]

The doctrine of the humours, as expounded by Hippocrates, came from the drawing together of a number of older concepts. These included such factors as the Pythagorean emphasis on the number four, leading to a doctrine of cosmic elements. The four Empedoclean elements (of fire, air, water and earth) were linked to the sun, sky, sea and earth, and were considered to be of equal value and power. Each had its own particular task and nature and in the course of the seasons, each in turn gained ascendancy. This concept of seasonal ascendancy of each element is found in sixteenth century writings in the form of the domination by the four humours, of different seasons of the year and even of certain times of the day and night.[17]

Philistion,[18] though a follower of Empedocles, added the idea that each of the four elements possessed a certain quality: "to fire belongs heat, to air cold, to water moist, to earth dry." These qualities came not only to form dual combinations (e.g. fire became hot and dry), but they could also be used as predicates of any other substances. Here then, through the qualities, was an apparent link between the original elements and some corresponding components of the human body. These components could not be regarded as pure fire, pure air, pure water or pure earth. The actual substances of the body which could be said to correspond with the four elements and with their four qualities were the four humours or body fluids, blood, phlegm, yellow bile and black bile. However, it must be remembered that these body fluids had long been recognized in a purely medical context as causes of illness and, if they became visible (in the form of vomiting, or the like) were considered as symptoms of illness. Also any part of nutritious materials improperly digested by the body were said to be surplus humours. Euryphon of Cnidus [19] had assumed an indefinite number of such humours which, he believed, could rise to the head and generate illness. Alcmaeon of Croton [20] believed that the predominance of a single quality could cause illness and that an equality between the qualities presented health. However, his list of qualities was long and included "moist, dry, cold, hot, bitter, sweet and the rest."[21] Tastes remained linked to qualities, sweetness was always hot and sourness cold.

From this brief indication of the background ideas, it can be seen that humours linked together, in an indefinable way, the cosmos, the four elements, the four qualities, materials of the human body, and could also provide an explanation for the cause of illnesses. Not only did the sequence of development of ideas about the humours lead to a number of different facets to the meaning of the word, but at the end of the sixteenth century another meaning was in use. Hertford and Simpson, in their comments on *Every Man in His Humour* by Ben Jonson (1573?-1637), explain that Jonson insisted on the stricter physiological and psychological doctrine of humours, of which he said

> . . . some one peculiar quality
> Doth so possesse a man, that it doth draw
> All his affects, his spirits, and his powers,
> In their confluctions, all to runne one way;

This (say the commentators) is in contrast to the loose popular meaning of the word humour which could be used to describe an "apish or phantastike straine," i.e. a passing impulse or caprice. In the Elizabethan period, humour had both the accepted "physiologiçal" meaning and also the more superficial meaning it can have today.[22]

Books in the vernacular describe the humours briefly, avoiding the complicated details referred to in Ogden's study "Guy de Chauliac's Theory of the Humors," which illustrates the ideas of Galen, Arabic and Mediaeval authorities.[23] Langton says there are eight humours. The four natural humours are blood, phlegm, choler and melancholy; the unnatural are the same four which have been changed "by putrifaction, or els som otherwyse from theyre owne natyve qualities."[24] The four unnatural humours are further subdivided by some writers to give a total of eleven, e.g. blood, two; phlegm, four; choler, four and melancholy, one. Elyot makes further subdivisions, i.e. nine kinds of unnatural phlegm. These are described in terms such as "watery" or "slimy" or "raw," "viscous like bird lime and heavy," or "salt that is mingled with choler."[25] Reference is made below to four natural and eleven unnatural humours. The unnatural humours were of particular importance in relation to disease, but are not examined in detail here, as the emphasis is on the preservation of health through maintenance of the natural humours.

The origin of the humours is referred to later, following the sequence suggested by Langton, who says that "the sprynge and well of humours maye then best be perceyved when the maner and waye how to nourish the bodye is declared." However, he reminds his readers that

> the same food whych is receyved by the wesant [throat] into the stomacke for the preservynge of the bodye, is the matter and substaunce, whereby, by the vertue of the liver they be made and engendred.[26]

Blood is hot, moist and sweet; phlegm is cold, moist and tasteless (the word used is "unsavoury") "lyke unto the pure water"; yellow choler is hot, dry and bitter; black choler or melancholy is cold, dry and sour. These humours are called hot, cold, dry and moist, because they are "so in power, and not in acte." There is a difference between things "hot in power" and "hot in act," Langton explains,

> For that thing is hot in acte which is hot alredy, and that is hot in power, which is not hot alredy, but may, and is apt to be hot afterward.[27]

Blood (hot: moist). Blood has pre-eminence over all other humours in sustaining living creatures because "it hath more conformitie with the originalle cause of lyvynge."[28] It is likely to have the right proportion of heat and moisture because it is part of the generation of new life. "Bloode and the seed of man be beginners of our generation, of the whych is the substaunce and matter wherof our body is made, and the seed of man is nexte under God."[29] Though other humours are carried with the blood "yet the especiall part of the noryshment is that that is properlye called blood." There is the humour Blood and also the liquid found in the blood-vessels. These two are not identical, for in the "liquid blood"* all the humours are mixed. This, says Lemnius, can be

---

*This term will be used to identify circulating blood when a differentiation is required.

plainly seen "when a veine is opened (for it is not all pure blood that gusheth thereout)."[30]

First, before the blood is cold it has an "ayrie fomy spirit." This disappears and then there is "an exact and pure liquor of most perfect and excellent ruddinesse, the which is pure and right blood." In this "swimmeth" choler and sometimes tough clammy Phlegm. Lastly, the "whole masse or lump" (clotted blood) is Melancholy, so that "sometime the blood that issueth out of the veines, liquifieth and is dissolved into choler or Phlegme, or clottereth and thickneth into Melancholy and retayneth either no colour or very little blood."

Blood is only natural in "the mixture in which it have the rule and dominion."[31] It can lose its natural qualities and degenerate into the unnatural humour in two ways. One is by putrefaction due to the "stopping of the pores" or other oppilations. The other change is caused by an alteration in substance. This occurs when blood is mixed with evil humours, as in dropsy where blood is mixed with water. When too much Choler, Phlegm or Melancholy is present, blood "taketh a newe name and is called eyther cholericke blowd, flewmaticke, or melancholy bloud."[32] Ogden says "Guy's statements always make clear whether he is referring to the *massa sanguinaria* or to the contained humor 'blood.' "[33] Elizabethan writers in the vernacular often make their differentiation less clear with the resulting apparent paradox between the view that those with less blood were more susceptible to illness[34] and the practice of blood letting.

Phlegm (cold:moist). "The excrement which falleth from the brayne into the mouth, can not properly be called flemme but rather muck."[35] The humour itself is described as a nourishment but "halfe boyled." It is thin and white, "not fatte nor coloured like blood,"[36] and it dilutes the blood, cooling any excess heat in it. When in the veins phlegm nourishes the cold:moist parts and "lubrifieth the moving of the joints." It is usual to describe four sorts of unnatural phlegm, though some writers subdivide them further. The four types are: *vitrea,* like glass (this comes from gluttony and idleness); the others are sweet phlegm, bitter (phlegm mixed with melancholy), and salt (phlegm mixed with choler).[37]

Choler (hot:dry). "Choler doth participate with naturall heate as longe as it is in good temperaunce." It is yellow or red in colour. There are four kinds of unnatural choler identifiable according to changes in colour. All are mixtures of natural choler with other humours. Authors do not agree in detail. The following descriptions are from Elyot. "Citrine" is a mixture of natural choler and watery phlegm; yellow (like egg yolks) is choler with congealed phlegm; green (like green leeks) has come from the stomach rather than the liver (where the humours are concocted); green "like to grene canker of mettal" is caused by the excessive adustion or burning of choler or phlegm. [38]

Melancholy or black choler (cold:dry). Natural melancholy is the dregs of pure blood. Part of it is carried with the blood, making it thicker and increasing "the power retentyve, in the veynes and other places where it cometh." [39] Also, natural melancholy nourishes melancholic parts such as the bones and spleen.

There are two sorts of unnatural melancholy, one due to a change in the natural humour by adustion or burning, and the other due to a mixture with other humours. Both produce symptoms of madness. The natural humour becomes unnatural when it "is burned as drye as ashes. For Hippocrates saith that bothe blood and red choler wyl be turned soone into Melancholye, when for lacke of ayre, they be smothered in the veynes." The stopping of the pores can change a sanguine or choleric body to melancholy. The person so affected will become sad and solitary. The dilution of melancholy with a little blood "maketh a manne merye madde"; mixed with a great deal of red choler he will become "starke woode." [40] If melancholy is mixed with phlegm the man will be slothful and without sense. The effects of unnatural melancholy received considerable attention from the Elizabethans, the most famous English work on the subject being Burton's *The Anatomie of Melancholy, what it is, with all the kindes etc.* [41]

Langton sums up the functions of the natural humours as follows:

The use of these forsayde humors, is such in especiall as foloweth. The bloud serveth to the nowrishment of the hole body, flewme helpeth the movying of the joynts, yellow chollar clenseth the intestines of their flewme and filthe melancholy healpeth the action of the stomake. . . [42]

The basis of a regimen for health was that foods of *similar* qualities and degrees should be taken to keep the balance of the humours normal. In sickness, when the normal balance has been altered, foods and medicines of *contrary* quality should be given. In childhood the natural dominant qualities are hot and moist. [43] In youth heat increases and moisture lessens; then, as ageing proceeds, heat and moisture are lost. This is the explanation for the fact that both children and old people require a hot, moist diet. The child requires similar qualities to maintain and develop the body. The old, who are becoming cold and dry, require contrary qualities to combat ageing.

Members or parts of the body

The method of classifying parts of the body varies according to whether the differentiation is made according to structure or function. Some authors combine these methods. The two main divisions used by sixteenth century writers are "similar" and "dissimilar." These definitions are given by Langton:

> For *similares* be such partes as be lyke unto them selves in all thinges, which they they be divided, or parted in sonder the leste of them kepeth the same name that the whole dothe whereof it is a part: and *dissimilares,* be such as are unlyke them selfes in all thinges, which when they be divided or parted a sunder, none of them can be called by the name the hole is, as in example.
>
> No part of the head, can (yf it be separat, and parted, from the head) be called an head.[44]

Langton includes water, blood, bone and flesh among the similars.[45] Lowe divides the parts of the body into five groups. First the principal members (brain, heart, liver and testicles) in which materials of importance to the body are engendered; secondly the parts that serve the principal members (the nerves serve the brain, the arteries the heart, the veins the liver and the spermatic vessels the testicles); thirdly parts neither govern nor are governed by others ("the Bones, the Cartilages, Membrains, Glands, Tendons, Ligaments, Fat, simple Flesh, and so forth"); fourthly those parts which have proper virtue of themselves (The Belly, the Kidnies and the Matrix [uterus]); finally there are the "Members called excrementous" (the nails and the hair).

Elyot agrees with this classification of the principal members, but calls the second group "Official members"; the third group he describes as *similares* and the fourth group are named "Members instrumentall" and are given as the "stomach, raines bowelles and all the great synews."[46] These of their virtue, he says, "do appetite meate and alter it."

Because sixteenth century writers in the vernacular use a variety of terms for classifying parts of the body, all derived from earlier texts, a summary of the main headings used is given. No attempt is made to disentangle the various classifications:

Henri de Mondeville (c.1306) used the main divisions of *consimilia* and *officialia*; under the heading *consimilia* he subdivided them into *consimilia simplicia* and *consimilia comporita,* made up of "simple similars." These compound parts are described in such a way that they could be equivalent to the "dissimilars" according to the definition given by Langton.[47]

Elyot (1541) lists principal, official, parts called *similares* and members instrumental.

J. Vigo (1543) refers to members "nutritive," members "spiritual," members "animal" and extremities of the body. These parts are divided into simple and compound.[48]

Langton (1547) uses similar and dissimilar.

Bannister (1578) says "These therefore are the words of *Vesalius.* All the partes of man's body are either similar or simple with sence as are Ligamentes, Fibres, Membrans, Flesh, and Fatte: or els Dissimilar, or Instrumentall, as the Veine, Artery, Sinew, Muscle, Finger, and other Organs of the whole body: which are made so much more instrumentall, by how much the greater store of similar partes with the instrumentall are compounded."[49]

Vicary (1586) uses simple and compound.[50]

Lowe's description (1612) of the five sorts of members has been given above. He makes a distinction between similars and dissimilars and under his chapter on Elements gives the twelve "sensible elements" (or similar parts) as bones, cartilage, flesh, nerves, arteries, pannicles (membranes), ligaments, tendons, membranes, the skin, the "fat Grease" and bone-marrow.

To sum up: the principal members are those wherein materials of importance are engendered. The official members serve the principals. The nerves serve the brain, the arteries the heart and the veins the liver. The similar parts are those which have the same nature throughout, and the instrumental parts are those which "of their vertue do appetite meate and alter it." [51]

It is necessary to know more about the brain, heart, liver and stones of generation so that the work of the powers and spirits can be understood more easily. In the following descriptions, detailed anatomical details, given by some sixteenth century writers, have been omitted.

The generation of man occurs through a mixture of seed and blood. In the seed of man there is more fire and air than water and earth. In the blood, however, "there is lesse of fyre and ayer, than there is of water and earth: and yet in the same there is more moysture then drynesse."[52] That is, the seed has more heat and moisture than does the blood. The characteristics of the brain, heart and liver differ because they develop from different mixtures of seed and blood. According to Langton, the hot boiling seed makes three little bladders, from each of which one of the three organs will develop.

The brain[53] develops from Langton's *third* little bladder when it is filled with seed which, itself, is filled full of spirit. The brain, therefore, is made only from seed and because of this the brain can be filled with the "most fyne spirites" which it conserves and alters, thus enabling the senses and the faculty of voluntary motion to operate.

All cogitation and imagination come from the brain. Langton dwells at length on the marvellousness of this organ. He likens it to the sky as both (it seems to him) are great heavy substances which hang unsupported but do not fall. He suggests that there is something divine and celestial about the brain.

The second of the three little bladders receives fine blood and spirit, and from this the heart develops. It is clear that the heart is considered the most important part of the body because of the way in which all other parts of the body adjust, however hurtfully to themselves, so that the heart will be protected. Langton describes it as being like the action of subjects for their prince, and says:

> yet in mans bodye though there be infinite subjects ther can be founde no disobedience to theyr lorde and governor, whyche is the heart: ... I praye you is not every parte readye to defend him; though it be to the utter destruction of them al for ever ... and to say truthe, he is worthy to have no lesse homage or servyce seyng he is auctor of lyfe to al the rest. ...[54]

The liver[55] developes from the first little bladder which draws up gross blood. This blood, when congealed and mixed with the seed, forms the liver. Langton says "for the very dutye and office of the lyver, is to engender blood for the nouryshmente of the body and therfore it is hote and moist accordynge to the nature of blood." Langton recognizes that some say the heart is the well-spring of the blood. "For the heart is the beginning and well of bloud and the first member that hath bloud. ..."[56] However, Langton himself follows Galen's view that blood is formed in the liver.[57]

It is "the fleshe of the lyver, which engendereth blood, althogh the lyver receyve both vytall heat, and spiryte of the hearte." During the alteration of juice into blood various impurities arise. Langton's description follows Galen's words and analogies very closely. The light superfluities or "flour of the wine" rise to the top and go to the gall-bladder as yellow choler. The dregs sink down and go to the spleen as black choler or melancholy. The two remaining humours are derived from blood and neither of these are described so precisely. The sanguine humour or "blood" is not clearly differentiated from blood itself. In this context[58] Langton does not refer explicitly to phlegm but to a "certayne watrye substance" still remaining, part of which may be further concocted and turned into blood and part of which makes the blood thinner so that it can pass more easily through the fine veins of the liver. Later Langton describes phlegm as a water humour, cold and moist, which has been incompletely altered into blood and which thins and cools the heat of the blood.[59]

Little mention is made of the stones of generation in books on health. The longest piece of information on these parts seems to be that given in *Batman uppon Bartholome*. Even so, most of this is taken up with the shamefulness of the private parts, the effect of gelding and the fact that those members which have the virtue of engendering children should be used only for the "lawful generation of children."[60] Constantine the African is said to have explained that the substance of the testicles is made of crude flesh, white and soft and designed to hold the "strong heat" which will boil blood and change it into "whiteness."

> Then the privie stones with other members that serve the privie stones be the head and well of the humour seminall, and first foundation [of] radicall [heat] thereof.[61]

To fit the act of generation into the framework of Aristotelian causes, the male is the formal cause, providing movement and shape, the female is the material cause and provides the matter. Lemnius puts it graphically, saying that man is generated from female blood and male seed, the one being "apt convenient and tractable matter like moyste claye or soft wax" which is ready to have fashioned from it anything the workman wishes. The wax is the female contribution; the workman is the male.[62]

On the whole, the functions of the principal members are not listed clearly by authors in their sections referring to each organ but are mentioned in the information given on the powers and the spirits.

Spirits*

The following descriptions of the spirits are almost direct transcriptions from Christopher Langton's *Introduction to Physick*,[63] with some modernisation and some repetition omitted. The sixteenth century phrases speak best for themselves.

The spirit is a subtle vapour of the blood which by virtue of the heart gives power to the body in all manner of works. Although there is but one source of all spirits they can be identified by their location. Three different spirits are mentioned. The Vital spirit is a flame in the heart made of blood carrying vital heat to the other parts of the body. The arteries (called pulses) carry this spirit, the importance of which can be judged by the fact that every part of the body has need of "vitall and lyevely heat" to conserve its substance. This vital or lively blood is preserved

> . . .by that same lytle sparcle of vitall spirit, whiche in olde tyme wise men dyd so mache marvel at, that summe thought it to be mannes soule, and summe the instrumente of mans soule.[64]

It was accepted by all that death is, as (Langton says) Aristotle had said, "nothing but the quenching and puttynge forth of lyvelye heat."[65] The Animal spirit is a spirit that by virtue of the brain is made brighter and convenient for the working of the senses and the stirring of the sinews. Though the heart is the originator of spirits, they take on a new nature in the brain. Indeed, Langton explains, there seems to be a certain affinity between vital and animal spirits, for the spirits that best temper the heart are those that will bring forth the most noble and excellent effects in the brain. For all that, there is a difference between these spirits because they have different effects. Vital spirit ministers to the heat of the body, animal spirit stirs the senses and causes movement. This is the general view, but some, such as Lowe, are more precise about the work of the animal spirit, saying it is that which "remaineth in the braines," of which a great part is sent to the eyes, some to the ears and divers other parts. Lowe explains that the animal spirit is not "brought through all the Nerves substantially . . . but only by the Nerves optickes, because they have manifest hollownes, and not the rest."[66]

There is some uncertainty over the Natural spirit. Langton explains that some people add this third kind of spirit called natural, which

---

*The sequence of powers and spirits has been reversed for the sake of clarity.

nourishes the blood in the liver. He refers to Galen as doubting this, saying:

> . . . id est si spiritus naturalis est aliquid, whiche is as muche to saye, as yf the naturall spirit be any thynge. For althoughe it can not be chosen, but that there muste be spirite in the lyver yet it is brought thyther by the pulses, which is a token that it commeth from the hert. . ."[67]

The arguments put forward in *Principles of Physick*[68] are based on the anatomical differences of the brain and liver and the lack of arteries coming to the liver. The points made are that if there was a natural spirit it would (like the animal spirit) have to be made from the vital spirit. But the vital spirit, made in the heart, is carried throughout the body by the pulses and there are no big pulses connecting the heart and the liver only "such as be with the smallest for such a pourpose."[69] Also the liver contains no cavity in the way that both the heart and brain do, wherin the natural spirit could be generated. Elyot has no qualms on the matter. He clearly describes the natural spirit as that "which taketh [h]is beginninge of the liver, and by the vaynes, which have noo poulse, spreadeth into all the holle bodye."[70] Langton withdraws from discussion, saying "but I wyl determyne or constitute nothynge of thys matter: leavynge every man to hys own judgement."[71] The most widely accepted view was that:

Vital spirit is made in the heart from blood and air by the force of vital heat and spreads throughout the body to maintain its vital heat.

Animal spirit is made from vital spirit in the brain and influences the senses and causes movement. It is spread throughout the body through the nerves (sinews).

Natural spirit is engendered from vital spirit in the liver and is required for natural operations, such as concoction and the making of blood. It spreads through the body in the veins.

Powers and operations

Three words are used interchangeably by many sixteenth century writers to describe powers. These are powers, faculties and virtues. No clear differentiation is made between powers and their operation. Lowe, in his chapter headed "Of Actions and Operations of Vertues," describes the actions in terms of vital, animal and natural, adding that it is unnecessary to go into the matter further, "seeing the difference is not great betwixt vertues and Operations of Vertues."[72]

There are the same number of powers as spirits. They are given the same names and are related to the same parts of the body. Elyot, Langton and Lowe describe them as follows:

Vital or spiritual power. Elyot describes the spiritual power as that which dilates the heart and arteries and likewise constricts them.[73] Where the spiritual power is stirred into action by external causes it produces anger, indignation, "subtilitie" and care. Lowe says the same sort of thing, but separates the vital power into its active and passive parts. The active dilates the heart, as in mirth and love; the passive virtue constrains and binds the heart and arteries as in conditions of melancholy, sadness and revenge. But all acknowledge that it is the vital power "which caryeth life through all the body."[74]

Animal power comes from the brain by the sinews, affecting all parts of the body. It has three main actions, described by Lowe in terms of three virtues — namely, the motive, the sensitive and the principall. The motive virtue is concerned with voluntary movement through the instruments of the muscles and nerves. The sensitive can be divided into the external and the internal parts. The external senses are: seeing, hearing, tasting, smelling and feeling. The virtue "sensitive interior" is "a virtue that corespondeth to the five externall virtues, by one organ only, and there is called sence common." The principal virtue consists of imagination, reason and remembering.

Natural power "is that which commeth from the liver and sendeth the nourishment through all the bodie."[75] The action of this power can be separated into that part "whiche dothe mynister" and that "To whom is mynistred." These divisions are separated further into the processes (or faculties) required for digestion,[76] assimilation and nutrition.[77] Natural power is the most important power in relation to nutritional theories and therefore will be further examined in detail.

Langton is quite discursive about the powers but makes these points in his writings. He talks about the "natural powers or actions" and does not confine his information to the one "natural" power. He explains that anyone who wants to know how many natural powers there are in the body must understand the natural workings of the body, "for every worke commeth of some action, and also every action of some cause."[78] He gives as examples the fact that a child, before it is fully formed, is the result of a "natural work" proceeding from the natural action of generation. After birth, another natural work is required to bring the child to its full growth. This is achieved through the faculty called auction. When a person is fully grown the nutritive faculty takes over. In order that a person "maye long continue and endure, nutrition onely doth make and bryng to passe."[79] Sixteenth century theory accepts this division of the faculties and (like Galen)[80]places the emphasis on different faculties at different stages of life, but recognizes that all are closely interrelated. The emphasis is such that generation dominates the period before birth and includes the period of growth to the complete infant. Auction is strongest from birth to maturity and nutrition is concerned primarily with the maintenance of the grown body. Langton elaborates further on the meaning of these three words:

Generation is not some simple action but is a compound of alteration and formation;

> For howe could eyther bone, sinowe or veyne be made without anye alteration of theyr substaunce: or how coulde they be well figured or proportioned except they were first out of all fassyon and ordre.[81]

The words generation, alteration and formation had elaborate philosophyical connotations for sixteenth century theorists, but Langton, in this context, does not define them precisely. He does say that alteration takes place in both generation and in nutrition, but explains that the alteration of generation differs from that of nutrition. "For in generation that is made fleshe, whyche before was none: but in nutrition, the meat or nouryshment is made lyke to that that is nouryshed."[82]

Auction is an amplification in the length, breadth and depth of all parts of the body. This can occur only when generation has fashioned the parts. The way in which every part can become bigger always seems to require some sort of explanation. Langton uses the same example as Galen,[83] namely that of children filling animal bladders with air and warming and rubbing them so that they expand. It will be seen that as the bladder becomes larger its walls have stretched and become thinner. The difference between this example and growth is that nourishment is brought to the part during growth. If nourishment could be applied to the bladder as it stretched, then its walls would not become thin and the bladder would grow in the same way as the body does. Langton ends his example by saying,

> Wherfore it is very evydent that nothynge can be encreased as it ought to be, without nouryshment: . . . and therfore auction is suche a thyng as can not possibly be without nouryshment.[84]

This clearly states that growth cannot occur without nourishment. The practical application of this fact is not carried through, as no direct link is made between any special need for nourishment and the growth of the young, though adequate heat and moisture are recognized as being essential for them (see also Chapter VIII Section II).

Nutrition. "Nutrition is the makynge lyke of that which nourysheth, to that, that is nourysshed."

Langton stresses the similarity of nutrition and assimilation, saying "seeing that assimulation is the onelye action of nutrition." He then points out how complicated a process this can be. Yellow can be made red in "one symple alteration or chaunge," but the conversion of blood into bone must go through the stages of blood thickening into flesh and then the flesh hardening and whitening into bone, for which "it muste both have long tyme, and moche alteration."[85] In some circumstances it is impossible to alter foods so that they can nourish a particular individual, for "nothynge can be made lyke, whyche in qualitie differeth, or be contrary." Therefore it is recognized that not all living things can be nourished by every food.

Another reason why not every food suits all living things is because of the amount of excrement involved. Langton illustrates his point by referring to the ability of animals to be nourished by grass, though man cannot be. Man's capacity for altering grass is not great enough; it has too many excrements for him. With difficulty man can be nourished by roots, though much of this food will pass into the intestines and only a little be taken up by the veins, and will still leave much exrement.[86] At the opposite end of the scale, man can very easily change flesh into good blood without the loss of a lot of excrement.

To make all these alterations requires the work of many powers and instruments in the body. Langton outlines the processes in this way. His description is given here at length, but with some modernization of spelling for ease of understanding.[87]

Therefore let no man marvel at the great number of instruments which God and nature hath ordained to the nourishing of the body: for some do prepare nourishment for every part as the mouth, wesande maw [stomach] and liver. And some do separate the excrements from good juice, as the small veins in the liver. Others do let out excrements as the nether [lower] mouth of the stomach and the great master vein of the liver, called the Cava. Others do receive the excrements, as both the bladders, as well that that is in the liver, [gallbladder] as the other beneath [urinary bladder]. And besides this the raynes [kidneys] milt [spleen] and guts. And others do thruste forthe excrements, as the muscles. And finally there be some prepared to carry the profitable juice throughout the whole body as the veins. . . . For after that the juice is fallen out of the veins, first it is dispersed abroad, and by and by, is joined or put into that part, which shall be nourished, and afterward fastened or glued to the same, and last of all made like. And then it may very well be called nourishment, and not before.

The differentiation between material that is nourishing, i.e. after it has nourished, and foods which are potentially nourishing, is a perennial and difficult question. Langton refers to Hippocrates and says,

Nutrimentum quod nutrit Nutrimentum quod est, veluti nutrimentum, nutrimentum, quod est nutriturum. Whyche is as muche to saye as nourysshement that doeth nourysshe alredye, and norysshmente that is lyke norysshement, and norysshement, that hereafter wyll noryshe.

That which is already made like, Hippocrates (says Langton) calls *nutrimente*. That which is "fastened onely, and not made lyke," he says, is like *nutriment*. All the nutritious material in the stomach or veins is called *nutrimente in time to come*, because if it is well digested, it will nourish. From this Langton believes it is "evydentlye proved, that noryshment is the making lyke of that nourysseth, to that whyche is nouryshed."[88]

Besides the three parts of natural power already referred to, that is, generation, auction and nutrition, natural power can be divided into that "whiche dothe mynister" and "To whome is mynistered."[89] The four virtues related to "whiche dothe mynister" are the Attractive, Retentive, Concoctive and Expulsive. Nature has endowed all the living parts of every living creature with these virtues and Langton stresses that for man's survival it is necessary for the four powers of attraction, retention, concoction and expulsion to be present in every part.

For it shall not be possyble for any creature that hath so many dyvers partes, sette so farre one from an other to lyve or continue a very short tyme: yf he lack the powers aforsayde.[90]

Langton explains that without the virtue of attraction there could be no admixtion* and therefore no agglutination.* No assimilation*

---

*Admixtion is the mingling of one thing with another; the addition of an ingredient. *Agglutination had a similar meaning to the present one, i.e. a glueing together or adhesion or cohesion. *Assimilation is the action of making or becoming like.

can occur without agglutination and nutrition depends upon assimilation. These remarks and later descriptions show that, as in Galenic theory, it was recognized that nutrition took place *in situ* in all parts of the body.

The Attractive Power. This is in every part and draws into the parts things of like qualities and those things which are "mete and convenient." The way in which the attractive power works is compared to the action that occurs when "the adament stone draweth yron, the jette stone chaffe or strawe."[91] Langton points out that the Epicureans do not believe in the power of the "stones" but explain the attraction as being due to little "mottes."[92] He rejects this view as being very foolish (it is of course contrary to the ideas of Hippocrates, Galen and Aristotle), and explains that the Epicureans have been shamefully deceived. In order to convince the reader of the reality of the attractive power Langton quotes a number of examples, e.g. the attraction of stones, medicines which will pull out thorns or draw out the poison of a snake or a toad, the speed with which men with short necks and wide throats swallow their food half-chewed (this is the attractive power pulling the food down from the mouth), and the separation of the watery substance from the blood through the action of the kidneys. Here it is said to be the attractive power of the kidneys acting rather than any expulsive power.[93]

Most sixteenth century physicians did believe, like Langton, that each part of the body had an attractive virtue which could draw into it suitable material for its own nourishment. Elyot refers to the attractive power as the one which "appetiteth."[94] Though appetite is mentioned frequently it is usually in terms of a factor which should regulate the taking of food. On the whole, sixteenth century authors are not very forthcoming with further information. Langton gives the most.[95] He is quoted below with a partially modernized spelling.

Appetite is provoked in the higher mouth of the maw when the parts, being very much wasted, doth lack nourishment, and endeavoureth to draw of the veins, the veins of the liver and the liver of the stomach or maw of his overmouth,[96] which is drawn together, and vehemently desires meat. This drawing together cometh of melancholy, which brought thither by a vein coming from the milt and of this fashion hunger or appetite is stirred up or provoked if it be long unslaked, it may turn to further inconvenience.[97]

The idea that melancholy from the spleen provokes appetite in the upper part of the alimentary tract is not the only theory. Langton himself offers an alternative idea, saying "Summe thynke that hunger cometh not as I have descrybed, but that there is a peculyar power in the nutrityve partes, as in the stomacke and lyver whyche doo provoke it." He adds the example of the pike which is reputed to eat so greedily that its stomach rises up into its mouth.

Though Elyot uses the word appetite in relation to the attractive power, he is really considering the three factors of hunger, appetite and attractive power. A point of interest which does emerge from Langton's remarks on appetite is his reference to the fact that when hunger is not satisfied the liver will act upon the stomach, "For in such case alwaye the lyver fylleth the stomake with excrementes."[99] This would explain why some stomachs are still full late in the morning despite the fact that the individual is fasting. This two-way traffic between stomach and liver was an accepted function.[100]

The Retentive Power. It is not sufficient for the attractive power to draw nourishment to the parts unless the nourishment can be held there. If the "juice" is not held at the place where the nourishment is required "but shoulde be caryed to some other parte"[101] then agglutination and assimilation cannot take place. Therefore each body has the retentive virtue in it. As proof of this virtue Langton explains that sometimes the retentive power can be perceived by the senses, sometimes its action can only be recognized by reason. The recognition of the power by the senses is said to be so obvious that it needs no demonstration.

Two examples of the retentive power recognized by reason are: a woman retaining a child within her for nine months before birth and the stomach holding food in it long enough for the food to be altered and concocted. An argument against this last example is that food is retained in the stomach only because the lower opening of the stomach is very narrow. Langton counters this by saying that not only food is held in the stomach but also drink, even though drink "which for his slypperness and subtillitie woulde passe through out a very lylte hole." He also points to the material found in vomit some two to six hours after a meal is taken. It will be appreciated that the significance of the pyloric sphincter was not clearly understood, as in animals examined after death the sphincter would be relaxed. Sixteenth century physicians were able to conclude that there is a strong retentive power in the body.

The Concoctive Power. The modern dictionary definition of concoction includes the following: "To make ready or mature by heat; digested refined or matured by heat."[102] Elyot says briefly that "concoction is an alteration in the stomacke of meates and drynkes, according to their qualities, wherby they are made lyke to the substance of the body."[103] The usual descriptions given by modern students of Renaissance physiology are similar to Sherrington's in *The Endeavour of Jean Fernel*.[104] The first concoction is the conversion of food into chyle: the second, or great concoction, is that in which blood is manufactured; the third, broadly speaking, is the alteration into flesh of the materials absorbed from the veins. This is the most usual type of description; however, Langton states that "there be manye kyndes of concoction" and describes four sorts.

(i) Concoction in the stomach. This is where food is altered and turned into "chile in the which the four humors are not, but potentially."[105] Concoction is sometimes referred to as digestion; in fact Elyot uses the word "Digesteth" when referring to concoctive power. Celsus, in *De Medicina*,[106] sums up what ancient authorities thought was gastric digestion. Erisastritus thought food was ground up in the belly. Plistonicus (a pupil of Praxagoras) thought food putrefied. Hippocrates believed that food was cooked up by heat. Celsus says that the followers of Asclepiades disagree with all the above notions, believing that no concoction takes place at all, but that instead material is transmitted throughout the body in the same crude form as when it is swallowed. Sixteenth century theory held to the Hippocratic and Galenic views — that is, that digestion in the stomach was like a cooking process, with heat from the liver like a flame under the pot.[107]

(ii) Concoction in the liver. Here the chile or "juice" is turned into blood, that is, the *masse sanguinary*.[108] The quality of the juice depends on the foods eaten. Some make good juice, others ill juice. Elyot gives lists of these.[109] From good juice comes good blood, and from ill juice bad blood. Elyot adds that "Cruditie is a vycious concoction of thynges receyved, they not beinge holly or perfitely altered."[110]

(iii) Concoction in the veins. Here blood is prepared for the nourishment of the whole body.

(iv) Concoction in the parts. Here the nourishing blood is made into the appropriate similar material to that which is being nourished, "And this kynde of concoctyng, dyffereth as moche from the alteration of the meate into the juice as nutrition from the chaungyng of the juice into blood."[111] The alteration of black to white (or vice versa) or blood into bone, require a number of stages from the one extreme to the other.

Another factor to be considered is the demand of all the parts for the material available. Langton compares a man's body with the household of a Prince, where every day a large number of meals are served in different places at different times of the day. Everyone (or all parts) cannot be fed at once and some must wait. In the body the stomach, liver and heart are fed first, then the veins, then "every parte as he is best able ... the weakeste parte goeth ever to the worst." However, sometimes "the weaker plucketh from the stronger as the stomacke from the lyver, when the lyver is ful of meate and the stomacke is empty and hath none."[112] (This does not mean that Langton thinks the stomach is the weaker organ but is so only in this situation where the full organ is stronger than the empty.) Langton points out that the weaker must not take anything from the stronger by violence.[113] Those parts which are naturally weaker will have an increased amount of excrement. The example given is the skin, which may break out in boils. In all concoctions, the changes that take place include a separation of what is needed from that which is to be rejected.[114] The removal of excrements is controlled by the expulsive power.

The Expulsive Power. In the same way that the attractive power draws toward itself the needed materials, so the expulsive power rejects hurtful and unwanted things. To prove this point Langton returns to the woman with child. As long as all goes well in the pregnancy the expulsive power rests (and the retentive power is dominant). If anything goes amiss then the child is expelled, this being entirely due to the action of the expulsive power. To make his case stronger Langton refers also to the separation of good juice and excrement in the stomach and the removal of water from the blood in the liver.[115] (The blood is considered to be "thickened" juice.)

Other writers do not refer in detail to the expulsive power. They do recognize that it may, frequently, need help and lists of methods of evacuation are given. Elyot describes the treatment under the headings of "Vomyte" and "Purgations by siege."[116] Meat or drink which is superfluous or corrupted in the stomach is best expelled by vomiting, provided the patient is well enough to bear it. Purges by siege means through the gut and expelled at the anus. The treatment to produce this evacuation can be with potions, electuaries or pills by mouth or via the rectum using suppositories or clysters.[117] Elyot describes the appropriate sort of conditions under which each sort of treatment may be given. The list of ingredients of purges is long and consists of varieties of herbs and fruits.[118] With his list of purges Elyot includes digestives, e.g. "Digestyves of Choler." Here the reference is to those plants "which of their propertie do digest or purge superfluous humours." There is a difference between "digestive" and "purge," though not defined. Purges remove and digestives break down. Elyot adds after his list of purges of melancholy "Melancholye for the thynnesse and subtylnesse of the humour, nedeth no digestive." The word "digestive" can also refer to any food which, if taken at the end of a meal facilitates the proper concoction of the meal. An example is cheese. In choosing a purge Elyot advises,

> This is a general rule concernyng excrementes, that the cause of retaynyng of them beinge perceyved, the contraryes unto that cause wolde be gyven . . . [e.g.] If the cause be of taking soure thynges or bytter than to use competently thynges sweet or fatte.[119]

Writers stress the characteristics of different foods with regard to their "causing oppilations" or their loosening effect; many descriptions of foods in the sixteenth century refer first to the quality and degree of the food and then add such things as "purges the breast and lungs." The help or hindrance a food could give to the retentive or expulsive powers was an important consideration.

For the other aspect of natural power, i.e. "to whom ministered," we agree with Elyot when he says

> All the resydue concerninge things naturall, conteyned in the Introduction of Joannicius, and in the lyttell crafte of Galene,[120] I pourposely passe over for this tyme, for asmoche as it dothe requyre a reder havynge some knowledge in philosophye naturall, or els it is to harde and tedyouse to be understande.[121]

Annexed to things natural are Age, Colour, Figure and Diversities of kinds. Elyot actually gives detailed reference only to age and colour.

Age is here divided into four sections, but it was frequently further subdivided (see Chapter VIII, Section III).

Colour can be due to inward causes (i.e. to a man's natural complexion) or to outward causes. These include hot and cold climates, the illustrative examples given by Elyot being "englyshe men be whyte, Moriens [sic] be black."[122] Other outward causes of colour are "accidental" things such as the emotions of fear, anger or sorrow.

Figure. Lowe says of Figure or habitude that "It is a thing that sheweth the temperature whereof the body is composed." He refers to four figures, namely Quadrature (of good temperature), Crassitude or thickness with excess heat and humidity, and Extenuation which is hot and dry, and the fourth Figure which "is very fatte, proceeding of exceeding coldness and humidity."[123]

Diversity of kind. Another word used for kind in the sixteenth century is "species," which refers in this instance to mankind in general and not to a particular individual. The meaning is Aristotelian. Cuffe, discussing the "perpetuall preservation of the species or kind," explains that species is a thing "existent onely in the imagination [and] not having any reall being."[124] Beyond listing "diversity of kind," authors make no further reference to it in relation to diet because all their remarks are concerned only with man.

Varieties of heat

The importance of heat to life and health is immediately apparent from any book on the preservation of health. However, most authors do not attempt to define or explain the many types of heat mentioned. The kinds of heat referred to include those that are described as:

accidental*	lively
actual	moving
elemental	natural
flowing and running	proper
gendering	putrefying
generative	radical
heat of the seed	rotten
heavenly	temperate
implanted	unnatural
innate	vital

In addition, there is the added differentiation between hot in act and hot in power, and also between the quality "hot" and the hotness of such things as pepper. A number of modern writers have written about the concepts of heat in relation to physiology in the period under consideration. Clagett discusses heat in relation to late Medieval physics[125] and Sherrington touches on the views of Jean Fernal.[126] Both Goodfield

*The list is given in alphabetical order. A number of the descriptions are synonyms for one another.

and Mendelsohn[127] include references to sixteenth century ideas in their studies of the theory of heat in physiology and Pagel comments on the views of Harvey's predecessors.[128] None of these works are designed to explain the meaning or derivation and interrelationships of the types of heats listed above. A sixteenth century work on health that makes some contribution towards this is John Jones' *Growing and Living* (1574), in which he tackles the subject of heat.[129] Some of the authors Jones refers to are:

Aristotle	Fallopius	Montanus
Avicenna	Fernelius	Moses
Cardanus	Fuchsius	Pliny
Chaucer	Galen	Rhazes
Cicero	Hermes Trismegistus	William Turner
Damascenus	Hippocrates	Zoilus
Drusianus		

A summary of Jones' information follows below, omitting his philosophical discussions, and with a minimum of comment. The object here is simply to indicate some of the ideas held in Elizabethan England about the relationship of heat to the body. Jones' style, unfortunately, is as obscure and complex as is his subject.

The Aristotelian separation of heavenly and elemental heats is followed.

Heavenly heat is related to celestial bodies, the supernatural and the soul.

Elemental heat is the beginning of all growing and living things and is God's instrument. Together with moist, cold and dry it makes the parts. Jones says "I say this taking the elementall force for the whole Element" and continues,

> But because this heate is not in acte, as *Fal.* affirmeth *li. de cal.* it cannot be touched or felt, albeit devisable in the compounds, that is although it be, it cannot be knowne by any sensible reason.[131]

It is contained "in very deede in the fleshe, bones and all the parts" but so altered that it cannot be recognized by any sense. Yet if you compare the parts of the body to the elements and compare the heat in living bodies to fire and the breath to air then "you shall finde a great resemblaunce of the second Elements." (This is taken to mean the corrupted, not the pure elements.) It is this *elemental* heat "which maketh our temperature with the other Elements" and is important in the formation and composition of the body. If this heat is changed, then

> all things are dissipated, or disservered, all things decay, which happneth not in other qualities and therefore this heate is as it were a knot or band of our composition.

Multhauf has pointed out that Fernel emphasizes the importance of distinguishing the "innate heat" of concoction from "elemental heat."[132]

Natural heat.

> We have another heate called naturall, which is known by sense as the unnaturall also. For ther is no man if he will feele that may not easely perceave heate in all living creatures, growing or not growing. . .[133]

This is recognizable by the senses (as also is unnatural heat) and is present in all living things, whether growing or not growing. It is present in different degrees in different species. Sometimes it is so weak that "it is knowne rather by reason than by sense." The strongest natural heat is found in lions; it is weak in fishes and "more slacke as in plants." Jones quotes a case to emphasize that there is natural heat in plants. (This is a point of some doubt and receives considerable contemporary discussion.) The example given is the fact that the snow which falls nearest to a tree melts first, thus showing that natural heat is present in the tree (and therefore in plants).

Accepting the notion that plants do have natural heat, the question is, how do they get it? The belief is that plants receive their heat from their seeds, which in turn have obtained it from the earth. It is asked how the earth, which is cold and therefore has no "actual heat" in itself, can provide the required heat? The explanation is that

> The earth truely waxeth warme accidentally, not naturally, nor actually, neither potentially, but either by the heate of the Sonne, and starres reflected, or else through their moving, heating and therefore the sommer is hot by reason of the beames of the Sonne which fall directly uppon us.[134]

It is pointed out that "the sonne hath not his heate in acte," nor does it provide *elemental* heat; the heat is derived "by reason of the rowling of the sonne and starres: for all moving is heating, as affirmeth Aristot."[135] This is the same as the heavenly heat to which Batman refers. Jones has a marginal note saying "Heavenly heate cause of earthelie increase," and points out in the text that it is this relationship between the shining and moving of the planets and the heat in plants which caused "that Astronomicall and Philosophicall saying of *Ptol.* and *Aristot.* that is that all inferior things are ruled by the superior, and that the sonne and moone engendreth man."[136]

Seeds in the earth can obtain heat from the warmed earth, but "when the earth hath conceaved these seedes" they can also obtain heat for growth from antiperistasis (the Aristotelian "reaction" of qualities).[137] This is defined in modern terms "as the intensification of a quality by sudden contact with its contrary quality,"[138] and here it would seem to be when the coldness of the earth, in the absence of warming beams, exaggerates heat already within the seed. Alternative names given to this heat by Jones and other authors are: the *heat of the seed* or *proper* heat, *generative* heat and also *implanted* heat. In man, natural heat is received either in the seed or in the blood. It is the first heat of the elements and springs "either of seede or else of blood by which the sperme is nourished or else of the wombe in which living creatures are engendered. And therefore is called generative, naturall, and proper."[139]

The first great change occurs about the sixth day by which time the seed and blood have been baked together with great heat and the chorion formed.[140] The development of *natural* heat in an embryo seems to have been accepted without undue criticism; doubts as to how this occurs in other situations persisted. Jones quotes things that are "briede without damme," referring to eggs incubated without the parents and the engendering of snails and eels. The heat for this engendering comes from rottenness.[141]

The natural heat in living things requires perpetual preservation. Plants and growing things have the earth to preserve their heat, "but in those living bodyes which are in the ayre, this heate is preserved of a commune cause, and what is that cause? it is a moving and shining."[142] However, because "ther is no shininge or lyght in our bodies causing heate," it must be preserved by moving.[143] Jones expands at length on how this heat is produced, describing the diastolic and systolic movements of the heart and emphasizing the perpetual movement.[144] (Jones' habit of running on question and answer without adequate punctuation is distracting at first.)

> Therefore by moving heate is preserved in living thinges by what moving naturall or voluntary, the voluntary movinge is not perpetuall, it wil be wearied, therfore ther was required a naturall movinge perpetuall as longe as liffe endureth, as testifie the *Arist. lib. de. mundo* and which is that, it is the movinge of the harte diffused or spreade by the arteries. . .[145]

The efficient cause of this movement is the vital faculty. The heart, then is the "Fier and hearth of naturall heate: For it of all the partes of a living creature is most hote."[146] Jones explains that the heart has received this heat from the sperm or mother's womb and

> of necesstie it hath this naturall heate in it selfe in acte, which stirreth up the heart, this stirring up and closing kepeth the heate, there is faculty of moving and heate, heate kepeth the faculty, faculty engendreth moving, moving heate as oft as the faculty or operation of the hearte ceasseth, by reason of poyson received or any otherwyse, furthwith the heate ceasseth and the moving is hindred, the heate ceassing the faculty is destroyed. . .[147]

The heat in the heart requires its efficient cause, the vital faculty, which in turn is dependent on heat to maintain the living body, without which all faculties are "destroyed." As will be seen from the discussion of the effects of the non-naturals on the natural heat the heat in the heart must be kept temperate. Too little natural heat will cause the body to decline. Normally natural heat is spread through the parts of the body, which anyhow have need of it, otherwise it will become too much in the heart and destroy itself. Jones explains that the preservation of this heat involves all parts of the body because heat cannot be preserved "except a vapour hote in acte did flow to the partes." The heat is said to be "infunded, flowing and running." Jones explains that these are the terms that

> Philosophers and Phisitions do use, for by the flowing and running heate, is always understoode that naturall heat which can no more containe life without the radicall moisture nourishing, then the light in a candle can remain without moisture cherishing the fyer.[148]

The analogy between the heat of living and the burning of a torch has already been referred to. It is commonly used by writers from Galen to the present day. Jones' description follows in full:

> . . . it standeth as heate in a torch, or cresset kindled, for as the heate consisteth of that qualitie, and of the matter subject, which is not but a whot [sic] and drye exhalation and fume kindeled, and of this fume and quality, the light in the torch or cresset is kindeled: so also such heate as I have named vitall hath a matter subject to which it is knit and if it is made one called natural heate. And as in a burning torch smooke is supposed, so the proper subject of this heate is breath, which Phisitions call the vitall breath, of *Moses* the living soul, *Gene. cap.2* and it of the Philosophers is sayde to be the true subject of this heate.[149]

The relationship between vital heat and the soul was an important point of discussion for theologians and philosophers.

The quality hot cannot exist alone; it requires a subject. Natural heat "hath a thin subject to which it cleveth," and this proper subject is breath. Here breath is related to the "spirit or airy substaunce of heate and faculty."[150] A number of modern writers[151] have commented on the use of the analogy of the heat for life and the burning torch, when discussing the place of respiration in early ideas of physiology and also, following Aristotle, have commented on the supposed refrigerating effect of breath on the heart. The Elizabethans thought of the breath as helping to keep the heart temperate, either by cooling air or by the lungs' preventing the heart from receiving air that was too cold.

> The breath is the moving of the hart and of the lunges, gendered through drawing in of colde ayre, to temper kinde heat, and expulsing out of the same ayre: for the heart by no means can suffer the lacke of drawing of aire. . .

Natural heat can also be destroyed by lack of moisture or "drowned by superfluouse moysture or else by moisture viciate and unnaturall the bodie dyeth by suffocation, putrefaction, or corrupcion."[152]

The differences between the heat of animals and man and the variations from person to person and at different ages, can be accounted for by the relationship between natural heat and radical moisture. Jones also discusses the relationship between heat and moisture in the body, in terms of alteration, transmutation and concoction. The first alteration is a perfect alteration, later ones being imperfect.[153]

Unnatural heat. This is a heat which is against or contrary to nature, and therefore may be "accidental" heat. The case of accidental heat quoted by Jones, who had a particular interest in it, was that of hot spa water. Water is cold by virtue, and the methods whereby it might have become warmed are discussed at length. The conclusion reached is the Aristotelian one — that water obtains heat from the fire under the earth. There is a passing comment on the fact that the water in waterfalls is cold despite its fall from high and craggy places,[154] though this movement might reasonably be expected to produce heat.

The effects of accidental heat in living bodies are secondary, since they already have natural heat in them. Here the result of unnatural heat is due to the clash of two heats. Heat against or contrary to nature may easily be perceived by the senses, "and this doth not differ in

qualitie from the former [natural heat] for there is the same fiery qualitie on some part." The two heats differ because they are contrary "And
the heate contrary to nature destroieth the naturall, and contrarily."
Jones asks why do these two heats destroy each other? He explains,

> It appeareth not: bicause both be hot. Heat consisteth in the intended
> degree, or in the purchased acquired or els in the matter subject: for
> in every growing and living thing the naturall heate hath in it self a
> certaine degree, which it cannot passe or exceede: according to the
> which life endureth.[155]

Natural heat has its own natural degree which must not be passed. This
natural degree varies from species to species and even between the different parts of each body. If there is an increase beyond the proper or
correct heat this will cause a clash of heats. "If this heate [the normal
natural heat] shal be kindled beyond the degree, then they [the normal
heat and excess heat] strive betwene them selves." This excess heat is
sometimes called *rotten* heat.

Unnatural heats can also be contrary because of their "matter subject." The temperate or natural heat resides in the pure spirits and the
unnatural heat in the corrupt. Here the clash between natural and unnatural heat is due (in part) to the fact that "the putrefying heate doth
seeke to corrupt the naturall and the naturall contrarily assayeth to
qualifie and amend the rotten." The differentiation between "rotten
heat" (supposedly an excess of heat) is not clear, the words rotten and
putrefying frequently being used interchangeably. Beside the margin
note "Rotten heat defined," it is described as

> defined of *Galen in Ther* to be an alteration of the whole body, putre-
> fiing of the substaunce to corruption, of outward heate, because it
> entiseth unto it selfe naturall heate, together with moisture, and
> bringeth it forth by the poores. . .[157]

There then follow references to the cause of tertian fevers which are
not apposite to this study, though one sentence is appropriate to the
subject of different heats. In the beginning of tertiary fever

> we have a double heate, one contrary to nature, which is in the cho-
> lericke humors putrifiing, worthely therfore called putrifiing heate
> and it may also exceede it, this is not the fever, but the cause of the
> fever. . .[158]

Further on Jones explains:

And the chefest cause of putrifying heate is inward stopping, and obstruction of the waies or meanes so that the moist vapours and the digested can not evaporate or out breath ... [references given to Galen and Montanus[159]] therefore do wax hotte.[160]

Jones sums up the causes of an excess degree of heat on the body as follows:

Inward cause of excess heat.
(i) The presence of rotten heat sending fumes to the heart; the heart passes them on to the spirits which in turn spread them through the whole body.
(ii) Antiperistasis of the hot spirits to the heart which are, there, made so "vehement" that heat of a greater degree is kindled. Here antiperistasis will have the meaning referred to by Pagel,[161] a movement of antiperistasis a reciprocal replacement of hot evaporating matter and the product of its condensation in the periphery.

Outward cause.
(iii) "Boyling about the heart" caused by anger.[162] Outward causes are listed together: quick movement, running, extreme labour, "fervent heate," watch (being awake), hunger, strong medicines and over-hot baths. Jones says it should be noted that "unlesses this heate contrary to nature, doe hurt the action in degree, and dissolve the temperature of the parts, it is not called sickness whether it tary short or long time." A differentiation was required between the obvious rise in temperature after heavy exercise and that occurring in the course of a fever.

To avoid or mitigate the effects of unnatural heat the individual should adhere to his appropriate regimen or diet, taking into consideration all the non-naturals.

The following groupings appear to fit Jones' descriptions:
Heavenly heat is celestial and essential for the growth of vegetation on the earth. It is gendering, and when the earth has "conceaved" the seeds their heat can be called *heat of the seed* or *implanted* heat or *proper* heat.

Elemental heat is the beginning of life and analogous to the "pure" elements. It is not hot in act and cannot be felt by the senses. It is gendering and acts first on the conception of the embryo which then develops vital heat.

Natural (vital, proper, innate, or *lively) heat* is the heat which, with moisture, maintains the life of the body. The term *radical heat* and moisture is sometimes used. Natural heat is hot in act and is recognizable to the senses. It requires an efficient cause — the vital faculty — and when attached to its "spirit or airy substaunce" can be *flowing and running* to all parts. It is essential in all parts of the body and for good health should remain *temperate.*

Unnatural heat occurs when the natural degree of heat in the body is exceeded or altered by inappropriate "subject matter." The unnatural heats in the body are called *rotten* or *putrefying.* They can be due both to internal and external causes.

In relation to all these types of heat the two Aristotelian ideas hold good: one, that *initially* all heat comes from movement ("all heat is moving"), the other that "hot" associates things of the same kind and dissociates things of different kinds, hence the importance of heat in generation, auction and nutrition.

Things against nature

These are considered under the three headings of: the malady, the cause of the malady, and the accidents or symptoms of the malady.[163] Treatment usually requires medicinable meats or medicines. The preservation of health is in the hands of the individual himself if he follows his appropriate regimen in relation to the "things non-natural."

CHAPTER V
THINGS NON–NATURAL

> Under the absurd name of the *non-naturals* (non-naturalia), the ancients included six things necessary to health, but which, by accident or abuse often became the cause of disease; viz. *air, aliment, exercise, excretions, sleep and affections of the mind.* These are now denominated hygienic agents.
>
> Jonathan Pereira (1854)

THE ORIGIN of the term non-natural is open to question,[1] though its use extended over many centuries. The non-naturals, also called not-naturals, are those things which are not part of the natural body but are capable of altering it. All are essential for the preservation of health. In this they differ from the three things which are "against nature" — namely, the cause of sickness, the illness itself, and its aftermath.

Though the non-naturals play such an important part in health, great care and temperance are advocated in their use because "the rashe takynge, or golotonus usinge of them, may bring many thynges to the utter destruction of the bodie."[2] The most common sequence of non-naturals is that termed "Galen's division,"[3] that is, the six factors of: Air, Meat and Drink, Sleep and Watch, Exercise and Rest, Emptiness and Repletion, and Affections of the Mind.[4] Some authors condense these by using the Hippocratic grouping ("avouched by Galen") of Labour, Meat, Drink, Sleep, and Venus. Cogan, not following Elyot in this instance, defends his use of this form, saying that it is "more evident for the common capacitie of men, and more convenient for the diet of our English Nation. For who is so dull of understanding that cannot remember these five words."[5] He further explains that all the non-naturals are so closely interrelated that all six non-naturals will be covered by the five he describes and emphasizes the importance of the sequence in which the non-naturals should be used, which is "to beginne the preservation of health with labour: after labour take meate: after meate drinke, after both sleep: and venus last of all."[6] Instructions given about the six non-naturals are not so precise as to sequence.

N.B. Footnotes to this chapter appear on pages 311-316.

Though contemporary sixteenth century English Dictionary references provide no direct link between diet and the non-naturals,[7] by 1633 James Hart was explaining that "Physitians do most commonly take it [diet] for all the sixe things called not naturall."[8] Whichever form Elizabethan authors used in presenting their information about the non-naturals, all advice is firmly based on the accepted theoretical concepts and is also related in a practical and commonsense way to the contemporary situation. In all cases the greatest proportion of information given is about Meat and Drink; of the other six non-naturals, "Emptiness and Repletion" will be referred to in Chapter VII, dealing with Famine and Surfeit,[9] while the remainder are considered below.

Air

Ayre amonge thinges not naturall is chiefly to be observed, for as moche as it doth both inclose us, and also enter into our bodyes, . . .
                                                                    Thomas Elyot (1541)

Experience clearly demonstrated that without air life is extinguished. This effect was attributed to a change in natural heat which required the influence of air to maintain it at the proper level. Air went to the heart and could act as a refrigerant on any excess heat. Alternatively the lungs, through which the air had to pass, could "preserve the hearte from choking by receyvinge the external ayer which least it should hurt the hart wyth cold commyng sodenly up on it is tempered ther before."[10] Also, according to ancient teachings the action of expiration helped to remove smoky vapours from the heart.[11]

English authors point out that whatever the weather, be it "never so foule," there is no escape from the air surrounding us. Therefore they stress how important the substance of the air is, as well as its quality. Bad air was the main aetiological agent in Hippocratic pathology and was still considered to be a basic factor amongst causes of pestilence. Corrupted air drawn into the body will, inevitably, corrupt it; therefore it is essential to avoid such bad air. For good health the surrounding air should be of good substance — that is, fair and clear, without mists or vapours. It should be light and open, not "dark troublous and close."

The four main causes of bad air are given as: the effect of certain stars (referred to by Bullein as "unfortunates" whose influence brings corruption),[12] standing waters and stinking mists, any marshy ground (particularly where hemp or flax lay rotting), carrion lying unburied and too many people living close together in too small a space.[13] Situations to be avoided included "being neare to draughtes, Sinkes, Dunghilles, Gutters, Chanels, Kitchens, Churchyards or standing waters."[14] There was danger too in cellars and vaults and "holes where mettels be digged."[15]

For those who had a choice, the proper placing of the house and the planning of its outbuildings should be carefully considered. Unlike their predecessors the Elizabethans did not have to think in terms of building for defence against their enemies. Homes were built for the comfort and pleasure of the family and friends with the full recognition that the appearance of the building was also important.

"For the commodysous buylding of a place doth not onely satysfye the mynde of the inabitour, but also doth comforte and rejoyseth a mannes herte to see it."[16] Books on the preservation of health give practical advice about the positioning and care of the home so that bad air can be avoided. The aspect of the dwelling should preferably be with the main windows opening on the east and west sides; failing that, northeast or southwest. The east wind is the best wind, being "temperate, fryske and fragraunt." The south wind is the worst of all, being corrupt and making evil vapours.[17] These directions are derived from the Hippocratic *Airs, Waters and Places,* though there the author is not quite so precise, but emphasizes the benefits of facing the rising sun.[18]

In planning the estate there should be no marshy lands or standing water near the house. Where this is impossible, as in the case of moats and fish ponds, these should be fed by a fresh spring. If no spring was available such areas of water should be cleaned regularly and no excrement or kitchen waste thrown into them. Bad smells indicated bad air; therefore, in general terms, all buildings which might contain odorous material — such as the slaughter-house, brewery, bakery, dairy and stables (except for a few of the Master's riding horses) — should be placed well away from the main residence. Boorde suggests a distance of a quarter of a mile.[19] If the common privy is not situated over running water, it too should be placed well away from the house. The need for general cleanliness throughout the household is stressed, including outbuildings, and special care should be taken in the dairy.

Within the main house rules of hygienic behaviour, particularly with regard to the use and emptying of chamber-pots,[20] should be enforced. The need for cleanliness in the kitchen, larder, buttery and cellar is clearly stated. Smoke or dust in the atmosphere made bad air, so the smoke from the kitchen should be as little as possible, and any sweeping which caused dust to rise should be done when the sweeper is alone.[21]

Much of this detailed advice is good hygienic practice by modern standards, but how closely the Elizabethans followed it is difficult to estimate. John Shute, described as "the first known English architect,"[22] believed that bedrooms should face east, studies to the north and winter living rooms to the west, adding "For what side is defended from the south windes which are grevous and contagious."[23] However, to judge by the grandeur of the south fronts of houses like Wollaston Hall and Hatfield House[24] the possibility of contagion from this quarter was not taken seriously. Similarly, directions to keep stables and slaughterhouses a good distance from the main house seems usually to have been disregarded.[25] Pearson, in her comprehensive work *Elizabethans at Home,* describes the farm dairy, dovecote, chicken house pigsty and stables as being "within easy reach" of the farmhouse.[26]

Cleanliness in the home would, then as now, have depended a great deal upon the attitude of the mistress of the house. In general the situation seems to have improved towards the end of the century, to judge by a comparison of the remarks made by two foreign visitors: Erasmus commented on the filth left lying among the rushes on the floor in England,[27] and Lemnius, the famous Dutch physician, wrote with praise of the English freshly strewn rushes and sweet smelling chambers.[28] Two new factors which must have helped to foster a greater appreciation of cleanliness were the widespread growth of pride in the home[29] and increased daylight in the rooms. Improvements in the home came with the new materials for furniture and furnishings, and the light was improved by the great increase in the number of windows now that more window glass was available.[30]

While the substance of the air was a matter of concern at all times, the quality of the air took on a special importance in times of illness. The normal temperate man is unaffected by slight variations from the natural hot:dry quality of the air, but if the balance of the qualities in the body was disturbed then air of a contrary quality was needed. If a cool air is required this can be obtained by sprinkling cold water on the floor, or by the "strawying of herbes and be settying of suche boughs as be colde and moyst."[31] If a really hot:dry air is required the house can be "perfumed" by suitable hot:dry things until the air becomes sufficiently changed. In diseases of long standing a complete change of air — that is, of location — is considered the best remedy.

The action of air was basically similar to that of food and drink, in that all affected the body through alteration in the qualities present. In later works on foods, such as Lemery's *Treatise of all sorts of Foods*

(1745)[32] air is classed as a food. This association of air with food continued until well into the nineteenth century.[33]

Sleep and watch

> And if by imagination thou didest perseve sleping and waking wayed in the balance together, there thou should see them equal in waight.
>
> William Bullein (1558)

The classical description of sleep as the image or brother of death is frequently quoted, as is the short definition, attributed to Aristotle, of an "impotencie of the senses."[34] A fuller explanation says that,

> Slepe is the reste of the animal vertue, whiche is whan that the profitable vapours of the nouryshment, be caried up into the brayne which do melte and waxe soft there, and runnying into the brayne, do stoppe the conduytes of the sensis and also the synnowes, whyche be the instrumentes of movyinge.[35]

While the animal power is at rest, the natural power works more strongly and natural heat moves inwards from the outer parts of the body. This makes possible perfect concoction of both the food eaten and of any superfluous humours present. From the concoction vapourous fumes reach the coldness of the brain where they congeal and prevent the action of the senses. Proof of this theory can be seen, it is said, in the fact that people become sleepy after eating and that "most vaporous" foods, such as wine and milk, produce drowsiness.

Sleep was recognized as being essential to life;[36] being awake too long cooled the natural heat, "like a fier which with too muche moovinge and stirringe is blowen abroade and dispersed."[37] This naturally harmed the body, whereas the proper amount of sleep had certain beneficial effects: strength was restored, body and mind refreshed, anger pacified, sorrow assuaged,[38] and the whole man brought to a good temperate state.

All advice related to sleep is based upon the realization that during this period the natural heat moves inward and requires material to concoct. This material must have moved into a proper position for concoction and be in a correct proportion for the individual's particular powers of digestion. Sleeping habits should be considered in relation to time, place, position of the body, and the quantity of sleep needed. The proper time for sleeping is quite clearly at night, between sunset and sunrise, for this follows the course of nature. The silence and moisture of the night lulls one to sleep, whereas in the daytime natural heat, spirits and humours are drawn to the outer parts of the body and sleeping in the day was "as it were a fighte and combat with nature." For the sick or weak who could not sleep at night, sleep in the first three hours after sunrise was allowed. Any afternoon sleep should be avoided; the superfluous humours, which would normally be dispersed if the person was awake, would instead remain in the muscles, veins and joints. If sleep during the day is essential it should be of short duration,[39] taken at least half an hour after a meal and in an upright position (to facilitate the movement of the food down into the stomach). Sitting up in a chair or even standing leaning against a cupboard are suggested.[40] The sleeper should be awakened gently. It is wrong to go to bed directly after supper. Time should be allowed "untill the meate bee well mingled and gone downe to the bottom of the stomacke."[41] This is facilitated by gentle walking for an hour or two after eating. This time should be carefree and merry because a good sleep required a quiet mind; otherwise dreadful dreams might come.[42]

The bedchamber should be clean and sweet smelling and situated upon an upper floor, but not directly under the roof.[43] Sleep was best in a dark room of moderate temperature, too cool rather than too hot, following the Hippocratic advice to "sleep in a cold place well covered."[44] Sleeping on damp earth or cold stones was for soldiers or prisoners but, says Cogan, certaintly not for students. The bed should be large, long, soft and well shaken and made rising toward the feet and "no higher than a man may easily fall into it standing upon the chamber flower." Cogan gives no reason for this requirement, though a number immediately come to mind.

The position to be taken during sleep is carefully described. Besides the raising of the feet "so that the bulke or chest of the bodie may be lowest," the head should be "somewhat high, well bolstered up," and the individual should start his sleep on the right side in a relaxed position with the body, arms and legs slightly bent.[45] All this is obviously designed to aid the mechanical movement of the material to be concocted. Sleeping on the back was to be avoided. For those with weak stomachs, sleeping face downward helped the concoctive action of the natural heat. The wearing of a head covering to keep the head warm is a good thing, but to sleep in shoes of any sort hurts the sight and memory and causes the whole body to become overheated.[46]

The amount of sleep required depends upon the health, age, digestive condition and complexion of the individual. For a healthy person seven to eight hours sleep was generally recommended. More sleep was required in winter than in summer. The healthy need less sleep than the sick, old people more than youth or middle age, those with poor digestion more than those with good digestive powers. The choleric who "are hotte and do eate lytell, and digeste quyckely,"[47] need only a little sleep, while the phlegmatic need more to counteract the moist humours they engender. Those with natural melancholy are comforted by a long sleep.

Sleep should end when digestion is complete and waking comes naturally when the body needs to get rid of its waste products. Sufficient sleep gives a feeling of lightness to the whole body. If the time is too short the head and eyes are heavy and an aftertaste of the last meal may be present. If there is doubt as to the completeness of the sleep a skilled examination of the urine can indicate if it has been sufficient.[48]

Clear directions are given as to the steps to be taken upon rising. These are an elaboration of the six given in the *Regimen Sanitatis.*[49] First is the admonition to "ryse with myrth"; the body should then be gently exercised to facilitate the downward movement of waste matter prior to evacuation. After going "to stool" rubbing of the limbs and trunk with the hands or a linen cloth was advised. This had to be done with care, avoiding the stomach, belly and kidneys.[50] The face, and particularly the eyes, as well as the hands and wrists, should be washed in cold water — not in hot water, which was harmful.[51] The teeth and mouth should be cleaned thoroughly and the hair combed. This was intended to open the pores and allow the unwanted vapours from sleep to escape.[52] After dressing in freshly aired and brushed clothes it was good to take exercise. Boorde suggests "a thousand pace or two" in the garden.[53]

Exercise and rest

For as the flowing water doeth not lightly corrupt, but that which standeth still: Even so bodies exercised are for the more part more healthfull, and such as be idle more subject to sicknesse.

T. Cogan (1584)

Cogan divides exercise into two parts, saying, "As man doth consist of two partes, that is body and soul, so exercise is of two sortes, that is to say of the body and of the mind."[54] Though all bodily exercise is movement, not all movement was considered exercise, "soft" or "light" moving being excluded.[55] Labour or exercise — the words can be used interchangeably — is defined as "vehement moving, the ende whereof is alteration of the breathe or winde of man."[56]

Exercising had three important functions. Firstly, it hardened the limbs and made those, such as labourers, who took exercise regularly, stronger and altogether healthier than people who were physically inactive.[57] Secondly, natural heat was increased, digestion speeded up and nutrition improved. Finally, exercise also quickened the movement of the spirits throughout the body, thereby helping to purge it of excrements.[58] Sixteenth century theory and advice follows a pattern in use from ancient times[59] and directions as to the type and timing of suitable exercise, in relation to the condition and circumstances of the individual are complicated and detailed. The following general summary gives the types of exercises referred to, though authors vary in their classification and the list is incomplete compared with records of contemporary pastimes.[60]

Vehement exercise. Elyot says that this is a compound of violent and swift exercise, but the exact differences are not clear.[61] Examples of *violent* exercise are: digging in heavy soil, carrying heavy burdens, climbing up a rope, hanging by the hands with the feet off the ground, wrestling, casting the bar, holding the arms outspread for a long time. *Swift* exercise would include: running, playing with weapons, going on the toes, throwing the ball (if the ball is chased after throwing, the exercise becomes vehement). *Vehement* exercise consists in: leaping, football, quoits, dancing, tennis, shooting, bowling in a field or alley, throwing of the javelin many times.

It was recognized that some of these violent exercises were actually "work" for husbandmen.[62] Most of the vehement exercises were banned by statute for the great majority of adult males in England on "military, economic, and to a lesser extent, moral grounds."[63] These restrictions did not apply to the social group from which the readership of books on the preservation of health was drawn. People of the upper ranks enjoyed their games.[64] However, Elyot, in the chapter "that shotyng in a longe bowe is principall of all other exercises," of *The Governour*, states that [nine-] pins, quoits and football should be utterly rejected by all noble men. The last is nothing but "beastly furie and extreme violence: whereof procedeth hurte, and consequently rancour and malice to remaine."[65] Tennis was commended above all other exercise by Cogan, who said "Galen most commendeth the play with the little ball which wee call Tenise."[66] Because it entailed stooping, which hurts the head, tennis was not considered to be suitable for grave personages busy with weighty affairs, or for those whose head is not temperate. Such stooping can be avoided, it is noted, by standing with the head held upright and striking the ball with a racquet.[67] Dancing was not prohibited by statute, but came to be condemned by Puritan preachers. It was an activity to be avoided by sage Magistrates and studious students as being too great an exertion.[68]

Moderate exercise is described as walking long distances or going on a journey.[69] If the long walks are often repeated they become a strong exercise. Gentle walking is a soft and light movement and as such is not considered an exercise.

Gestation is the situation "where one is caried and is of another thyng moved, and not of himself."[70] This is particularly suitable for the weak and those suffering a long illness. Modes of travel referred to include a horse-litter, coach, waggon, and being rowed in a boat or barge. To be carried on rough waters was a different matter, for the emotions induced and the physical difficulties endured made this type of gestation into violent exercise.

Exercises for parts of the body. There are obviously many different types of actions which will exercise special parts of the body. Examples are: running for the legs, shooting for the arms and shoulders, playing bowls for the back and loins, while the "stomacke and entrals, and thighs and reines of the back are chiefly exercised by ryding."[71] The chief exercise for the breast and trunk is "vociferation." This makes the natural heat "fine and stable," strengthens the parts of the body and improves resistance to disease.[72]

Cogan stresses the importance of playing instruments and singing to overcome the "dumpes of melancholie." He points out the way in which the singing and whistling of ploughmen and carters lessens the tediousness of their tasks.[73] The physical action entailed was also of importance. Finney has shown in her study of vocal exercise in the sixteenth century that music was good not only for enjoyment but it also had an important physiological value in the regimen for health and disease.[74]

Frications or rubbings. Sixteenth century writers refer in some detail to the frictions and unctions used by the ancient Greeks and Romans.[75] Though, as noted above, Elyot found rubbings in the morning beneficial, the general attitude, in England, of describing but not advocating, is summed up by Cogan when he says,

> And of fricacies they [the Ancients] have made generallie three sorts, first hard rubbing to binde or consolidate, then soft rubbing to loose or mollifie, and lastlie meane rubbing to augment and increase flesh. But this kind of preparation whereof Galen hath written abundantly in his seconde book *De Sa. Tuen.* is not used in England. . . .

Cogan concludes with a "merrie tale" of rubbing: the Emperor Augustus, seeing an old soldier rubbing his back against a pillar, gave him money to hire a servant to do the rubbing, and soon found all his soldiers rubbing their backs against walls.[76]

Baths, it is said, "sometimes supplieth the office of Labour, and standeth in steede of exercise, beyng either ayrie or waterie in sweete water."[77] This statement is from the translation of Gratarolus, who is referring to Galen's advice and gives a special section on bathing. Despite the increasing interest in the use of mineral baths,[78] which were considered to be of benefit to the sick, English writers on the whole make few references to the use of baths by the healthy. Bullein, however, is quite explicit:

> The best bathing is in a great vessel, or a little close place with the evapuration of divers sweete hearbes wel sodden in water, which have vertue to open the poores softly, letting out feeble and gross vapors, which lieth betwene the skinne and the flesh.[79]

This sort of bathing, with the use of sweet oils as an unction, is particularly good during times of pestilence. Gratarolus considers baths especially suitable for those who "have fat and corpulent bodies or else bee replete with aboundance of humours,"[80] but always they must be used in moderation and avoided completely in very cold weather or in the hot summer. The effect of baths on the natural heat and the humours could be very damaging. Washing in cold water must be avoided by all who were not accustomed to it. Adults could become accustomed gradually by starting their cold baths in the warm weather. Cold baths should not be taken by those who were still growing, because the effect on the natural heat could inhibit growth.[81] Vaughan recommends cold natural baths for those subject to rheumes, dropsies and goutes, and asks "How shall a man bathe himselfe in winter time when waters be frozen?"[82] Here he refers to the healthy man and the answer he gives includes a recipe containing turpentine and butter mixed with herbes to be used with linen cloths.

The washing of the head was a matter for comment. The old saying "Wash thy hands often, thy feete seldome, but thy head never" appears to have been accepted by many. This is contradicted by physicians with the advice that the head should be washed with warm water which contains a variety of substances of a "cold nature." The head should then be dried quickly.[83] The primary object of all sorts of baths was to remove superfluous material from the body; the greater importance of baths for the sick was due to the fact that they produced more super-fluous humours. For this reason references to bathing are sometimes given in the section on purging.

Exercise of sight, hearing, smell and taste. The emphasis placed on the need for pleasant surroundings reflects the belief that the senses were strengthened by such a situation. Gratarolus explains that,

> Moreover it is expedient, temperately to recreate the senses, as for example, the sight with viewinge and beholding faire shewes and beautifull things, the hearing, with harmonicall and melodious Musicke. . . .

For smelling, the sweet smell of rose-water is suggested and for taste, a mixture of sugar, pomegranate or quince juice, thickened by boiling, is recommended.[84]

For all bodily exercises the individual has to choose the appropriate type, duration and strength of the exercise he should take, always bearing in mind the heating/drying effect exercise will have on him. The obvious example is that a man of choleric complexion should be most careful of how much exercise he takes.[85] As well as the advice already given, in regard to specific types of exercise unsuitable for special groups, the general rule was that "sick folkes, leane persons, yong children, women with childe may not much travaile." The body should not be exercised if any ill humours are present because the increased movement of the spirits may disperse the bad humours to parts previously unaffected.[86] One rule that should be applied to everyone was the Hippocratic saying, as referred to by Cogan, "Let labour goe before meate."[87]

The best time for exercise is when both the first and second concoctions are complete. Exercise too soon and the mass of material in the stomach will be improperly concocted, causing the body to become filled with crude humours; exercise too late and yellow choler will be increased. The proper time for exercise can be determined from an examination of the urine, which should be a "temperate" colour.[88] Cogan notes that students in Germany and England neglect this advice which accounts, he says, for students being often troubled with "Scabbes." The fact that workmen are able to go back to work after their meals without ill effect is explained by the fact that "Greate labour overcommeth all things."[90]

Though Cogan describes the time of day and season which the Romans thought proper for exercising, he adds, "I restraine no man to

the houre," provided exercise is taken "after the excrements bee avoyd-
ed, in an wholsome ayre, and before meate." For a healthy man the
amount of exercise to be taken could be judged in this way. Exercise
produced four clear changes: (i) the flesh swells (ii) the body becomes
red (iii) movement becomes easier (iv) sweating occurs. When any of
these changes stop, such as "if the lively colour stirred up by exercise
shall vanish away," then the exercise should be stopped. Of the four
points, the two most important are sweating and "abating the fleshe."
Rest, as such, is not emphasized, though the best time to rest is "whan
the body is weried with labour."[91]

Mental exercise or study is the "naturall nourishment of the mind and
wit," for it is in man's nature to want to exercise his mind, as is shown
by the mental activity of young children. For a learned and skillful
man, to study is to live; idleness is not only against nature but also dulls
the mind. Study is defined as "A continuall and earnest cogitation applied to some thing with great desire,"[92] and this should not be undertaken in a haphazard way. Most English books on health limit their
advice to the warning that too much study is even more harmful than
too much bodily exercise. Cogan is an exception and gives quite detailed advice to students. This is one of the few occasions on which he
refers to the influence of the "planetes (as the Astronomers teache)
most favourable to learning." These are *Sol, Venus,* and *Mercurie,*"[93]
which come together in the early morning. The morning is definitely
the best time for study, not only because of favourable planets, but also
because the rising sun clears the air, which in turn helps the blood and
spirits of the student. The day should begin with prayer, followed by an
hour's meditation and study. This should be interrupted by a brisk
combing of the hair (forty times) and teeth cleaning, both intended to
stimulate the head. Studies should then continue until around noon,
with short breaks every one or two hours. Afternoon study is not considered good, but two hours work after noontime is permissible. However, this period should be used to reconsider the matter already read
and not for new studies. Mental exercise at night is bad, for the same
sort of reasons that staying awake at night was not recommended: the
spirits go to the brain, leaving the material in the stomach undigested.
Cogan then rather undermines his argument by giving examples of such
famous "diligent students" as Pliny and Galen who were said to have
worked both night and day.

The conditions under which study is best done are described. A quiet
"closed" room, or gallery, is best for concentration.[94] The light should

come from the side opposite to the "pen handle." Standing, leaning on
a pillow, is advocated for study, as this is better for the movement of
the blood and humours and avoids sitting down all the time. Those who
exercise the mind should also have proper recreation, though this
should "not bee dissolute nor unsober, but honest and pleasant."[95]
Music is particularly recommended, because it not only gives "solace
and recreation, but also because it mooveth men to vertue and good
manners, and prevaileth greatly to wisdome."[96]

Throughout the advice on Exercise and Rest, the need for a balance
between the two is stressed, but if this balance is not maintained then it
is less damaging to have too little exercise than too much, remembering
always that "sluggyshnes dulleth the bodye"[97] harms the mind and
that idleness of body or mind can lead to sin.

Affections of the mind

Passion is a violent motion of the soul in the sensitive part thereof.
                                        Pierre Charron, trans. Lennard (1601)

The Elizabethan belief that a passion of the mind, such as great joy,
could cause death[98] was founded on the acceptance that there is "a
verye great connexion or knittinge together between the bodye and the
mind."[99] The instrument of passions was the "sensitive soul." At this
time theological discussion of the soul took place against the background of the traditional theory of the soul with its threefold aspects.
These consisted of the vegetative soul which gives life but no feeling,
the sensitive soul that gives life and feeling, and the rational soul (ex-
clusive to man) which gives life, feeling and reason.[100] Discussion of the
soul and its influence was not strictly limited to theological works;
moral treatises in the vernacular, such as the translations of the works
of La Primaudaye, Charron and Thomas Wright, *The Passions of the
minde in generall*, went through many editions.[101]

Wright describes passions and affections or perturbations of the mind
as the actions which are common to man and beast (both had the sensitive soul) and discusses the meaning of these three terms.[102] The difficulty of defining each term has been summarized by Anderson in her
study of *Elizabethan Psychology and Shakespeare's Plays*.[103] In general,
passions and perturbations suggest a more violent response than affections though the distinction is not clear cut.

Writers on health use all three terms to describe the four main emotions of anger, fear, sorrow and joy.[104] The physical reactions to these

responses are described. In anger the natural heat moves from the heart to all parts of the body, "getting the body on fire." However, if natural heat is feeble then it will not go out to the parts, with the result that they are cold and trembling.[105] During anger the pulse increases.[106] Harmful results of anger include: fevers, apoplexies, forgetfulness, loss of reason, fancies of the mind, deformity of the face, lack of appetite, poor digestion, and insomnia. The angry person is likely to swear and blaspheme [107] and become uncharitable and undutiful. Anger does not kill because it does not cool the natural heat[108] or dissolve the strength.

In fear the blood and spirits are drawn inward, leaving the outer parts cold and trembling and the pulse weak.[109] The action of fear is sudden and immediate. Sorrow comes little by little. It too "draws in" the heart and exhausts the natural heat and moisture. The action is far reaching. The wits are dulled, reason lost,[110] the body extenuated; it "drieth up the bones"[111] and can lead to death, for "sorrowe hathe killed manye."[112]

Elizabethan writers touch on the "heaviness of mind" or depression, which is the greatest enemy to life; but this, as part of the illness of melancholy, is best discussed in treatises devoted to melancholy.[113] Joy or gladness of the heart prolongs life, the body becomes fatter, the temperament more equable and there is a drawing of natural heat outwards.[114] It is this outward movement of natural heat which can cause death if the shock of joy is too sudden. Advising against "inordinate gladness" Elyot reminds the reader that "the extreme partes of mundaine joye is sorrowe and hevinesse."[115]

Though each of these passions produced characteristic physical reactions, there was some uncertainty as to whether all passions arose from a common centre or whether certain kinds of emotion originated in particular parts.[116] Most generally it was held that all passions reside in the heart, though other organs are related to them in a special way, as Shakespeare associated the liver with love and the spleen with irascibility. Many writers on health confine themselves to describing the physical reactions due to anger, fear, sorrow and joy, and offer no specific treatment. Others try to get to the root of the problem and explain that affections of the mind "not onely requyre the helpe of physycke corporalle, but also counsayle of a man wyse and well lerned in morall phylosophye."[117] Elyot gives counsel along these lines.[118] The angry man was advised to contemplate the patience with which Christ bore His sufferings.

The effects of sadness were considered to be particularly serious and much advice was given on ways to counteract it. Firstly, the ingratitude of a friend should be counteracted by the realization that "thou arte delivered frome a monster of nature,.that devoured thy love." Secondly, the death of a child could be softened by considering the many children who caused their parents more pain than is caused by a child's death. Thirdly, when goods or authority are lost it is good to remember that this is seen to happen frequently to those who seem to work hardest at increasing their goods and enforcing their authority. Fourthly, where promotion is withheld, reassurance comes from the fact that if this is done against the opinion of good men, then it is obvious that the authorities are blind; however, if it is due to personal folly, then this is what must be changed. In general it is good to dwell on possible adversities, for from the contemplation of miseries can come a contempt for the chances of fortune, which in turn gives one a quiet mind.

Medical advice for counteracting sadness recommends that surroundings be pleasant in all aspects. Unpleasant sights, sounds and smells should be avoided. Because of the movement of the natural heat towards the heart, temperately hot and somewhat moist foods should be taken; they should be easy to digest and be boiled rather than roasted. Unsuitable foods include hard cheese, salt fish, large oily seafish, cabbages, beans, garlic, red wine and old salt, sour, fried or burnt meat. Elyot adds items which are specifically "Confortatives" of the heart when it was hot, cold and temperate. The list is mostly herbs, but unusual items included are "the bone of the harte of a redde deare" (for the hot heart) and a "unicornes horne" for the heart that is cold.[119] Things to comfort the temperate heart are predominantly jewels or minerals.[120]

Venus

For those authors who use the "Hippocratic five" non-naturals, the last matter to be dealt with is Venus or "carnall copulation." The desire for copulation was recognised as being God-given, so that "by procreation the world might be replenished with people."[121] From a physiological point of view it was believed that after

> the third and last concoction: which is doone in everie part of the bodie that is nourished, there is left some part of profitable bloud, not needefull to the partes, ordeyned by nature for procreation.[122]

As food was concocted and new blood formed every day, material for procreation was continually produced. This inevitably gave rise to bodily lust which required relief, lack of relief being the cause of many illnesses. On the other hand, the dangers of immoderate Venus were also many. Hippocrates is said to have likened the effects to those symptoms present in the falling evil[123]and Avicenna is credited with the statement that if the loss of seed is "above natures measure it doth hurt us more than if forty times as much blood were avoided."[124] However, "the commodities which come by moderate evacuation thereof are greate."

Unlike the other non-naturals which are common to all ages, "Venus is chiefly used in lusty youth." This period is somewhat narrowly restricted, in a statement attributed to Galen, to the ages between 25-35 years. The question is asked whether Venus is necessary for all men, and as might be expected, Biblical texts are used to reconcile the natural lust in man with the wickedness of uncontrolled indulgence in it. Cogan discusses the advantages and disadvantages of marriage at some length and states his belief that "The single life is more convenient for Divines."[125] For the single student he gives special advice, warning that because of its abundance of blood the sanguine complexion is most given to Venus. A number of unctions and drinks are recommended, but basically the methods of avoiding or subduing lust are those given in the Bible. Cogan places great emphasis upon the dangers of evil women. Students should either forego the company of women altogether, or

> if they be in companye with them, stoppe their eares, that is to say, bridle their senses, or binde themselves to the mast, that is to say: pray unto God for grace, least they bee intangled ere they be ware.[126]

All the non-naturals act upon the body by affecting the amount of natural heat and radical moisture present. Sometimes this is by a direct increase of natural heat, as in exercise; sometimes the concentration of heat is transferred to a different part of the body, as during sleep or in emotion; sometimes the natural heat is affected indirectly because of an alteration in the balance of all the humours or a loss of material from the body. The amount of detailed information given by sixteenth century authors about each non-natural is not surprising when it is remembered that books of that period devoted to the preservation of health are basically books on the subjects which later came to be put under the headings of nutrition and hygiene. The advice given can be summed up by this verse:

> Ayre, labour, foode, repletion
> Sleepe, and passions of the minde,
> Both much and little, hurt a like,
> Best is the meane to finde.[127]

CHAPTER VI
CRITERIA FOR ESTIMATING THE VALUE OF FOODS

> Jo. Aliment, is that which augmenteth and nourisheth our bodies.
> Pe. How many kinds of aliments are there?
> Jo. There are divers sorts . . .
> Pe. Are they all used after one intention?
> Jo. No, they are of divers natures, and must be used in divers man-
> ners, according to the temperature of the body. . . .
>
> Peter Lowe (1596)

IT IS IMPOSSIBLE for a man ever to be totally unaware of food. The importance and emphasis he places on it in his life varies with his ideas about the relationship of food to himself, his social conditions, and his personal idiosyncracies. A study of the ways in which the value of food has been assessed through the centuries shows that the basis of estimation of food values mirrors the generally accepted contemporary concepts of the life processes. Modern concepts are biochemical; sixteenth century concepts were "elemental," in the Aristotelian sense, to match the traditional acceptance of ancient teachings.

The division of physick into diet, medicine and surgery required that some differentiation be made between food and medicine. Sixteenth century authors attempt to make a distinction, but this is difficult because of the inevitable overlapping of the two groups. Bullein gives a fairly precise definition, saying

> Those things that overcome and gouverne the body as purgations, expulsives etc: these be called medicine and those things that nourish and augmentith the bodie be called meates.[1]

Today, as traditionally, the basic distinction between aliments and medicaments is that aliments provide substances which nourish the body, whereas medicines are capable of changing the state of the body. But difficulties of differentiation remain, as in the case of vitamins.[2] Often the division between aliments and medicaments is a pragmatic

---

N.B. Footnotes to this chapter appear on pages 316-319.

one, dependent on the reasons for prescribing the substance and the conditions under which it is given rather than the individual characteristics of the substance itself.[3] Cogan is necessarily vague, saying "And nowe shall I speake of herbes and fruits I mean of these that appertaine to diet, as they be used for meate and not for medicine." He adds that he knows that "there may be as *Hippocrates* sayeth medicinable meate," giving the examples of pepper and garlic as being "hote and drie farr above the meane."[4] The general view seems to have been that "medicinable meats" and medicines were those things with qualities in a high degree above the temperate, but this rule was not strictly adhered to.[5]

The foods which nourished could be identified more precisely because only those things which have themselves been nourished can nourish. Jones elaborates on this.

> Now, all nourishmentes, whereof Dyete consisteth, spring of the first commixtion of Elementes, and they bee eyther of seedes, plantes, or living thinges. For as Fernelius[6] saith, *libro secunde, de abditis rerum causis.* Nothinge can nourishe us, which is not itselfe nourished, and endued with lyfe, as these bee. Certayne of these be simple, certayn compound: Some doo worke in matter, some in qualitie, and matter, as sayeth *Dioscorides, de medica materia.*
>
> Of these, the one sorte be simple meates of meane temperature, endued with no especiall qualitie.
>
> The other be mixed, and are called Medicinable: by cause although they nourishe, yet in qualitie they do alter and chaunge the body of the receyver: Whereuppon there is of nourishments a double facultie: One by which they alter, the other by which they nourishe.
>
> The former [with the "altering facultie"] is knowen of colour, smell, and taste, and also of those things, which doo excell, applyed outwardly, or receyved inwardly.
>
> The latter [with the "nourishing facultie"] is knowen by no reason, but by experience onely; because the whole nature of the thing nourished is a certain propriety to their substance, of *Galen* called likenes 3 ther.7 By which reason nourishment is sweete and pleasant in taste, and as the familiaritie of them, is by pleasantness perceyved so in the contrary by unpleasantness tryed, if so be that those things which do differ from nourishment of their whole nature are unsaverily eaten.[8]

In relation to nourishment Fernel explains the difference between flesh and stones in terms of the *vita* and *calore* in living things. He does not comment on the fact that flesh as eaten is dead and has therefore lost the "life and heat" it had when alive. He is judging the nourishing properties in the light of experience.[9]

From the dietary point of view all foods were distributed within three main groups or "orders." The actual divisions are rather vague and sometimes inconsistent. Also it was recognized that there were great differences between the dietary value of foods within a single group.

The first order includes: bread corn,[10] which "is of greate power and strengthe"; all domesticated four-footed beasts; "great" birds, such as goose, swan, peacock and crane; honey and cheese. Langton notes that there is not only a difference in the dietary value of beasts themselves according to age, but also in the various parts of an animal.[11]

The middle order, giving a "lower degree of nouryshmentes," includes roots, all wild fowl, and fish, especially those which cannot be salted and dried.

The lowest order includes all sorts of salads and "whatsoever groweth in a little stauke," such as cucumbers and gourds, also fruit.

Henry Buttes, in his charming *Dyets Dry Dinner*, presents his foods in this sequence:[12]

(i) Fruits	(v) White meats (dairy produce)
(ii) Herbs	(vi) Spices
(iii) Flesh	(vii) Sauces
(iv) Fish	(viii) Tobacco

As he deals only with the "Dry Dinner," all drinks are omitted. Buttes explains his choice of sequence in this way:

Fruits come first because Adam and Eve first fed on them. Then, after the exile from the Garden of Eden, they "fell to herbs and roots" and man, says Buttes, lived for a long time like hogs on beechnuts and acorns. Because man would not, or could not, be a husbandman he turned to eating flesh and, after flesh, fish was the next easiest thing to get. White meats were more difficult, and required the "help or art of man's invention," so they came later. Gradually man's appetite wanted more than "necessary" food, so he added spices for his "voluptuous delight." Because honey is included in spices, the excess sweetness soon cloyed and condiments or sauces were required to restore the appetite. Finally, according to Buttes, tobacco was valuable for "airying" the body to counteract any putrefaction which would come from excess.[13] This sequence is not as fanciful as it might seem; sixteenth century writers had constantly to try and reconcile Galen's advice on food with teachings from the Bible.

The sequence used by Cogan, which is more practical and more usual, is: cereals (including beans and peas), herbs and vegetables, fruits (including nuts), spices, meats (including birds), fish, dairy produce, salt, vinegar and mustard, i.e. "sauces" and drink.[14]

The six characteristics to be considered when estimating the value of any foodstuffs are: Quality, Substance, Quantity, Custom, Time, and Order. The value of a food had always to be estimated in relation to the circumstances of the individual who would take the food. Quality and Substance are discussed in this chapter; the other factors are referred to in Chapter VIII, Section 5 and Chapter IX.

Quality

In general, the use of the word quality (standing alone) by sixteenth century writers, refers to the hot, cold, dry and moist qualities of the elements or of the humours. However, it is also used to describe some other characteristics of foods, which will be referred to later.

Of the four elemental qualities, heat and moisture have already been referred to in detail; cold and dryness are not given such attention. Elyot describes some effects of cold and dry in this way.

A. What distermperaunce hapneth by the excesse of sundry qualities in meates and drynkes.

B. What commoditie happeneth by the moderate use of the said qualities of meates and drinkes.[15]

Quality	A (excess)	B (moderate)
Cold	Do congeal and mortify	Assuages the burning of choler
Dry	Sucketh up natural moisture	Consumes superfluous moisture

Qualities of foods. Most authors refer to the qualities of specific foods; these were generally accepted and fairly standard. Buttes tabulates both the qualities and degrees of his "dry" foods. A number of foods are included in Newton's *Approved Medicines and Cordiall Receipts,* where the items are classified under their qualities and degrees.[16] Cogan and others do not always refer to the actual qualities, but sometimes only describe the effect of the food.

Degrees of a quality. As has been pointed out in relation to heat, the degree of all the qualities was of the greatest importance, not only to keep the normal balance of the body's temperament but also as a guide to the recommendation of certain foods. Each quality has potentially four degrees. This system was used by Galen, and Temkin points out that just as he had a quantitative scheme for the potency of drugs, so also he had a quantitative scheme for foods:

> If a person's temperament deviates to one side, being too warm by three (imaginary) units, the food must deviate to the same degree in the opposite direction, i.e., it must be three units too cold. Then, and then only, will it have a purely nutritional effect without increasing the abnormal deviation.
>
> Admittedly, these units *(arithmoi)* of which Galen speaks are purely imaginary and cannot be measured. [17]

In succeeding centuries the emphasis on quantification of the qualities and humours was posological. The attempts of Richard Swineshead, Thomas Bradwardine, Arnald of Villanova, Walter of Odington and Antoine Ricart to provide precepts for such a quantification have been examined by a numer of modern scholars. [18] Sixteenth century writers on the preservation of health make no attempt to suggest rules whereby the appropriate intake of qualities from foods can be met. John Dee's advocacy of the use of arithmetic in his "Mathematicall Praeface" to Billingsley's *Elements of Geometrie* [19] gives the following two rules in relation to the mixture of medicines of different qualities and degrees. He refers to the work of Roger Bacon and Lully.

The first rule is that when you have an equal weight of two mixible things whose degrees "are truely knowen," whether their forms are of contrary qualities of the same, but of different "intentions and degrees," or of a temperate and a contrary sort, "The forme resulting of their Mixture, is in the Middle betwene the degrees of the formes mixt."

The second rule applies to two mixible things of different weight, and different qualities and degrees of qualities and says:

> What proportion is of the lesse quantitie to the greater, the same shall be of the difference, which is betwene the degree of the Forme resulting, and the degree of the greater quantitie of the thing mixible, to the difference, which is betwene the same degree of the Forme resulting, and the degree of the lesse quantitie.

Using "the rule of Algiebar," Dee calculates that when 2 lb. of liquor, hot in the fourth degree, is mixed with 1 lb. of liquor hot in the third degree, the degree of heat in the resulting mixture is hot in 2/3 of the fourth degree, the form resulting being 3 2/3 degrees. To use these rules correctly two things were necessary: first, an exact knowledge of the qualities and degrees of the materials involved and secondly, as Dee stresses, they must be mixible. It would be impractical to use Dee's rules when attempting to achieve precision in diets for the preservation of health, because neither of the two rules could easily apply to foodstuffs. Also, the wide range of variation within which the changes of humours could be considered temporary or harmless made these rules inapplicable to individuals.

The method of ascertaining the degrees of a quality are not usually explained in books on health. However, Jones, discussing the quality hot in relation to the benefits of natural Baths, says:

> The just degree (as sayeth Montanus. . .) sensiblie changeth. The second, a feeling payne, payne [sic] bringeth. The thyrd effectuallie changeth, with manifest signe of greefe. The fourth, both sence and temperature fynisheth.[20]

The way in which qualities and their degrees are applied to foods is illustrated by an arbitrarily selected range of examples.[21]

Strawberries Cold and dry in the first degree, "the riper the tempera-
                tur"
Dates   Hot in the second degree, moist in the first.
Pheasant   Temperate in all qualities.
Hare   Hot and dry in the second.
Milk   Moist in the second, temperately hot.
Pepper   Hot and dry in the third and almost in the beginning of
                the fourth. (This is about the highest degree of qualities
                given for any food.)

Despite the fact that Batman, in his presentation of the work of Bartholomaeus Anglicus, sometimes makes very precise alterations in the description of a degree of a quality of a food given by the original author,[22] Elizabethan physicians in general, who derived their information from the observations and records of earlier writers, do not appear to be so precise. It is not at all clear why certain qualities and degrees were applied to foods. But some of the apparently contradictory information given is due to whether the description is related to the sensory reaction felt, or if it is according to the "power" (or effect) of the substance. Both brine and vinegar are called "dry" despite the fact that they appear moist; "yet experience hath proved them drye because they consume the superfluous humours bothe of flesh and also of other things."[23] The osmotic effect of a strong salt solution in the process of preservation, referred to by Batman under his section on heat, is an example of the "drying effect" a moist substance can have. He says,

> For the heat of the salt dissolveth the parts that bee earthy, watery and airely; and so by slackening and softening of the heate is induced moistnesse. Heate bringeth in drinesse, for the heate working in moystnesse dissolveth it first, and when it is dissolved consumeth it.[24]

Other characteristics sometimes called "qualities" of foods. Though of less importance than the elemental qualities a number of these characteristics had also to be taken into consideration. In modern dietary planning the main characteristics to be considered are nutrients, texture, taste and colour. The present concept of nutrients is derived from the new ideas and techniques developed in physiological chemistry in the nineteenth century. There is nothing exactly comparable to nutrient in sixteenth century theory. Modern nutritionists consider the texture of foods in terms of the effect of the blandness or roughness of the food on the digestive tract — e.g., bland for cases where there are lesions of the tract, and roughage to prevent constipation. Elizabethan theory was much concerned with the laxative or binding effects of foods. Today the effect of the taste of foods is considered to be limited to pleasant tastes encouraging good digestion and bad tastes warning of danger. Tastes are not considered to be specifically linked with the functions of nutrients in the body. Colour is considered in the planning of a meal in order that it will be more appetizing.[25] As has been indicated, under "things natural" the taste, smell and colour of food played a significant part in their value for Elizabethans.

(a) **Taste** is defined by Batman "as properly a vertue of knowing sauvours."[26] In order to taste, three causes are necessary: the effective cause, which is the animal virtue, and the material and instrumental causes, which are the tongue and the arteries in it, respectively. The tongue is hollow, moist and unsavourie (tasteless in itself). It receives in the hollow part the humours that come from the thing to be tasted. The tongue is full of holes so that something from the material tasted can enter, whether it is thick or thin. The tongue is moist so that it helps to dissolve the thing to be tasted.[27] The action of tasting occurs by the animal spirits coming down, the sinews of the tongue meeting the material to be tasted and taking on the properties of that substance

"afterwards it presenteth to the high perserverance of the soule." Taste
is necessary for life, for "if the tast be corrupt or faile: the vertue of
feeding faileth." The tongue is unable to distinguish flavours if a single
humour has mastery in the substance of the tongue. An example given
is of red choler making everything taste bitter. "The taast hath lyking in
sweete things, for that lykenesse that it hath with sweetenesse." Both
are hot and moist.[28]

Elizabethan writers derived their classification of tastes from the
Greeks, with some modifications.[29] Jones describes Greek tastes as
being classified in this way:

Calid: Dulcis, Salous, Amarus, Acris.
Frigid: Acidus, Austerus, Acerbus.

The degrees go from 1-4 for hot tastes, and 1-3 for cold tastes. These
are the seven simple tastes — four hot and three cold. The eighth taste
(the *apoios* of the Greeks) is tasteless, without quality.[30]

(b) **Hot Tastes.** 1. Sweet. This is pleasing to the senses, moderately
warming, not very moistening or drying and can "easely be turned to
nourishment." This virtue always comes from the simple sweet taste.
This is altered if sweetness is mixed with, say, bitter or sharp tastes.
Examples of sweet taste are: Sugar, honey clarified or distilled, honey-
suckle, etc. Jones says, "as for wine and fattie tastes they are applyed
to the sweetest."

2. Salt. A hot salt taste brings a certain kind of feeling of heat because
of earthy dryness in a watery moisture. It may heat and dry to the
depth. Salt taste comes from "salt, salt peeter, sal gemme, salt water
bryne, the salt sea etc."

3. Bitter. A hot bitter taste seems to "shunne away from the tongue."
It produces a greater diminishing of earthy substance through heat than
does the salt taste, and therefore has greater force in heating and drying. Bitter taste comes from "Aloes, wormewood gaul etc."

4. Sharp. A hot sharp taste heats, dries, and thins. It can also burn
and consume. Sharp taste comes from "pellitorie of Spayne (pyre-
thrum), Brimstone, Arsemart otherwyse called water pepper, etc."

(c) **Cold Tastes.** 1. Sour. This manifests an earthy substance not completely overcome by heat, resulting in a cooling and drying effect. Sour
taste comes from "unripe grapes, sorell, vergis [verjuice is the acid of a
sour fruit], cider made with wild appels etc."

2. Rough. "Temperatly set on edge and stoppe..." It is cold and dry,

but less so than harsh. Rough taste comes from "Mirtilles [berry of the myrtle], unripe gaules [oak-apples], and the rind of pomegrantes."

3. Harrish. There is unevenness in this taste. It seems to consume the moisture of the tongue (dries the mouth). It is cold and dry. Harsh taste comes from "unripe hedge pears, unripe medlars, sloes etc."

There is good agreement between the quality of the tastes and the qualities of the examples given. There are only minor discrepancies, e.g. sugar (hot:moist) is given as an example of sweet (hot:dry); honey is also given and is hot:dry. Sorrell is cold:moist according to Buttes, and cold:dry in Cogan,[31] where it is an example of a cold:dry taste (sour). Almonds are an example which shows the agreement on qualities and the difference between sweet and bitter: they are hot and dry (Batman, *Uppon Bartholome*), hot and moist (Elyot, *Castel of Helth*), hot and moist (Cogan, *Haven of Health),* and in Buttes, *Dyets Dry Dinner,* sweet almonds are hot and moist, whereas bitter almonds are hot and dry.[32]

Thus taste itself is a factor in the effect of a food on the body because of the qualities it disseminates. Jones gives not only the effects of simple taste, but also of tastes "adjoined" together. Examples are harrish joined to bitter or sharp, and rough joined to sharp. It is important "always to understande that the one or the other is done more or lesse according as the one or the other have preheminence, which rule in every taste ought to be kept."[33]

If the tongue has a predominant humour, this humour will determine the dominating taste, e.g. a red choler makes everything seem bitter; a salt phlegm makes everything salty.[34]

Elyot describes the effects of excessive and moderate amounts of various types of foods.[35]

Bitter food: in excess it does not nourish. In moderate amounts it "Cleanes and wipeth of [off] also mollifies and dispells phlegm."

Fat and oily (unctuous) food: in excess it "Swimmeth long in the stomach and brings in loathsomeness." However, in moderate amounts it nourishes and makes things soluble.

Salt food: in excess salt foods "Do fret much the stomach"; in moderate quantities it "Relenteth phlegm clammy and dries it."

*Harrish/Stiptike** food: in excess such foods "Do constipate and restrain," whereas in moderation it "Binds and comforth the appetite."

Sweet food: in excess it "Chausseth [chafes] the blood and causes oppilations and stopping of the pores and cundytes [conduits, natural

---

*Harrish and Stiptike described as "rough on the tongue," seem to be used here as alternatives.

channels] of the body." In moderation it "Cleanses, dissolves and nourishes."

Sour food: in excess it "Cools nature and hastens age," (Elyot does
not tell us what effect sour food has when taken in moderate amounts.)

Clammy[36] food: in excess it "Stoppeth the issue of vapours and urine
and engenders tough phlegm and gravel." In moderation it "Thickens
that which is subtle and persynge [piercing]."

Sometimes a more detailed comment is given about the effect of a
certain taste, as in *Regimen Sanitatis:* "A sower thynge, as Avicenna
sayeth in many places, hurteth the seniwes, for the stomach is a member full of senowes."[37] In his study of Van Helmont's ideas on gastric
digestion, Pagel points out:

> What is sharp and acid contracts the stomach and may thus help
> digestion by inducing the organ to retain and digest food for a longer
> time and more thoroughly than normal. Black bile that is acid and
> excreted by the spleen into the gut and stomach can therefore pro-
> mote gastric digestion.[38]

In the context of sixteenth century theory the effect of food being
delayed in the stomach was somewhat different. It was recognized that
black bile from the spleen could reach the stomach. Batman's description of the functions of the spleen include a phrase describing the
placing of the spleen on the left side for "cooling of the lefte side, and
for to save the heating of the stomacke, to whom he is joyned."[39] Black
bile brings melancholy humour with it, but the digestive effect of acid
black bile is not emphasized. The extensive use of vinegar, wine and
verjuice in the diet must have provided sufficient acid for it to be recognized that such acid was not harmful, but any beneficial effects are not
particularly stressed. Any action of an acid in extending the time that
food was held in the stomach was not always considered beneficial, for
the delay could lead to putrefaction.

"Fat and oily" are linked with sweet, and seem to aid concoction and
nourishment in a mechanical way. Butter taken before meals helps food
to slide down. If taken in excess the oily material floats on the top of
the stomach contents and inhibits the proper concoction of the contents[40] and "brings in loathsomeness." This effect is produced by foods
which are fat or oily, e.g. butter, cream or vegetable oils. Foods are

classed according to whether they appear oily or greasy rather than by their actual fat content. Recommended methods of preparation often produced an oil-like substance during distillation; this was called the oil appropriate to the name of the material distilled. Oil of Honne is described as "Not an unctuous oil but certain element which is neither oil nor water."[41] It is produced when honey has been heated (twice) and all the fumes driven off. The residue is the oil. Thus references to oils may mean either the actual oil or fat, or refer to the "oily" products of distillation of a food which contained no fat.

Unlike the modern view, which limits tastes to those identifiable by the tongue, and which recognizes the interaction of the senses of taste and smell, sixteenth century theory separates taste from smell.

Smell. This is described by Batman as: "this power of smelling through the subliltie thereof if it be well disposed comforteth the vertue animal and cleanseth superfluous from fumositie." The smell of a substance played an important part in its value. The instrument of smelling also helps to make perfect the virtue of the spirit and helps and strengthens the virtue of life that is in the heart. Pleasant smells are comforting: "the beautie and fragrant savour of roses is verie comfortable to all the senses." If the smelling is corrupted or infected, the value is lessened. However, strong unpleasant smells are not always harmful; "fox-stink," for example, is said to be good against the palsie.

Substance

No clear definition of the word substance has been found in the sixteenth century works studied. It is probable that the word has nearly its modern meaning of "stuff," with some overtones of such things as bulk and texture.[42] Form also is explained in practical terms: Elyot says, "By fourme is understand grossenesse, fynenesse, thichnesse or thynnesse."[43] Therefore a wide variety of characteristics can be placed under this heading, the main ones being those characteristics which Elizabethan authors themselves say require consideration. Here, only those factors have been included which appear in their descriptions of the effects of foods.

A very important characteristic of a food was the type of juice it engendered. "Aliment, is that which augmenteth and nourisheth our bodies. . . . That which nourisheth well ingendereth good juices." Later, in answer to the question, what is aliment which engendereth good juice?, Lowe replies, "It is that which is light of digestion that nourisheth well, maketh little excrements and ingendereth good bloud."[44]

Making good or ill juice. Elyot gives three separate lists of foods which make good juice, ill juice, and thick juice.[45] Other writers more commonly confine themselves to those things making good or ill juice.

(a) *Good juice* is on the whole made from the lighter, pleasanter foods. They include: bread "of pure flour somewhat levened, well baked not too old or too stale," eggs new and soft, new milk and soft cheese, all birds of the "middle order" and some of the bigger ones (such as pheasant, peacock, curlew and capon), fish from stony rivers (those between tender and hard, such as pike or perch), sweet fruits and a variety of herbs, wine and ale of the right age and properly made, the flesh of young animals and fat or "clammy" flesh, the liver and brains of poultry.[46] Elyot adds mirth and gladness to his list of those things engendering good juice.

(b) *Ill juice* comes from old flesh and foods of poor quality such as unripe fruits, "moche used" apples and pears, hard cheese, raw herbs (some are listed), "grayne lyke" peas (probably chick-peas), fish from muddy waters, and the offal and entrails of "almost every great beast." A very significant point made by Langton is that ill juice is made by "all poudered" (salted) fleshe and also "alle salte fyshe."[47] Considering the amount of food that had to be preserved by salting, this must have been a distinct disadvantage. Elyot does not specifically mention salted food. Langton also links ill juice to certain tastes, such as "al thinges that be sharpe, tarte or bytter." As regards herbs, a list is given of those that will cause ill juice if taken in too great a quantity. Elyot ends his list with "Feare, sorowe, pensyfenesse."

The difference shown here between foods making good or ill juice seems to depend on what we should now call good or poor quality. Quite clear descriptions are given for the foods making good juice, indicating exactly what sort of food was needed. No particular emphasis is placed on any special type of foods, e.g. grains or flesh, for making either good or ill juice.

Elyot's foods making *thick juice*[48] are difficult to classify. He includes other sorts of bread, great sea fish and shell fish, beef, offal, much-boiled milk, sweet and deep red wines, cheese, fried or hard eggs, unripe figs and apples, "all round rootes" and a variety of herbs, vegetables and chestnuts (the only nuts mentioned). It is difficult to see any clear pattern of selection in this list.

The connection between juice and blood is very close. Therefore those things which form good juice will help towards making good blood. For good blood to be produced foods must contribute qualities (elemental) similar to those of blood, namely hot:moist. Elyot's list seems to contribute at least one of the two required qualities from most foods. For example, soft cheese (for good juice) is "cold and moist in the second,"[49] but the hard cheese, making ill juice, might be considered to have lost moisture and so would not contribute either of the needed qualities to make good juice. No clear explanations for the choices are given, but they follow the basic theories regarding the qualities of a food.

Ease of digestion. How easily or with what difficulty foods can be digested are other important factors. Lowe has mentioned the importance of foods being of light digestion for good juice. The frequently used terms gross and fine can only be understood by indirect references. For example, Elyot in referring to the diet for a choleric man (see Chapter V, Section 1) explains that choleric men can eat foods of a grosser type, without harm, than other people can, and a piece of good beef is recommended for them rather than a leg of chicken. From reading the sixteenth century texts it seems as if grossness and fineness were probably estimated by appearance and texture, as they might be today, together with the traditional classification for that period.

Fine food, though of easier digestion, was not necessarily the most nourishing, says Langton:

And for the mooste parte, this is alwayes trewe, that every thynge, as it is of strongest substaunce, so it is hardest to be digested, or altered into good juice, but where it can be altered, it nourysseth more then that, that is moche fyner.[50]

Elyot explains:

Of them [foods] whiche do nourishe some are more grosse some lyghter in digestyon. The grosse meate ingendereth grosse bloude, but where it is well concocte in the stomake and well digested, it maketh the fleshe more fyrme and the officiall members more stronge, thanne fyne meates.

Elyot adds that those who labour hard and those with very choleric stomachs, "here in England," can eat gross food in great quantity, "for as moche as in a hotte stomacke fyne meates be shortly aduste and corrupted."[51] Ease of digestion was not therefore simply a characteristic of the food alone but rather the joint characteristic of the appropriate type of food and the action of the stomach it went into.

Proper concoction is also influenced by the length of time the food remains in the stomach. Passing through too quickly produces too much excrement and so some of the value of the food is lost. Too slow a passage will cause burning up or putrefaction. The length of time food stayed in the stomach depended in part upon the order in which it was taken and what foods were eaten together (see Chapter IX: Quantity, Time and Order). Medlars, for example, are slowly concocted and hinder the concoction of other foods.[52] The other factor to be considered was whether the foods would have a loosening or a binding effect upon the body.

Costive or laxative effects. Much concern was felt about the speed with which food passes through the alimentary tract. Reference has already been made to the use of purges and emetics to clear out the system. The expressions costive and laxative, or binding and loosening, appear frequently in descriptions of the characteristics of foods.

Langton has a chapter on each aspect.[53] Those things that "bynde the bellye" include: unleavened rye bread, hard roasted eggs, tame (and inactive) small birds (also cranes), hare, goat, beef, hard cheese and well boiled honey, unripe pears, oranges and quinces, white olives and sharp wine. He sums up: "finally al thinges that be harde, leane, tart, or sharpe, and of flesshe that is rosted, sooner than that that is sodden, have power to bynde the belly." Things that "do leuse the bellye" are unleavened barley bread, lettuce, purslane, oil, onions, mallow beets, cucumbers, cherries, mulberries, garlic, raisins, dry figs (and some other vegetables and fruits), all manner of shellfish, young tender fish, fat flesh in soups or boiled, those birds that swim (these usually have oily flesh), milk, raw honey, sweet wine, "al that is dronke luke warme, and all fatte or swete meates, doe make the bellye laxatyve."

A modern list of laxative foods would certainly include figs, prunes, oils (but of the mineral variety), possibly pulses, and whole wheat bread — always, of course, related to the digestive powers of the individual concerned. It was recognized in the sixteenth century that brown bread "with much bran" can make those that have been costive, "soluble."

The length of time that food stays in the stomach will influence the chances of it putrefying there, but the characteristics of binding or loosening do not seem to be directly connected with the characteristics of "putrefying easily" or not putrefying in the stomach. Langton's two lists are as follows:[54]

Putrefy easily	*Do not putrefy easily*
Leavened [wheat] bread	Unleavened [wheat] bread
All other unleavened breads	All wild fowl of the middle order
Milk	Beef
Honey	Hard and lean flesh
All sorts of cheese	All salt meats
Wines which are over sweet or else "over thynne"	Sharp wines

A comparison of the two groups suggests that one of the criteria used to determine whether or not a food would putrefy easily in the stomach was whether it putrefied easily at all, or rather whether an obvious change occurred in the food after a comparatively short time. Milk, cheese and breads are likely to change noticeably, whereas hard lean flesh (if it is somewhat dry), salt meats, and unleavened bread (which was then probably virtually a lump of flour paste dried hard) could all be considered to "keep."

Langton also has a chapter on foods that cause the belly to swell.[55] These are not related to foods that cause putrefaction in the stomach, but can be classed under the lists of foods (referred to later) which affect an organ of the body. Langton stresses that even if foods make good juice and good blood this does not necessarily mean that they will not affect another part of the body — in the case of the belly — adversely.

Causes oppilations (blockage or obstruction). Elyot, referring to the diet of old men, describes oppilations as follows:

> let them beware of all meates, that wyll stoppe the pores, and make obstructions or oppilations that is to saye, with clammy matter stop the places, where the naturall humours are wrought and digested.[56]

He gives a list of things making great oppilations; they are thick milk, all sweet things, rye bread, and sweet wines. If such things are by chance eaten in abundance (Elyot advises), then things which will resist or resolve oppilations must quickly be taken, as for example white pepper, garlic, and onions.[57]

Phrases like "stoppeth the liver" or "causeth oppilations" (in various parts of the body) are frequently used. It was essential in contemporary dietetic theory that there be free and easy movement of the spirits and nutriments throughout the body. This movement was considered to be much more diffuse than in modern concepts, where gross movement is restricted within the circulation of the blood and lymphatics. Theory allowed the phlegm (for example) to move easily between brain and breast and fumosities could move upwards from the stomach into the head, affecting the sight and causing headaches.[58]

The production of excrements. The loss of any material from the body was of considerable importance according to sixteenth century theory. Therefore the following characteristics need to be considered under this general heading.

Foods which cause sweating. These would include food which opened pores (the opposite of a form of oppilation). Most sixteenth century writers on diet do not dwell on this aspect. Boorde says that figs "do provoke a man to sweate; [but adds] wherfore they doth ingender lyce."[59] This comment needs some amplification. Figs were traditionally associated with lice. Boorde is suggesting here that figs cause lice because of the sweat produced — that is, because the lice come from the sweat.[60] Foods such as hot pepper and spices which, in fact, can cause sweating, are not included under this heading.

Foods which provoke urine. Langton describes them as, for the most part, all things that smell fragrant including, as would be expected, a number of sweet smelling herbs. Others are onions, wormwood, thin wines, long peppers, mustard seed, and "pyneapples."[61] The basis of choice does not seem to be a dietetic one; the only liquid referred to is the wine, though possibly many of the herbs were automatically taken boiled and so added fluid to the diet.

Foods that incite Venus. Too great loss of seed was a serious depletion of the body, so that foods which had an aphrodisiacal effect should be avoided on both dietetic and moral grounds. Many examples of foods which provoke Venus are given by Buttes. Four of these are listed here to illustrate the range of foods involved: saffron, crab, pistachio nuts and pigeons.[62]

Cogan advocates cold apple for celibate students. Boorde says cucumbers "restrayneth verneryousness."[63] But otherwise antidotes to Venus are mentioned very infrequently in descriptions of foods, but may be found under sections headed "Venus." Cogan advocates herbs, especially parsley and rue, to be eaten daily.[64] Plasters of herbs to be applied to the back or reynes are said to subdue Venus. Harrington in his *School of Salernum* says that "sharpe vinegar lessens sperme," but other authors do not seem to stress this view.

Foods which cause ventosyte. A number of foods are described as likely to produce wind. Flatus was considered to be excrement and had to be got rid of. Boorde in his instructions to be followed upon rising each morning stresses the importance of not holding in "your egestion or your uryne or ventosyte."[66] Harrington put it this way:

> Great harmes have growne and maladies exceeding,
> By keeping in a little blast of wind:
> So *Cramps* and *Dropsies, Collickes* have their breeding
> And *Maized Braines* for want of vent behind.[67]

Peas, beans, and grapes are some of the foods causing wind. Still today pulses are often considered as "windy," though this is usually due to poor preparation. Under primitive cooking conditions, the fear of wind from eating pulses is often a deterrent to groups of people taking extra peas and beans which would provide protein that they need. Onions, leeks, and garlic are not (as might have been expected) included as causing ventosyte, though Boorde says that radishes "doth breke wynde."[68]

Maketh excrements. This is a term met with in texts but without a precise meaning. It seems to include other meanings such as foods which cause crudities or putrefaction or turn humours into harmful conditions or make evil juice. It does not seem to have been applied to foods which are recognized now as laxative or bulky and so could cause a greater amount of faeces.

Besides the main characteristics listed above there are innumerable vague terms which are used over and over again. Some are given below:

> "Strengtheneth principal parts"
> "Stays fluxes"
> "Cleanseth the breast" (or stomach or lungs, etc.)
> "Comforteth the heart"
> "Preserveth health"
> "Restorative . . ." (to an organ)

Authors also provide lists of foods which help or hurt particular organs of the body. These include foods which affect the brain (wits and memory), the eyes, the heart, lungs, liver, spleen, kidneys, stomach, and teeth. Examples from Elyot are:[69]

Meates whiche do hurte the tethe. Very hotte meates, Nuttes, Swete metes and drinkes, Radyshe roots, Hard meates, Mylke, Bytter meates, Moche vomyte, Leekes, Fyshe fatte, Lymons, Colewortes.

Thynges which do hurt the eyes. Drunkennesse, Lecherye, Muste [new wine], All pulse, Sweet wynes and thycke wynes, Hempe sede, Very salte meates, Garlyke, Onyons, Colewortes, Radyshe, Reedinge after supper immediately.

Thynges good for the eyes. Eyebryght, Fenell, Vervyn [*Verbena officinalis*], Roses, Celandyne, Agrymonye, Cloves, Cold water.

It is impossible to determine the basis of choice for these foods. Obviously practical factors, such as hard foods and nuts hurting teeth, were an important consideration.

It is clear that, according to sixteenth century theory, there were a large number of characteristics to be considered when evaluating a food, but from a modern point of view one important term is missing. Today a food can be evaluated according to its *nutritive value* (that is, proportion and content of chemical elements which will benefit the body); this can be ascertained from food tables. Thus a food can be described as nutritive in its own right, quite unrelated to the circumstances of the individual who will eat it.

In the sixteenth century the term "nutritive" is used, but nearly always in terms related to digestion: "Veale is [a] nutrytyve meate, and doth nowrysshe moche a man, for it is soone dygestyd";[70] and elsewhere, "The tunge of beestes be harde of dygestyon, and of lytall nowrysshement."[71] "Grosse" foods were, in general, less easily digested than "fine" foods, so the latter were likely to be more nutritious. But, and this is frequently stressed, if the gross foods were concocted properly due to the strength of the appropriate powers in the body, then a gross food was more nutritive than a fine one. The explanation is that the firmer material of a gross food was more like the firm parts of the body.

A striking difference between sixteenth century theories and our own is their evaluation of foods and drink by the conjunction of the characteristics of the food, together with those of the individual consuming the food.

CHAPTER VII
FAMINE AND FASTING, SURFEIT AND PESTILENCE

Famine

Hunger setteth his first foot in the horse manger.

W. Harrison (1577)

THROUGH THE CENTURIES, upheavals due to war, plague and changing social conditions, as well as the susceptibility of agriculture to unfavourable changes in climate, caused fairly frequent shortages of food. Penkethman in *Authentic Accounts of the History and Price of Wheat, Bread Malt etc.* makes reference to the years 1521, 1526, 1527, 1553, 1556, 1558, 1573, 1586, 1594, 1595, and 1596 in discussing dearths.[1] These references, together with Howe's descriptions in Stow's *Chronicles,* indicate that shortages in the sixteenth century were not aggravated by simultaneous epidemics of disease, in man or beast, such as had magnified the disastrous dearths of the fourteenth century.[2] The descriptions put less emphasis on the horrors of famines and more stress on the impact of food shortages in terms of food prices, which rose too high for the poor to pay.

Historians of many periods have referred rather generally to the "starving poor," but how many people at subsistence level actually starved to death is impossible to estimate. It was reported that in 1527 the scarcity of bread in London was so great "that many died for want thereof."[3] Goubert, in his painstaking demographic study of the people of Beauvais from 1600-1730, considers that French peasants did die of starvation in periods which he calls *crises démographiques,* – that is, when the foodstuffs available were inadequate for the population, due either to poor harvests in relation to a fairly static size of population, or an increase in population without the necessary increase in agricultural production.[4] Though such crises are close at hand for all people who live at subsistence level, it is possible that late sixteenth century England was in a better position than France because despite increasing numbers England was still less populous; also, contemporary descrip-

N.B. Footnotes to chis chaper appear on pages 319-322.

tions suggest a plentiful supply of fresh and salt water fish, meat, game, fruits, and wild herbs.[5] Without underestimating the consequences of poor nutrition to health, happiness and working ability, it is probable that few died of starvation, though certainly many may have gone miserably hungry in town and country.

The main reasons given for dearths in the sixteenth century were, firstly, excessive rain which ruined the harvest. The effect of this was, of course, particularly bad when poor harvests recurred in a sequence of years, such as 1594-1596. Secondly, blame was put upon the "transportation of grain out of the country."[6] This alteration in distribution, together with changing commercial practices and the striking increases in the growth of towns and villages (a phenomenon which did not pass unnoticed; Giovanni Botero's work on the development of towns was translated into English in 1606[7]), caused the impact of any widespread food shortage to fall heavily on the urban poor.

Two groups of people whom we today would expect to be particularly concerned over famine are the doctors and the government. The advice on health published by physicians was directed to a section of society fairly well protected against food shortages. No chapters were written on what might have been entitled "the regimen against the dearth." In fact, the words dearth and famine hardly ever occur in books giving dietary advice. The word starvation is never used because the verb to starve originally meant to die and the old phraseology was to starve of hunger or cold. In *Coriolanus* the *First Citizen* says that the patricians ". . . suffer us to famish and their storehouses crammed with grain." Starvation with the meaning of too little food to sustain life, came into use in the eighteenth century. Sixteenth century physicians were aware of the bad effects of "much hunger and emptiness," but related their advice to individual readers. Though it is obvious that doctors must have been aware of food shortages it would appear from their writings, or rather from their lack of references to the subject, that the effects of famine were not considered to be a dietary problem. This is understandable when it is realized that people dying from acute starvation show general, rather than particular, symptoms of weakness, emaciation and lethargy leading to a state of coma. In less severe but more prolonged shortages hunger oedema may appear, giving a "plump" appearance; this would have been too difficult a diagnosis for an Elizabethan physician. Besides this, the group who would feel the effects of shortages first were believed to have stronger stomachs than the nobility and gentry, and were considered quite capable of digesting the harsher foods which had to be eaten when grain was scarce. As Harrison puts it, in time of famine "the poor doo fall to horsse-corne,"[8] — that is, to eating beans, peas, oats, tares (vetches), and lentils. In England generally these grains were considered mainly as a food for animals, though Cogan does note the habitual use of oats in northern counties and Cornwall, and when writing of beans, says "in Leycestershire they make breade. I mean not horse breade [which is commonly done throughout England] but for their familie."[9]

However, it had to be understood that only those who had become accustomed to this fare would find it wholesome and beneficial, for "Beanes are a windie meate, and hard to digest. Wherefore they are meate for Mowers, as the Proverbe is, and for ploughmen but not for students."[10] This differentiation between the digestive powers of various social classes of people is significant because of the attitude, discernible at all times, which follows from it. It was accepted that the lower orders of society were capable of eating harsher foods and therefore in time of dearth "Rustics" could exist on beech-nuts and acorns.

The government took a different attitude from that of the physicians. Reference to the Statute Books shows that the authorities were always concerned about supplies of basic foodstuffs for the community. Comprehensive regulations for the food markets of London have been described in detail by McGrath in his study of marketing in the London area from 1600 onwards.[11] Obviously the position and administrative structure of the City made London a special case, but it is indicative of the general attitude of the authorities. The subject of greatest concern was the staple food, bread. Regulations to protect its sale were laid down in the *Assize of Bread*, which also referred to "Ale wyth all manner of wood and cole, Lath, Boord, and Tymber, and the weyght of Butter and Cheese."[12]

These regulations applied to normal times; in times of crisis special orders were promulgated by the Privy Council.[13] Gras, in his study of *The Evolution of the English Corn Market,* refers to *The Booke of Orders,* which laid down a practice of restraint in corn policy for abnormal times, "aimed at discovering the corn surplus of the country, and then controlling the sale of that surplus in the interests of the consumers."[14] Gras has summarized the orders under thirty-three points. This number of different points indicates a minute system of regulation requiring too much zeal and vigilance for its effective enforcement.[15] Hampson, discussing the treatment of poverty in Cambridgeshire, when referring to Cambridge in 1596-1597, says the

[Privy] Council positively bombarded the justices with Orders concerning the maintenance of food supply yet profiteers took advantages of disputes between Town and Gown, and engrossing and forestalling were rampant.[16]

If this was the case in a town in close touch with the central government, no wonder there is such emphasis on the neglect of the regulations in Sir Hugh Platt's *Sundrie new and Artificial remedies against Famine* published in 1596. This book was written "uppon thoccasion of this present Dearth" and seems to be the only English book available on the subject.[17] Platt was a realist with a practical approach and reveals the attitudes of mind of a humane imaginative man of his time. He begins by giving five points concerned with moral behaviour and administrative efficiency in relation to food shortages. He advises prayer to God for relief, more "charitable and religious care" by the junior officers enforcing the regulations related to the shortage of grain, and calls for greater cooperation among officers of all ranks. Attempts should be made to curb the "coveteous and unmerciful" lords who set high prices directly there is a threat of scarcity. Platt hopes that the Christian virtue of abstinence will prevent the rich feasting while the poor are famished. One meal from an Epicure, he comments, would serve as a whole week's provisions for a poor man. Finally he suggests that, in the long term, the prevention of dearth rather than its relief would benefit the country most.[18] The rest of the book contains a variety of recommendations. These are presented in a somewhat confused sequence but can be classed roughly under the following headings:

How to make unpalatable foods acceptable. Example: "Howe to take awaie a great part of that ranke and unsavourie tast of Beanes, Pease, Beechmast [the fruit of the beech tree], Chestnuttes, Acornes, Veches, and such like." This was to be achieved by boiling the seeds, more than once if necessary, and drying them. Bread could then be made from their flour.[19]

How to use the foods available more economically. Example: "Howe to save much flower, or meale that is lost in all our usual corne mils, that grinde either with winde or water."[20] This could be done by the use of Platt's "boulting Hutch," which had previously been illustrated in his *Jewell House of Art and Nature.*[21] Another example is how to make starch for stiffening garments without using corn. He advocates Aaron roots and gum arabic,[22] as these are not desirable as foods.

In a section on "Substituting new foods for the accustomed ones," Platt wanders a little from the subject of dearth and discusses the preservation of foods to prevent shortage. These include dried sweet parsnip roots (or carrot or turnip roots) ground into a powder and added to flour to make cakes without spice or sugar. He refers to a way of preparing a food in the form of "hollow pipes or wafers" which are suitable for long sea voyages. This "cheape fresh and lasting victuall, called by the name *Macaroni* amongst the Italians," was provided by Platt for Sir Francis Drake's last voyage.[23] The value of this food lies in the fact that it keeps well, is light, easily prepared, fresh, cheap, serves as both bread and meat, and can be improved by the addition of oil, butter, or sugar or such like. Other examples of substitute foods include instructions on how to make cheap liquor when malt is extremely dear, and breads made from unusual foods such as gourds and pumpkins.[24]

The second main section of Platt's book is "An abstract of certain frugall notes or observations in a time of dearth or famine, concerning bread, drink and meat, with some other circumstances belonging to the same." This is said to be taken out of a Latin writer, "intituling his booke *Anchora famis & sitis.*"[25] There are forty notes in this section. To modern eyes not all of them seem particularly frugal or suitable at times of famine. For example, Note 36 advises that bread made from eggs is both wholesome and more filling, especially if kneaded with yeast from strong beer; Note 38 gives the recipe for an excellent bread made with milk, either leavened or unleavened, very nourishing and even better if fried bacon is added. The smell of bread is also considered nourishing and refreshing to the spirits, though Platt interjects, "I thinke hee meaneth that, which is new and hot from the Oven."[26]

No book on famine would be complete without advice to those who find themselves without hope of obtaining their usual food. Platt entitles his section, "Certain strange and extraordinarie waies for the relieving of a prisoner, or other poor distressed creatures, when al hope of usual victual is taken from him." Examples include the drinking of a man's own blood or urine and Paracelsus' idea of applying a clod of earth to the stomach to keep from famishing, for a few days. The story is quoted of soldiers, imprisoned by the Turks, living for thirty days without food by sucking a "small piece of Allom." Platt gives the source of this tale as Dr. Grindal, Archbishop of Canterbury, but he himself is somewhat sceptical:

> For though we might suppose that the salt of nature might receive some strength or vigour from this minerall salt, yet howe the guts should be filled with so small a proportion I cannot gesse much less determine.[27]

Other methods of alleviating hunger are chewing tobacco or liquorice root.

In the last section of his book the prevention of dearth is emphasized and Platt deals with a subject in which he has a great interest — that is, "A new and extraordinary meanes for the enriching of arable grounds." He writes of *Compost* and offers to provide personal advice and the appropriate material to the Gentlemen and Farmers of England who wish to learn his secret.[28]

Despite the different social and nutritional attitudes in the sixteenth and twentieth centuries, the basic approaches to the alleviation of hunger have many similarities, whether the shortage is due to natural dearth or to rationing, as in the Second World War. In both cases advisors tried to learn from past experience, the Elizabethans from the difficulties of mariners on long sea voyages and in modern times from the lessons of rationing in the First World War. For success both depended on the proper regulation of food supplies, through statutory regulations, with the prevention of profiteering. A comparison at a more simple level shows that some of Platt's attempts to provide familiar dishes made with substitute foods, have an uncanny similarity to some of the recipes put out by the U.K. Ministry of Food in the Second World War.

Fasting and abstinence

Not that which goeth into the mouth defileth a man but that which cometh out of the mouth. . . .

Matthew 15 v. 11

In the sixteenth century the words fasting and abstinence were used interchangeably; the present distinction between not taking food and abstaining from a particular food was not observed by English Roman Catholics until the end of the eighteenth century.[29]

Physicians advising on diet discussed the value of abstinence to the individual. The benefits were considered in relation to repletion and as a part of the treatment for disease. In some cases abstinence could replace purging. Boorde describes abstinence simply as the "moste best and parfytest medysone that can be"[30] against a surfeit. Others reiterated the theme that "Ther is nothyng, that so muche profiteth ether the sicke, or the hole, as doth abstinence, yf it be taken in due tyme and orderly";[31] but a note of warning was sounded about the harm of too much hunger, as this damaged the whole body and particularly hurt the stomach, for the natural heat finding no material there to work on "turneth his violence and power to the radicall and substantiall humour,"[32] with the result that moisture was withdrawn and the body made lean and debilitated. As most readers of works on the dietary for health had no problem in satisfying their hunger, the matter is pressed no further and the general view was that abstinence was beneficial when used in the proper circumstances.

From the religious point of view the object of fasting — and it was frequently emphasized that this included abstention from other things beside foods — was said to be: (i) to chastise the flesh — that is, to bring the body into subjection to the spirit, (ii) to enable the spirit to be more frequent and earnest in prayer, and (iii) to give a testimony and witness of submission before God through "the affliction of our bodyes."[33] The important part of the fast was the discipline it imposed rather than the actual act of fasting "whiche of it selfe is a thyng merely indifferent."[34]

If the action of avoiding particular foods had no great merit in itself, then did it matter which foods were taken or avoided? The strict laws of the Jews were well known from the Old Testament and some felt it necessary to explain that these rules, even though recorded in the Bible, need not be adhered to. A tract which showed that "we may at al times eat such meates as god hath created for the sustenaunce of man. . . ." emphasized that Jew and Gentile were one in Jesus Christ, that faith in Christ gives forgiveness of sins "and deliveraunce from the curse of the lawe, and maketh us lords over the creatures of god to use them for oure nede at all tymes with thankes gyvyng."[35] The idea that some foods are unclean is rejected. All foods received into the body with thanksgiving are sanctified by prayer and the word of God. Though considerable controversy did arise over the actual significance of food in the doctrine of the Church of England, the basic tenet of fasting was the abstinence from all those things which were delectable and gave pleasure.

Customs of fasting have varied greatly in different parts of the Christian world through all ages. Before the Reformation the principles of fasting followed by the Church in England kept strictly to the seasons and days of fasting inherited from the Primitive Church. The weekly fast days, on which fish was taken, were Friday and Saturday. Following the Reformation the discipline of some of the clergy became very slack; it was noted in 1547, for example, that the Archbishop of Canterbury had eaten flesh openly during Lent.[36] The following year an Act of Parliament ordered "abstinence from flesh meat on all days formerly accounted fasting days," giving as a reason that it is "for the better subdueing of the body to the soul and the flesh to the spirit."[37] The Act refers to Lent, Ember Days, Vigils, Fridays and Saturdays. The subsequent Act of 1552 included, in addition, any other days appointed to be kept as a fasting day, adding that "no other even or day shall be commanded to be fasted."[38]

From some points of view the Reformed Church found itself in something of a quandary regarding fasting. If all the ideas from the Old Faith were to be rooted out, then it could be argued that fasting, which was such an inherent and widely practised part of Catholic devotions, should go too. But there were at least two reasons why the habit of fasting should be retained. Firstly, the discipline and self-denial involved were a part of all Christian teachings; secondly, fast days could be used for the economic regulation and betterment of the Realm. What resulted were arguments for and against what was basically the same thing. The influential theologian Thomas Becon, writing in the early fifteen-sixties, felt it necessary to condemn "the popyshe and supersticious fast" as serving "the custome only, and is done at the commaundement of man wyth a grudgying and unwyllyng mind. . . ."[39] Catholic fasting, it was claimed, was undertaken for the following reasons: because of custom, so that the individual fasting could be considered a devout Catholic; to honour some saint, and finally in order to deserve the remission of sins for everlasting life.

Concurrently with these condemnations, Ecclesiastical directions and Acts of Parliament were laying down rules of fasting in England. Both religious and secular fast days are explained to the people in the second book of *Homilies* (1563). Here a different aspect of fasting is emphasized, namely that good works (fasting is classed as a good work) do not bring grace but are brought forth by grace. "So no man doth good workes to receyve gráce by his good workes: but because he hath fyrst receyved grace, therfore consequently he doth good workes."[40] Good works are good because they show the doer to be an obedient child of God; they act as a testimony to his belief and an example to others. Care was taken to point out that no man should do good works with the object of "purchasing heaven." This type of argument, and more, were used to support the moral value of fasting in the face of statements of even lay writers like Cogan, who said that fasting had previously been "superstitiously abused."[41]

The second part of the "Homilie of Fastyng" sets out, naturally enough in view of its origin, to show that secular laws controlling fasting were equally acceptable. The argument is presented along the lines that

> no constitution of lawe made by man, for thynges which of theyr own proper nature be meere indifferent can binde the conscience of Christian men to a perpetuall observation and keeping thereof, but that the higher powers hath full libertie to alter and change every such lawe and ordinaunce eyther Ecclesiasticall or politicall when tyme and place shall require.[42]

The Homilie then points out that laws made or changed by the Ruler for the benefit of the people have the approval of God. This combination of religious and secular reasons for fasting was acceptable to the consciences of English Protestants. Referring to fish days, Cogan says,

> And that flesh might be more plentifull and better cheape, two dayes in the weeke, that is Friday and Saturday, are specially appointed to fish, and now of late yeres by the providence of our prudent princesse Elizabeth, the Wednesday also is in a manner restrained to the same order. Not for any religion or holinesse supposed to be in the eating of fish rather than flesh, but only for a civil policie as I have said.[43]

These policies were publicly recognized as being intended to conserve the cattle of the country, encourage the fishing trade and reverse the decay taking place in some east coast fishing villages.[44] Cogan comments that no doubt the price of fish and flesh would be lower if all the fish days were properly observed, as they would add up to one half of the year.[45] Strype, in his *Annals of the Reformation,* suggests that despite the fact that Justices were empowered to punish those who did not comply, the extra fish day "was not over-well regarded in most parts of the realm."[46] It is impossible to estimate how well the rules of fast days were observed, but both Catholic and Protestant churchmen complained of their neglect. The secretly printed *A Treatise with a kalendar* was sent into England to encourage the Catholics to fast. The author comments on "so great a decay of devotion both in the common people and others," the explanation being that people did not fast for "fearing they should be accounted Papists."[47] The Protestant author of *The Holie exercise of a true Fast* complains "how few there are, of those which beare the name of Gospellers, that have so much as the knowledge of this exercise, so far are they from any lawfull and right practise of it. For a great number as a needlesse thing, reject it altogether." This neglect was said to be due (in part) to the prejudice felt against the Popish fasting.[48]

In the Church of England much was left to the conscience of the individual, no Tables of the "Days of Fasting and Abstinence" being provided until the *Prayer Book* of 1662.[49] For some, fasting meant going without all food for twenty four hours; for others total abstention from food and drink was maintained until sunset, when a limited amount could be taken. To some, fasting was the strict limitation of the type, quality and times food was taken in the day; others thought the substitution of different foods was adequate, while in other cases fasting was interpreted as a reduction in the normal intake of food.

Becon had explained that "The true and christen fast during the tyme of fasting is to abstain from al kynde of meates and drinkes (except very necessiti requireth the contrari. . . .)."[50] The phrase "except very necessiti requireth the contrari" was to be taken seriously, for no fasting should be undertaken which would be harmful to the health.

This is illustrated by the directions for a public fast,[51] given in 1563 "duryng this tyme of mortalitie, and other afflictions, wherwith the Realme at this present is visited."[52] People between the ages of sixteen and sixty years were to eat only one "competant and moderate" meal, which was to be "without varietie of kyndes of meate, dyshes, spyces, confections or wynes but only such as may serve for necessitie, comlynesse and health." The meal could include either flesh or fish as long as the quantity was small. Besides the young and old, those exempted from this rule included "sicke folkes" and labourers when at harvesting or at some other great exertion. Rules of fasting were formulated with due consideration for the health of the individual. Though proclamations in 1559-61 forbade butchers to sell meat in Lent, sick people were excused and licences were issued in the period 1564-1650 by local clergymen,[53] allowing such persons to take meat in Lent if their condition so warranted. The licences were quite specific about the types of flesh which could be eaten.[54]

From the nutritional point of view no damage was likely to come from the substitution on fast days of fish and dairy produce for meat; consequently both rich and poor should have gained both spiritually and physically from the rules of fasting. By reducing the amount of food eaten, an individual would be following the advice of the physicians for the preservation of his health, and if the rules were strictly followed, the food "not eaten" by the rich should be given to the poor.

Surfeit

> They are as sick that surfeit with too much,
> as they that starve with nothing. (*Merchant of Venice,* Act I,ii)

Elizabethan literature abounds with references to the bad effects of surfeit or repletion and books on dietary advice repeat over and over again warnings against excess of food or drink. The words surfeit, repletion, fullness and excess are used somewhat imprecisely in the texts, though chapter headings most usually refer to repletion, one definition of which is, "a superfluous abundance of humours in the body: and that is in two maner of wyse, that is to say in quantitie and in qualitie."[55]

The quantity can be too much in two ways. One is when the vessels are so full that they can take no more, as in the case of the stomach being full and distended, or when the veins are filled with blood. The other sort of repletion is when the vessels may be only half full but the "power is loded to muche," – that is, when more has been taken in than the individual can digest, or the power for making blood is inadequate.

Damage from surfeit comes because the stomach is so stuffed with unconcocted material that the liver, which is the "fire under the pot," cannot cook the food properly. "Fumosyties," resulting from the overloaded stomach, will rise up to the head, causing headaches, dimness of sight, inability to speak, dullness of the wits, and sluggishness of the body, as well as reduced appetite. The effect on the brain will in turn affect many other parts of the body. These symptoms are merely the precursors of many infirmities to come which will shorten a man's life.[56]

Though it was recognized that slothfulness and an easy life can cause a man "to waxe wonderous grosse fatte and corpulent,"[57] fatness is not stressed as a result of overeating. Portraits of the period, with some notable exceptions, such as Henry VIII in his later years, show few fat people, even bearing in mind the amount of padding in their clothing. It is possible that the common saying "fat paunches make lean pates"[58] made it unfashionable to be depicted as fat, but nevertheless no impression is given of a generally overweight group of people. Obesity does not seem to have constituted a problem despite the large quantities of food available to the rich. In comparison with our present situation, where obesity is a recognized hazard among the well-to-do, the sixteenth century use of purges and the unavoidable amount of exercise taken by even the most sedentary may have balanced any excess intake in a way that does not occur in our society.

Though "Twelve things that breede fatness" are listed by Cogan,[59] other writers do not bother to give a list but scatter occasional references to "fattening foods" throughout their texts. In general, foods which fatten include:

Wheaten bread	Sweet wines	Nuts
Milk	Raw eggs	Cherries
New cheese	Ripe figs	Bone marrow
Beasts' testicles	New grapes	Raisins
Pork	Beer	"Delicious meats"
Brains	Pears	

Foods that cause leanness are given as black pepper, cloves of garlic with bread and butter, and decoctions of fennel. There seems to be no consistent common factor which would account for this selection of fattening foods, but the distinction between foods which "fatten" and those which nourish was not a clear one. The section in *Regimen Sanitatis* which lists the fattening foods end,

> . . . These appeare
> To make the body fat, and nourish Nature,
> Procuring corpulence and growth of stature.[60]

A distinction is made between people who are "naturally fat," as are those of the Sanguine complexion, and those who are "properly fat." The Sanguine man has an abundance of flesh and requires an abundance of blood. Proper fat is said to be a token of a cold complexion. In Batman's translation of *De proprietatibus rerum,* "Fatnesse" is discussed in terms unchanged from those of the medieval writer. "Fatnesse is a moyste thing, and sitteth upon the small celles and places as sayth Constantine."[61] The word "celle" was commonly used and referred to a small enclosed space such as the cell of a honeycomb. The more precise modern biological connotation arose later, with the development of the microscope. The explanation of fatness continues,

> For subtill bloud and unctuous gathereth no fatnesse in hot places, there it may enter and pearce. But when it commeth to places, that kindlye are colde, there it congealeth at last, and tourneth into fatnesse.

Taking the word unctuous to be an adjective describing blood, an interpretation of the quotation is as follows. In hot conditions (e.g. where natural heat is present) subtle and oily blood does not form fat but enters the substance of the body. Where this sort of blood comes to naturally cold places it congeals and forms fat. The body needed its fat so that the sinews and cells would be tempered with the moisture of fatness; this fat also protected the internal organs against damage and insulated the body against cold. The fat round organs and the areas beneath the skin were said to be of the same type — that is, they were "all in one touching theyr substaunce."[62]

The recognition of a relationship between movement and fatness was of long standing:

> And *Aristotle. liber 2.* saith, that fatnesse is bread in the bodies of beasts, of bloud undigested and undefied (sic), and namely for scarcitie of moving . . . moving wasteth and destroyeth fatnesse, and so doth heate also.[63]

The heat produced by movement was required to dissolve unnecessary congealed fat. If too much fat remained it could affect the ability to conceive in women and beasts, and because it was believed that the fatter the man or beast the less blood they had, it made them more susceptible to illness, lengthened the time of healing, and increased the possibility of sudden death.[64] The end results of overweight are described in terms similar to our own, but the warnings are given within the whole framework of avoidance of surfeit and with an emphasis on the appropriate exercise rather than abstinence from a particular type of food.

Drunkenness

> Cas. Is your Englishman so expert in his drinking?
> Iago Why, he drinks you with facility your Dane dead drunk; he sweats not to overthrow your Almain; he gives your Hollander a vomit ere the next pottle can be filled. (*Othello,* Act II, iii)

There was a tradition, which persisted beyond the sixteenth century, that it was good from a medical point of view to become drunk once a month so that the vomiting which followed would act as a purge. The advice was attributed to Hippocrates, but this is questioned by Cogan, who says it is the advice of some Arabian physician, not Hippocrates.[65] It was generally agreed that drunkenness for pleasure should be avoided. Platt gives the same sort of advice as is given today on how to avoid getting drunk. He suggests drinking some oil before taking wine. The oil "will floate upon the Wine . . ., and suppresse the spirites from ascending into the braine."[66] Another much quoted, but admittedly un-proved, method was to place a live eel in a bowl of wine. After the eel is dead the wine should be given to the drunkard to drink. This "will re-clayme [him] from his bibacitie" and make him loath the beastly vice.[67] Like Platt, books on dietary advice concentrate on the dangers of taking too much wine. They refer particularly to the danger of stu-dents doing this. Immoderate wine-drinking is given as a reason "why fewe young men that be students, come to profound knowledge and ripeness in these days:"[68] for the harmful effects of drunkenness include damage to the liver, dullness of wits and the destruction of the mem-ory. They were also believed to cause dropsy, leprosy, and palsy.

Shakespeare suggests that the English had strong heads for drink, a characteristic they may well have developed through drinking ale and beer from childhood. Apparently many kept in good practice to judge from the increase in licences for alehouses, inns and taverns which by the year 1577 came to 19,759 for England and Wales. Monkton esti-mates this as one licence per 187 of the population.[69] The true extent of drunkenness in England at that time is impossible to estimate and opposing views are put forward. A nineteenth century commentator on the satirical palmphlet, *Bacchu's Bountie,* by Philip Foulface of Ale-foord (1593), makes the point that drunkenness was not a vice peculiar to the Elizabethans but one which had continued through the ages.[70] However, Henderson in his *History of Ancient and Modern Wines* tries to support the idea of sobriety among the English by quoting Camden and Fynes Moryson. These authors suggest that the English learnt their drinking habits in the Netherland wars and that "in generall, the greater and better part of the English held all excesse blameworthy, and drunk-enness a reproachful vice."[71]

This was not the aspect of England seen by the puritanical Philip Stubbes. He thought drunkenness was a horrible vice and "too too much" practised in England. Every county, city, town and village had an abundance of inns, taverns and alehouses "which are so fraught with maultwormes, night and day, that you would wonder to see them." Stubbes continues to expound, in colourful phrases, for another five pages on the wickedness, harmfulness and disgusting habits of the drunkard.[72]

The authorities were also concerned by the increase of alehouses and taverns. The Act of 1552 gave to Justices of the Peace the power to licence and suppress alehouses, a power they have held ever since.[73] One of the attitudes behind this legislation is illustrated by a Report of the Queen's Council in 1591 dealing with conditions in Lancashire and Cheshire which pointed out that attendance at the numerous alehouses and in the streets nearby was so great that the churches were empty.[74] The tone of the Acts changes under James I who passed legislation to "restrain the inordinate Haunting and Tipling in Inns," which, it was stressed, were designed for the traveller. However, on working days labourers were allowed to be there one hour at dinner time. In 1606 further restrictions on the sale of ale and beer were made and the individual drinker was included under *An Act for Repressing the odious and loathsome Sin of Drunkenness,* which was said to be the root and foundation of many other "enormous sins as Bloodshed, Stabbing, Murder, Swearing, Fornication, Adultery and such like . . . ."[75] Those convicted of being drunk were fined 5/ – to be paid within the week, the money to go to the poor of the Parish. The alternative was the stocks for six hours –a sobering period.

Undoubtedly, there were many opportunities for gluttony amongst a select section of the population. An examination of the banqueting menus for ecclesiastical enthronements, masks and city celebrations, shows this.[76] Archbishop Cranmer had tried to restrain the eating habits of the senior clergy by limiting the number of dishes to be provided at one meal. The extravagance of some church dignitaries was such that foreigners made jokes about it. The regulation (which proved ineffectual) provided a sliding scale with due recognition of status. An Archbishop must have not more than six flesh dishes (or six fish dishes on fast days), followed by not more than four second dishes. The scale went down to minor orders, who were permitted three flesh and two second dishes.[77] Elyot comments that he had been somewhat carried away writing about the laws and ordinances aimed at preventing gluttony in England. He says that rather than being directed towards bodily health, these ordinances are intended to provide "agaynste vayne and sumptuous expenses of the meane people. For the nobilitie was exempted and had lybertie . . . to lyve lasse while than other men."[78]

A more unorthodox method of putting people off their food is given by Mizaldus and quoted by Thomas Lupton. "Lute stringes or harpe stringes, cutte in lytle pieces and cast upon flesh newly sodden or roasted wyll seem to be woormes, whereby they that knowes not thereof wyll refuse the same meate."[79]

Pestilence

> Item, paid to Inglysshe's wief, of Anstye, for kepynge Kyrckame's
> house, beying visited with the plage for x weeks, at xvjd. a week,
> xiijs.iiijd. (The chamberlains' accounts: Leicester, 1564)

The impact of epidemics, at all levels of society, was sufficiently
familiar and disrupting for advisers on diet to include sections on how
to avoid the pestilence. Elyot gives "A diete preservative in the tyme of
pestilence."[80] Boorde includes a chapter which "treatyth of a dyete and
of an ordre to be used in the Pestyferous tyme of the pestylence of
swetying sycknes." The advice given is mostly concerned with what
actions should be taken to avoid epidemics.[81] Advice for those already
infected can be found in his *Breviary of Helth.* It is notable that Boorde
refers to the pestilence and "sweating sickness." The latter is the "sudor
Anglicus" which struck England five times between 1485 and 1551. Its
incidence was comparatively insignificant on the Continent and it seems
to have died out in England in 1551/52.[82] Cogan appends "a Preservation from the Pestilence: With a short Censure of the late sicknesse at
Oxford" to his main work of the *Haven of Health.*[83] Modern studies
illustrate how difficult it is to identify the various epidemics in England, including "famine-fevers" which contemporary writers class under
the general terms pestilence or plague.[84] Kellwaye's *A defensative
against the plague* (1593) gives the instructions incorporated in the current Plague Orders under the chapter heading which "teacheth what
orders magistrates and rulers of Citties and townes should cause to be
observed." These summarize proper sanitary practices.[85] The streets
and rivers should be kept clean and sweet; no excrement or filthy thing,
such as the blood from the surgeon's bloodletting, should go into them.
No animals should be allowed to roam the streets, "for they are very
dangerous and apt to carry infection from place to place." On hot days
the streets should be cooled morning and evening by having cold water
cast upon them. Where there already is infection, fires should be lit
morning and evening and frankincense or some other sweet smelling
thing burnt there. No hemp or flax should be kept in water near the
city, for it will cause a very dangerous and infectious savour. If a few
persons are infected they should be isolated from the rest and all the
bedding and clothes used by the sick should be burned. Those who attend on the sick must identify themselves by a badge or other means.
Special care was required to see that wholesome food was sold in the
markets and to make sure that those who could not afford adequate

food did not go short, because "there is nothing that will more encrease the plague than want and scarcity of necessary food."[86] The affliction of the plague was recognized as a community problem and both the cost of the burnt goods and the food needed by the poor were to be paid for by the rest of the community.

The portents preceding a plague were clear. It would come when the air of a place had changed from its natural temperature and become hot and moist, when the weather was cloudy and dusty, with strong hot winds, or when a foggy mist came over the fields and ponds. A general climate of putrefaction would be apparent; toadstools and rotten herbs would be plentiful; fruits, wines and beasts would all be in a bad condition, and other diseases such as smallpox and measles would be rife. People would notice that many women were being delivered of their children prematurely and both young and old would be afflicted with worms. Finally, Cogan says, a warning of pestilences is "when cruell warres and monsters against nature, or such like strange things do appeare."[87] But he does not place great emphasis on this; more concern is felt about changes in the normal pattern of climate, though in relation to the English climate one feels that there may perhaps have been a number of "normal conditions" which could be interpreted as a portent of plague.

The "one principall or generall cause" of the plague is the wrath of God for our sins. A particular cause is "certaine venemous vapours in the ayre contrary to the vitall spirit." It was well known that the plague was contagious. Cogan writes that the pestilence was brought to Oxford from London twice in twelve years, once by clothes and once by a stranger lodging in the city. He expands on the necessity of purifying households and household materials, for they can keep their venom for years. Woollen clothes are especially dangerous, "For as oyle feedeth the fire, so wooll above all things fostereth this infection and doth not only preserve it, but encrease it and fortifie it."[88] The movement of people who had been in contact with the disease was also a serious matter. Some said that those who go about spreading the plague could be considered guilty of murder.[89]

Preservatives against plague are prayer to God and avoidance of corrupted air. If this is not possible, the air should be purified and those foods and medicines should be taken which will strengthen the heart and vital spirits and so enable the individual to withstand the "poison."

The people most susceptible to infection are those of a sanguine temperament, then the choleric, the phlegmatic and lastly the melancholic,[90] but the disease is common to men of all complexions. Everyone should avoid anything which will inflame or open the pores or cause putrefaction. This means such things as hot:moist foods, heat from the sun, from a fire or from too many clothes, and exercise after meals. Close, cloudy weather should be avoided as should winds from the fens and moors. All crowds should be shunned.

Advice is given about suitable foods to take during the plague. The following table is derived from Elyot and follows his combination and sequence of foods.[91]

Foods to be taken or avoided during the times of pestilence

Forbidden or to be avoided	Recommended or permitted	Elyot's qualifying remarks
Foods which inflame or open the pores. Hot herbs, tart things.		
	onions, chicory with vinegar───────────────	because they resist against the venim
Very "fumishe" wine, New wines, Milk────────────────────────────────────		milk can be taken in small amounts with sugar
	Cold:dry fruits and herbs which are sour or bitter.	
	Figs, grapes, sweet cherries──	If eaten before an onion with salt
	Cold:moist things like cucumbers, melons, soft	
Mushrooms, much purslane, gourds and all things which will soon putrefy	fresh fish and damsons──────	If eaten before fennel and orange with salt and taken with a draught of good wine.
	Lettuce with mint or cinnamon. All sour things──────	Sometimes (as in the case of a weak stomach) they should be tempered with sugar, salt, almond milk, cinnamon, pepper, fennel, saffron, eggs and something that is fat and unctuous.
	Capers and vinegar	
Cheese that is fat and salty, colewortes, pulses────────────────────────		"Chittes" (chicken peas) are an exception.
Peas, rapes, spinach, rokat, mustard, much wine and eggs────────────────────		unless they are eaten with sorrell sauce, vinegar or orange juice.
	Parsley and parsnips	

On the whole these recommendations conform to the general advice of avoiding hot:moist foods, especially where the degree of moisture exceeds that of heat. When cold:moist foods are recommended they should be taken before or with hot foods. Elyot stipulates that the quantity of food taken should be more than the drink and the usual advice of avoiding too great hunger or thirst is repeated. Specific preservatives against the plague are given in the form of "Triacles," which were well known preservatives against poison.* They varied considerably but always contained a large number of ingredients. Also, recipes were given of powders for sprinkling on food (e.g. ½ oz. red sandalwood, 3½ drammes cinnamon, ½ dramme saffron)[92] and sweet smelling liquids for rubbing on the body or for drinking. These last mixtures consisted mainly of rose waters in vinegar, or a good wine with added herbs. The composition differs slightly according to the temperature, but all are sweet smelling. Of all the advice given on how to avoid the pestilence the most important and most frequently reiterated is to "Fly quickly from the place, abide farre off, and returne not soone againe."[93]

---

*See also Chapter XVI.

CHAPTER VIII
ADVICE TO SPECIFIC GROUPS

And therefore sayth Galene, even as a shoomaker cannot make one shoe to serve every mannes foote, so neither can a phisicion describe and appoint any one generall order and dietarie for all manner of persons.

G. Gratarqlus, trans. T. Newton (1574)

ACCORDING TO MODERN nutritional theories foods can be roughly classed as Energy-giving, Body-building, and Protective.[1] Everyone of whatever age or condition requires some foods of all these sorts. The changing needs of individuals during life and under a variety of circumstances alters the emphasis on the need for foods of a particular type.[2] When advising on the choice and allocation of foods, modern nutritionists give priority to the so-called "vulnerable groups," – that is, those who would be permanently harmed by lack of proper nutrition. This refers to those individuals who must be provided with material for growth and healing – namely, pregnant and nursing women, infants and children, and convalescents. Other members of the community are considered as requiring nutrients for maintenance (ie. the natural day-to-day repair and maintenance of the body). This selection of particular groups is based on the recognition that the provision of materials for proper growth is essential from the very start of life if the individual is to fulfill his or her physical and mental potential.

Though Galen's ideas regarding the importance of the growth and nutritive faculties were accepted and his statement "It will now therefore be clear to you that nutrition is a necessity for growing things"[3] was acknowledged, the idea of children (or pregnant women) having *particular* dietary needs as a group was outside the ideas of sixteenth century physicians. There was, however, recognition that a lactating woman required special treatment and that children must not be underfed. Except for the clear-cut divisions of the four complexions, writers are not inclined to classify people into specific groups but it is possible

---

N.B. Footnotes to this chapter appear on pages 322-328.

to consider sections of the population under the following general headings:

1. The four complexions
2. Children
3. Old people
4. Students (mention is made of diets for those labour as a contrast with those who use their minds)
5. "All manner of men and women"

This grouping is based on physiological theory and a rough classification of people who were in familiar and obvious groupings. Writers do not always place their information under appropriate headings. There are, for example, usually separate sections on diets suitable for people of each of the four complexions, but any information on children's diet is found scattered haphazardly through the texts. Many writers also devote considerable space to the diet required and remedies advocated for a number of diseases. The diseases commonly referred to are these:[4]

(i)	Pestilence	(ix)	Consumption
(ii)	Fever	(x)	Asthma or short-windedness
(iii)	Colic	(xi)	Palsy
(iv)	The Stone	(xii)	Madness
(v)	Gout	(xiii)	Dropsy
(vi)	Leprosy	(xiv)	Lassitude
(vii)	Falling Sickness	(xv)	Sicknesses at various times of
(viii)	Pain in the head		the year

Diets are also suggested for those "ready to falle into sycknesse" as well as diets affecting the sight, memory, or teeth. These have not been analysed here as they go beyond the scope of this study.

Section I
Diets for the Four Complexions

The word "complexion" is used by Shakespeare in at least five different ways. It can mean the bodily habit or constitution, the habit of mind or disposition, the appearance of the skin, the face or countenance, or a visible aspect or appearance of things or qualities.[5]

Besides these different meanings, when used in the context appropriate to this chapter, the four complexions of man are also loosely referred to as humours, temperaments, tempers, temperatures and constitutions.

The authors themselves are fully aware of the difficulties which arise from the imprecise use, or many meanings, of the words they had to use. When writing about melancholy both Bright and Du Laurens are careful to point out that the word melancholy can refer to: one of the four humours, or the normal constitution or temperament, or the disease. They emphasize that a person may be of a melancholic constitution without suffering from a disease of the mind.[6] Bright is careful to point out that despite the similarity in name, the complexions are not derived from the condition of the humours. He says, "A bodie of sanguine complexion (as commonly we call it, although complexion be another thing then condition of humours). . . ."[7] Complexions result from the balance of the qualities of the four elements; as Lemnius says, "[the complexion] proceedeth from the powers of the Elementes and not of the Humours."[8] Elyot's description is quite precise:

> Complexion is a combynation of two dyvers qualities of the four elements in one bodye, as hotte and drye of the Fyre: hotte and moyst of the Ayre, colde and moyste of Water, colde and dry of the Erth. But although all these complexions be assembled in every body of man and woman, yet the body taketh his denomination of those qualyties, whiche abounde in hym, more thanne in the other. . .[9]

The body in which "the Ayre has preeminence" is called *sanguine*. Despite this clearly stated separation of the complexions from the balance of humours, the exact usage of "complexion" is not maintained in the English texts, where there is often an ambiguous use of terms, the word humour frequently being used when complexion would seem to be the correct term. This leads to apparent differences between writers and to contradictions within a single work.

Sixteenth century writers differed in their definition of a "distemper." All agreed that a distemper occurred when the balance of qualities was wrong, but they disagreed upon what was correct. Langton, describing "nine temperatures," says that eight "do excede" and the ninth (which contains all the qualities in equal amount) is "wel tempered."[10] Elaborating on this he explains that "wel tempered" is the same as the "Arithmetricion's" *temperamentum ad pondus* or a complexion measured by "weyght," because all the degrees of the qualities are equal. Distemperate conditions cannot be measured by weight but only by "dignitie," for the qualities required in one part differ from those in another – e.g., "in the heart wel tempered, heate doth excede." This is called *Temperamentum, secundum justitiam distributativam.*[11] He believes that there is a "temperate meane" or "Eucraton" against which all other variations can be measured and suggests that the suitable standard to measure against would be a temperate man whose qualities are "keeping a meane without all excesse."[12] Though Lemnius suggests that Christ could be taken as the example of a perfect temperate man, it was generally agreed that such a man did not exist.[13] Du Laurens puts it this way:

> for even as it is not possible to finde the partie in whom the foure elements are equally mixed; and as there is not that temperament in the world, in which the foure contrary qualities are in the whole and every part equally compounded, but that of necessitie there must be some one evermore which doth exceed the other; so it is not possible to see any perfect living creature, in which the foure humours are equally mixed, there is alwaies some one which doth over-rule the rest, and of it is the parties complexion named. . .[14]

Though no man could have an equal mixture of qualities, this condition could be found in a part of men:" among all naturall things there is but one so tempered which is the inner skinne of the hand, chiefly in the extremitie of the fingers."[15]

It was accepted that every individual had a dominant quality or complexion and that this was his natural temper. A distemper occurred when this natural balance was thrown out. Many factors, external as well as internal, influenced an individual's natural complexion. These included: country of origin (the climate was a factor to be considered), parents, time, age, and diet or regimen. Lemnius, discussing the subject of complexions, divides nations according to their characteristics. He describes Englishmen as of comely stature, capable of notable achievements if they apply themselves to the task, not good in studies of the humanities and arts; they are also thick spirited, they hold grudges and become very angry.[16] In general it was believed that men in the South are melancholic, cruel, vindictive, and always fearful; those towards the North are phlegmatic, faithful, and true, but because they have grosser wits they are more cruel and barbarous.[17] This fits the general pattern of thought because the identification of an individual's complexion by his characteristics was part of the theory of complexions. Each complexion was linked to a set of characteristics of appearance and behaviour.[18] A sanguine man, for example, was "perceyved and knowen by these sygnes."

> *Carnositie or flesshynesse,*
> *The vaynes and arteries large.*
> *Heare plentie and redde.*
> *The visage white and ruddy.*
> *Sleape moche.*
> *Dremes of blouddy thynges, or thinges pleasaunt.*
> *Pulse great and full.*
> *Digestion perfecte.*
> *Angry shortly.*
> *Siege urine, and sweate abundant.*
> *Fallynge shortly into bledynge.*
> *The urine redde and thicke.* [19]

In general the characteristics to be considered when identifying an individual's complexion can be classed under these headings:

Fleshiness or leanness
The colour, quantity and distribution of hair
Colour of face
Need for sleep
Dreams experienced
Sharpness of the wits
Temper (emotion)
Pulse
Digestion
Ease of bleeding
Quality and quantity of excrements

Besides these characteristics it was accepted that the dominant complexion influenced a man's behaviour. For example, "The Choleric [man] is hastie, prompt, and in all his affayres envious, covetous, subtill."[20] As envy and covetousness were sins against God's Commandments it seemed as if the behaviour of the individual was already determined by his complexion. Thus his propensity towards sin and his chances of salvation were affected by influences outside the individual's control. Much controversy arose from this deterministic concept. The compromise argued by both Catholic and Protestant clergy and physicians was that the faculties of reason and will are placed in man to rule the flesh. With the help of God's grace the will can overcome natural tendencies.[21] Besides this effort of will, an alteration of diet could sometimes be of help.[22]

> Thus if a man throughe aboundance of humours, and stoare of bloude and Spirites, feele himselfe prone to carnalitie and fleshlye luste, let him by altering his order and diet, enjoyne to himselfe a more strict ordinary* and frame his dealings to a more stayed moderation.[23]

Lemnius does not mention any particular foods to be taken or avoided in this context, though he does note that one would be affected by (for example) oysters, which "exciteth appetite, and Venus; [and] nourisheth little,"[24] so one should avoid them.

Accepting the notion that an individual must try to live as good a life as possible by adjusting himself to the conditions of his natural complexion, it is of interest to know whether theory held that a child was born to its adult complexion or not. No clear-cut answer emerges. Bullein writes of the "temperate state of children, which beginneth at the birth. . . . Their temperaments or complections, be hot and moist, very like unto the seed whereof they bee procreated."[25] The father's seed was considered hot and thick while the mother's was more temperate; both are moist.[26] Children therefore will be of varying degrees of hot:moist. Elyot, on the other hand, says,

> And therefore late practisers of phisike are wont to call men, accordynge to the myxture of their complexions, whiche man receyveth in his generation, the humours, whereof the same complexions do consyst beinge augmented superfluously in the body or members by any of the sayd thinges callid not natural, every of them do semblably augment the complexion, whiche is proper unto hym, and bryngeth unequall temperature unto the bodye.[27]

It would seem from the above that Elyot writes as if he thought the child is born with its balance of adult complexion. Considering that as men of all complexions get older they become colder and drier, it would seem that sixteenth century theory allowed children to have their own particular complexion together with the hot:moist condition of youth, the degree of the hotness and moistness depending on the balance of all the elements naturally present in the child.[28]

Fernal compared the elements in the temperament to notes in a musical chord, each note persisting in its individuality though merged in a chord. He believed that the cardinal qualities did not disappear but

---

*"Ordinary" refers to the type of meals taken.

were latent and could reappear, as in old age, when the cold and dry of the temperament reappear and dominate.[29] Other writers of the period think in terms of a continuous change. Cuffe says, when defining age, "An age is a period and tearme of mans life, wherein his naturall complexion and temperature naturally and of its owne accord is evidently changed." He explains that the "interchangable dominion and continuall combat of the ever-jarring elements" cause a change. Even if there were no outward causes of transmutation, there is an inward ("home-bred") cause which will in time alter the temperature. He stresses that this is a gradual change and that the resulting slight changes in the proportion of the four qualities do not completely change the temperature. Therefore, despite all these influences it can be said that "a temperature or complexion is a firme and standing habit of the body."[30] Whatever viewpoint authors took on this point, great care was advocated in the feeding of infants to prevent the balance of qualities being adversely affected.

Ageing has a continual influence on the complexion. The loss of heat and moisture affects each complexion differently. This is illustrated by Elyot's description of the effect of age on sanguine and choleric men:

> And therefore the man, whiche is sanguyne, the more that he draweth into age, wherby naturall moysture decayeth, the more is he colerike, by reason that heate, surmountynge moysture, nedes must remayne heate and drithe.

As a choleric man grows older more natural heat is abated and dryness surmounts natural moisture, and the man becomes melancholic.[31] From the advice given on diet in old age it seems that "more" is really the operative word, i.e. that a man's complexion will tend more toward the choleric or melancholic as described above.

The measure of an individual's complexion had to be made by comparison. Sometimes this comparison was between known individuals, each of whom was himself distemperate. For example "Socrates compared with Aristotle, is hote because he is hotter than he, but in respecte of Aristippius, he is colde because Aristippius is muche hotter." Langton explains

> thus one man compared to dyvers, maye be bothe hote, colde, drye and moist: And some by comparynge distemperate bodyes of dyvers kyndes lerne to know their constitution, as a dogge compared with a man is hote, with a lyon is cold . . . or a flye is moyste. . .[32]

Alternatively the measurement was made against an imaginary temperate man.

It is very frequently stressed that it is essential for an individual to know his own complexion if he is to adjust his diet and regimen so as to maintain his health. As has been shown, the number of factors to be considered, and their variations, were very large. Nevertheless a skilled physician was considered well able to give a decisive diagnosis, and it was generally accepted that individuals did know what their complexion was.

From the diets advocated for the various complexions, it is not clear what degree of imbalance, from the mean, the individuals are considered to have. Elyot advises that where a sanguine or phlegmatic man or woman feels that, due to the action of some non-natural, they now have an excess of choler, then the diet to be followed is that advised for the person of a naturally choleric complexion, and similarly for other complexions.[33] On the whole, foods recommended are those with opposite or different qualities from the complexions; the advice given also refers to quantity, frequency of meals and digestibility.

The traditional comparison of the four complexions with four planets is not stressed in sixteenth century works on health. The reference is more frequently made in the seventeenth century.[34] It is noted by Lemnius that the "Humours [are] of more force then the Planets."[35]

(i) *Diet for a Sanguine man* (This complexion is hot:moist) [Jupiter].
To be avoided: any excess of food or drink, as this will make the sanguine individual become too gross and fat.
Any foods which have an excess of heat, cold or moisture.[36]
Foods to be taken with caution: old flesh, stale flesh, "too young flesh," marrow from backbone, brains and udders, fish from muddy places. Any excess of unripe fruit, raw herbs, onions, leeks, garlic, old figs.

The term flesh covers a wide range. Buttes lists twenty-two examples of flesh of varying qualities.[37] Old or stale flesh, in general, is not to be recommended. It is difficult to decide exactly what is meant by flesh of beasts "too young," because young pork and suckling calves are said to make good juice, and in other contexts young meat is frequently recommended.

Brains should be treated with caution, but the brains of capons and conys (rabbits) are an exception. The belief in the special value of chicken brains occurs frequently in the literature and is inherited at least from Arnald of Villanova.[38]

The avoidance of fish from muddy places has a long tradition, being mentioned by Hippocrates, and was generally advocated in the sixteenth century and after.[39]

The keynote of this diet is caution in the selection of foods. Boorde advises circumspection: "consyderynge that the purer the complexon is, the blode may be the sooner infectyd."[40]

(ii) *Diet for a Phlegmatic man* (This complexion is cold: moist) [Luna].

Under this heading Elyot notes the difference between pure phlegm and salt phlegm (which is phlegm mixed with choler) and is not as cold or moist as pure phlegm.[41] When advising on suitable foods Elyot does not differentiate between the two kinds. Boorde refers only to "Fleumaticke men" and makes no differentiation between the types of phlegmatic conditions.[42]

Foods to be avoided: all foods in which the cold quality predominates. Viscous, slimy and slippery foods, e.g. eels, fatty foods (Lemnius warns against eating animals which take little exercise as these grow fat but provide little nourishment),[43] foods near putrefaction, foods which are hard or slow to digest, foods which engender phlegmatic humours, e.g. fish, fruit, white meats (dairy produce), especially new cheese and raw herbs.

Foods to be taken in moderation: onion, garlic, pepper, ginger, salt, sour foods and drinks. The salt referred to is qualified as "especially dried." This refers to the use of powdered salt as opposed to the use of brine.

Foods recommended: all foods which are hot and dry, various "purges of the phlegm," including such things as nettle, elder, maidenhair, and candied ginger.

(iii) *Diet for the Choleric man* (this complexion is hot:dry) [Mars].

Unless accustomed by habit to eat fine foods, the choleric person is able to eat grosser foods than people of other complexions can do. Elyot says "better shall they [choleric men] digest a piece of good biefe than a chykens legge."[44] An individual's habits are of very great importance when prescribing diets. This is referred to again in Section V of this chapter.

Choleric people should eat more often in the day than other people do. They should never fast too long, as abstinence is dangerous to them. During long abstinence the choler in the stomach, finding nothing to concoct, becomes "burnt" to the sides of the stomach, causing damaging fumes to rise up to the head. Elyot compares this effect to a little soup or milk in a large vessel placed over a hot fire so that the contents get overcooked.[45]

Foods to be avoided: hot spices, wine, and such "choleric foods" as garlic, onions, rokat, kale, leeks, mustard, pepper, honey and sweet foods.

Foods recommended: cold foods, and foods which are digestive of choler. Elyot lists twenty-eight items for this.[46] With the exception of "clarified whey" and vinegar, all are of plant origin and include a high proportion of those with predominantly cold qualities.

(iv) *Diet for a Melancholy man* (This complexion is cold:dry) [Saturn].

The whole subject of melancholy received a great deal of attention from writers in the sixteenth and seventeenth centuries.[47] Much was written about the origin, significance and treatment of the melancholic condition. Authors give more details about the foods advocated or forbidden for this complexion than for any of the others. The information given below is gathered up from the works of Elyot and Boorde and the specialized writings on melancholy by Du Laurens and Bright, as being representative of the diet then advocated for the complicated and somewhat vaguely defined condition of a melancholy man.

A summary of the advice given is provided at the end of this section. Each of the four authors approaches the subject in a different way. Elyot discusses the varieties of the melancholy humour and then provides rather general advice and refers to his lists of foods which engender and purge melancholy. Boorde deals briefly with the subject; his advice regarding foods to be avoided is generalized, but he lists a few foods which are good for the condition, and eleven which will purge melancholy. Du Laurens discusses good and bad foods in some detail under the following headings: meats (i.e. food in general), bread, flesh, fish, pottage, pulse, fruits, drink and artificial wine.[48] Bright does not always agree with Du Laurens and is not so clear-cut in his advice. His approach is, rather, to say which of a group of foods would be the best, e.g. "of those [fish] that are defended with a crust the shrimp and crayfish go before the rest."[49] He makes the point that foods which are not suitable for melancholy people can be corrected by the methods of preparation and cooking. "Their [melancholic persons'] meates ought not only to be chosen such as if their [the foods'] own nature do ingender to[o] pure and thinne juice, but if the nature of the nourishment be otherwise the preparation ought to give correction to that fault."[50] Elyot says that for the melancholic complexion boiled meats are better than roast, and that burned and fried meats should be avoided, because burned and fried foods will be drier than boiled and therefore unsuitable for the melancholic cold:dry complexion.[51]

Following is a summary of the advice given on food for a melancholic person:

Foods to be avoided

Foods in general: Gross, slimy, windy, melancholic, burnt or dry, sour or bitter, fried, oversalted, and those hard of digestion.

Flesh: Old beef, pork, hare, waterfowl and all wild beasts, especially boars and harts. Also brains (despite the fact that the Arabs recommended them).[a]

Fish: Du Laurens forbids fish from still waters, those which have gross melancholic flesh, i.e. tunny, dolphin, whale, seal,[b] as well as fish with scales, and salted or powdered fish.[c]

Milk: Cow's milk and cheese, particularly if made from cow's milk.

Soups (pottages) and sauces: Do not use cole, blites, rocket, cresses[d] turnips, leeks or any bitter herbs in the making of pottages.

Pulses: All kinds of pulses, especially peas, beans, and vetches.

Fruits: Dry figs, medlars, cervises, chestnuts, nuts, artichokes, thistles, and old cheese.[e]

Herbs and vegetables: Du Laurens only gives a list of the herbs to be avoided when making pottage. He does not make it clear if they should be avoided altogether.

Drinks: One must avoid drinking anything between or directly after meals.

Foods permitted

Foods in general: Those which engender a pure thin juice, moist, soft or sweet foods.

Bread: From good wheat without bran, if possible made with rain or fountain water. Bright advocates "cheet" bread[f] which may have added barley, oats, or millet flour.

Flesh: Young flesh, calf, kid, mutton, rabbit, pullet, partridge, pigeon, young turkey. The gelded are better than the entire beast. Pork stuffed with sage, which dries up the moisture, is good. Brawn and muscle are the best, then the tongue. Of liver the pig's is the best. Fowl are better than beasts, especially those fowl which "useth much the feete, and lesse the wing."[g]

Fish: Fish from clear bright waters and running streams. Bright says fish in general are not wholesome, but "If the partie desire fish," the following are the best — white, of "brittle substance," of medium size and weight. Of shellfish only oysters are permissible, of "fish with a crust," shrimps and crayfish; from the rocky places of the sea, gilthead, whiting, sea perch, etc. [sic] mullet, lacie, haddock, sole, plaice. Of the fresh water fish, river fish are the best — e.g. perch, pike, gougon and trout. Many of these fish need "correction from the kitchen."[h]

Eggs: New, soft poached, and eaten with vinegar or verjuice[i] are very good. Bright, however, says roasted eggs are best, especially from hens, pheasants, and turkeys.

Milk: Whey if drunk with sugar or fresh butter. Mare's milk with sugar and a little salt taken two or three hours before other food.

Soups (pottages) and sauces: Pottages and broths are very good, especially with herbs such as borage, buglosse,[j] endive, succory, hops and balm, also with barley or blanched almonds. Gruel is good (this is usually made from fine flour meal, often oatmeal or other farinaceous substances). Sauces should be made from sour juices such as orange or lemon juice with added sugar or sweet butter.

Fruits: Plums, pears, sweet pomegranates, almonds, raisins, pineapples, citrons, melons, damsons, cherries, figs, grapes, apricots, and new walnuts.

Herbs and vegetables: Parsnip, carrots, skenet roots, salad herbs,[k] lettuce, mallows, endive, tarragon, sorrel, purslane, parsley, chervel and fennel. These should be taken with a little vinegar and plenty of oil and sugar. Capers washed from the salt and vinegar, and eaten with sugar and oil, are better than olives.[l]

Drinks: There was a recognized difference of opinion regarding the taking of wine. Some wine with sugar was permitted. Claret was preferable to white wine. Artificial wine made with herbs was recommended by Du Laurens.[m] Also permissible were ale or wine heated with a hot metal rod, and beer.

Notes (a through m) to above Summary (pp. 146-148)
[a]Du Laurens, p. 105. See also under sanguine complexion.
[b]Of the "fishes" listed only the tunny is classified as a fish today; the others are mammals. However, all four have flesh rich in oil.
[c]The term "powdered" can mean salted, but here refers to spiced or cured fish.

[d]Cole refers to coleworts or a type of cabbage; blites are spinach; rocket a plant of the crucifer family, a term sometimes applied to cresses; cresses, these may refer to water cresses or a type of nasturtium.

[e]Cervise refers to service *(pyrus domestica)*; old cheese refers to the fruit of the common mallow *(malva sylvestris)*.

[f]Bright, p. 258. "Cheet" bread is second in quality after "manchet," which is the finest.

[g]Bright, p. 259.

[h]Bright, p. 260. Gilthead is a name given to various fishes marked with gold on the head. Examples are the striped tunny and the dolphin *(Coryphaena hippuris)*. Lucie was probably a form of lucius, meaning pike. Gougon is an obsolete form of gudgeon.

[i]Verjuice, the acid juice of a sour fruit —e.g. green or unripe grapes or crab apples. It is frequently used as a condiment.

[j]These two herbs are referred to very frequently in the literature. Cogan says (p. 35) that Galen used the two names for the same plant. Buttes (Sig. G1[v] and G2[r]) says buglosse is the old name for borage. In the sixteenth century the two words are used to describe two different but somewhat similar plants. Borage was commonly called "borago" *(Borrago officinalis)*. Bugloss was popularly called ox-tongue or langdebeef *(Hycopsis arvensis)*. There was considerable confusion over the two names. See *Of Herbs and Spices*, by Colin Clair, 1961.

[k] Salad herbs are discussed in Chapter XII.

[l]Capers are the tiny pickled flower buds of *Capparis spinosa,* a small shrub growing in Mediterranean countries. The buds are placed in vinegar soon after picking and require no further preparation except renewal with fresh vinegar.

[m] Du Laurens, p. 106.

Section II
The Feeding of Children

No sixteenth century book is available which deals exclusively with diets for children.[52] The two most important English books of the period, related to children, are:

The Byrth of Mankynde, London, 1540. This is in part a translation by Richard Jonas of the *De Partu Hominis* by Roesslin,[53] and is the first printed book in English on midwifery.[54] Its main interest, in relation to diet, lies in Chapter II of the third book, which deals with the nurse and her milk.

The Boke of Chyldren, London, 1544,[55] by Thomas Phaire. This was published as an addition to Phaire's translation (from the French) of *Regimen Sanitatis Salerni,* which he called *The Regiment of Life.*[56] *The Boke of Chyldren* is said to be the first book on paediatrics ever written by an Englishman.[57] The book is mainly concerned with "the thyngs necessary, as to remove sicknesses, wherwith the tender babes are oftentimes afflicted."[58]

A number of authors make reference to infants and children but do not devote separate sections to their needs. It is said that Celsus was the first writer to state that children should be treated differently from adults,[59] but the particular nutritional needs of children are not specified. However, Phaire approaches this when he says in the opening section of the *Boke of Chyldren* that

> I entend to write somwhat of the nource, and of the milke, with the qualities, and complexions of the same, for in it consisteth the chief point and summe, not only of the maintenaunce of health, but also of the formying of infectyng eyther of the wytte or maners. . .[60]

It was recognized that "comely tallnesse and length of personage commeth and is caused of the abundance of heat and moisture, where the spirit is throughly and fully perfused."[61] The effect on children of inadequate food resulted not only in short stature and poor proportions, but worse still,

> for that in their tender and growing age, being kept under by famine and skanted of common meate and drinke, their nature moisture which requireth continuall cherishing and maintenance, was skanted and debarred of his due nourishment and competant allowance whereupon, the vitall juyce being exhausted and spent, they arrive to old age sooner than otherwise they should do, and are snatched up by death long before their time.[62]

This plea for sufficient food to be given to children is included in an attack on the behaviour of certain schoolmasters who did not fulfill the bargain they had made to look after their pupils and boarders.

In relation to children's diets the greatest emphasis is placed on the qualities and effects of breast milk on the child. For ease of presentation the material has here been divided up into the modern classifications of pre-natal, post-natal (breast feeding and weaning) and childhood.

Pre-Natal. Under the heading "Of the creation of the childe," Batman deals with the conception of the child and its uterine growth. The "generation" of a child requires heat as the efficient and working cause. "The matter of the child is humour *Seminalis,* that is shedde, by working of generation, and commeth of both the partes, of the father and the mother."[63] There are a number of differences in the ideas of Hippocrates, Aristotle and Galen regarding the respective contributions of each parent in the generation of the child,[64] but Batman explained that the "digested" blood of the father and the mother must be "medled togethers by working of kinde heate."[65] Blood from the male is hot and thick, but this is tempered by the woman's blood, which has contrary qualities. Because the preponderance of heat is on the right side, if the "matter gathereth in the cell of the right side" of the mother a male child results; if to the left side a female child.[66] If the virtue of the father's blood has mastery the child will be like the father; if the virtue from the two parents is equally strong the child will resemble both. This theory agrees with modern ideas in so far as it allocates an important part to both father and mother in the formation of the child's characteristics.

Most authors on the diet for health do not elaborate further on the basic information given by Batman. All agree that the child before birth is nourished by blood; "he is fed and nourished in the mothers wombe with bloud menstrual."[67] No specific reference is made regarding the diet needed by a pregnant woman in relation to the welfare of her child. Two ways in which food can influence the actual birth of the child are given by Huarte and Raynalde. Huarte explains that when an individual remembers any "delicat and savourie meat" the vital spirits "straight abandon the rest of the body, and flie to the stomacke and replenish the mouth with water." This action is so swift that if a woman with child longs for any sort of food and holds the idea in her imagination "she looseth her burthen if speedily it be not yeelded unto her."[68] Raynalde lists a number of things which will cause a "great hinderaunce to the byrth." If a woman is in the habit of eating foods which will dry, constrain or bind her, such as meddlars, chestnuts and all sour fruits, and sour sauces with rice of millet, these can hinder the birth. The use of cold baths in water containing certain minerals is also bad. The pregnant woman must not be allowed to become too hungry or thirsty, nor must she take, just before labour, anything "of great odour, smel, or savour, for such thynges (in manye mens opinions) attract and draw up the . . . matrix" and this hinders birth.[69]

It was recognized, in a general way, that the parents' diet before conception could influence the child. Hippocrates believed it could affect the sex of the child.[70] Huarte takes this idea further and suggests that the parents' diet before conception can influence the wit and behaviour of their child. This is elaborated in his *Examination of mens Wits*,

which is subtitled "In which, by discovering the varietie of natures, is
shewed for what profession each one is apt, and how far he shall profit
therein."

Huarte's thesis is that every individual is born with a certain proportion of wit. This intelligence should, because of the limitations of a
man's natural ability, be directed at only one aspect of science (sic) in
an individual's lifetime, if he is to succeed in this thing. Rules are given
on how to determine an individual's aptitude, and the author is concerned to see that as many children are born with aptitudes as possible.
The interest of the book, for the purpose of this study, lies in the suggested diets to be taken by parents, by which they can influence the
abilities of their children before conception has taken place. Huarte
says that "the parents who have a will to beget verie wise children, must
drinke waters, delicate, fresh, and of good temperature; otherwise they
shall commit error in their procreation." Other factors also have to be
considered; these include the direction of the wind at the time of generation, and the kind of air breathed: "yet it [the effect on the child]
standeth much more upon to use fine meats appliable to the temperature of the wit: for of these is engendred the bloud and seed, and of the
seed the creature."[71] In order to engender children of great understanding (which, Huarte comments, "is the ordinarie wit for Spaine") the
following foods are recommended. These should be taken at set times
before the child is conceived.

To engender children of great understanding.[72] White bread made of
fine meal seasoned with salt. The meal is cold, dry, subtle and delicate.
Salt is important because "it is so drie and so appropriate to the wit."[73]
Partridges, kid and muscatel wine are recommended.

Children with a good memorie.[74] To be taken eight or nine days
before conception — trout, salmon, lampreys and eels.

Children with great imagination. Pigeons, goats, garlic, onions, leeks,
rapes, pepper vinegar, white wine, honey and all other sorts of spices
make the seed hot and dry and very subtle and delicate in its parts.
Children engendered from these foods will have great imagination, but
not equivalent understanding, and they will lack a good memory.
Huarte does not trust those with great imagination, as the "heat inclin-
eth them to many vices and evils." However, if they are kept under
control he believes that the country will receive more service from their
imagination than from the understanding and memory of other men.

*Children of reasonable discourse, with reasonable memory and reas-
onable imagination.* Hens, capons, veal, weathers (sheep) of Spain, are

all foods of moderate substance and will engender children moderate in the qualities listed above, "wherethrough they wil not be verie profoundly seen in the Sciences, nor devise ought of new."

Foods to be avoided by potential parents. Cows' flesh, Manzo bread from "red graine," cheese, olives, vinegar and water alone. These foods will engender "strength like a bull; but with all, [they will] be furious and of a beastly wit."

For a "sonne, prompt, wise and of good condition." For this the parents should take goats milk and honey six or seven days before conception.

Huarte acknowledges that (despite his advice) foolish children may be born of wise parents and vice versa. He discusses this problem at length, rejecting the possible effect of the imagination (with frequent references to Aristotle's views on this subject). Huarte's argument [75] follows two main lines: there will be variation in the male seed because seed comes from blood, and different foods will produce different blood as the diet varies. There is "no child born, who partaketh not of the qualities and temperature of the meat, which his parents fed upon a day before he was begotten." He also argues that both parents contribute to the child and stresses the part played by the woman, giving her influence as the explanation for the birth of a perfect child, which was said to have been begat by a fish leaping on the woman from out of the river. With less credulity [76] it is also pointed out that the child of one white and one negro parent (regardless of the sex of the white or negro parent) "will partake of either qualitie." In the shaping of children Huarte puts the greatest emphasis on the relative strengths and qualities of the seeds of both parents. As far as the effect of the food eaten by the parents is concerned he has to acknowledge that there can be

> found a certain sort of man, whose genitories are endowed with such force and vigour, as they utterly spoile the aliments of their good qualities, and convert them into their evill and grosse substance. Therefore all the children whom they beget (though they have eaten delicat meats) shall proove rude and dullards. . .[77]

However, in some cases the innate qualities (in the modern sense) of the parents may overcome "grosse" meats and they can eat "porcke, yet make children of a very delicate wit." This proves, he continues, that "there are linages of foolish men, and races of wise men and some born blunt and lacking in judgement."

Following the chapter of what parents must do if they are to engender wise and witty children, Huarte writes about "What diligences are to be used for preserving the childrens wit after they are formed." When the creation of the child is finished "there remaineth not for the creature, any part of the substance whereof it was first composed." This continuous change in the infant from the time "he beginneth to be shaped" required foods, for "it little availeth to have engendered a child of delicat seed, if we make no reckoning of the meates, which afterwards we feed upon."[78]

Post-Natal. Breast feeding is the aspect of child feeding which has by far the greatest importance in the sixteenth century. Most books, whether they deal with the nursing woman or not, give advice on how to increase the flow of milk.[79] One author suggests the following:

> Item take two drams of Crystall beaten into a fine powder, and devyde that in foure equal partes: one of these partes geve unto the Nourse, the space of foure dayes to drynke, with broth made either of Cicer (*cicerarietinum*) or elles of peason (*peas*).[80]

Phaire lists the following: dill, aniseed, fennel, cristal, horehounde, fresh cheese, honey, lettuce, beets, mints, carrots, parsnips, the udder of a cow or sheep, goats milk, blanched almonds, rice porridge, powdered dried cow's tongue, poached eggs, saffron and drinking the "juice" from roasted veal.[81]

Much is written on the ideal characteristics of human milk and of the nurse who will provide it. Milk was thought to be formed from the menstrual blood which was further concocted in the breasts to form milk.[82] Human milk was considered the best type for children and was given to adults in periods of convalescence.[83] Unquestionably it is best for the mother to feed her own child, Phaire says "Wherfore as it is agreing to nature so it is also necessary and comly for the owne mother to nource the owne child." By "agreing to nature" he refers to the generally accepted belief that if lambs are nourished with goats milke they will develop goat's hair instead of sheep's wool, "Wherby it doth appeare that the mylke and nourishyng hath a marveylous effect in chaunging the complexion."[84] Because of this belief the choosing of a wet-nurse was an important procedure with many factors to be considered, any of which could influence the sukling child.

Characteristics of human milk. The general characteristics to be avoided or sought are described: milk is evil if it is too thick or too watery, blackish-blue, reddish or yellow, or is bitter salt or sour to the taste.

Good milk is white and sweet and its consistency can be tested as follows:

> when ye droppe it on your nayle, and do move your finger (it will) neither fleteth abroade at every stering nor will hange faste upon your nayle, when ye turne it downewarde, but that which is betwene both is best.[85]

It is said that Soranus was the first writer to mention this test, which continued in use for over sixteen hundred years.[86]

The choice of the nurse. The whole subject of nurses and their regimen, breast feeding, and weaning, are dealt with at some length by John Jones.[87] Jones' ardour for religion and his patriotism dim the clarity of his exposition because he interpolates sections on these subects within the main discourse. The information regarding nurses can be roughly classed under two headings: (i) how to choose a nurse, and (ii) how she should behave.

For a male baby it is best to choose a woman who has recently borne a son, for a female baby one who has had a daughter.[88] She should be of medium build. The best age is between twenty-three and thirty-three years. Preferably the nurse should have borne two or three healthy children and breast fed them herself. The nurse must be chosen according to the temperament of the baby to be fed, "according to that principle which teacheth, that the healthy are to be kept by the like, the unhealthy with unlike." The appearance must be pleasant to look at "without gogle eyes or loking a squint, say I, as she that is not separated from goodnesse."[89] Nor should nurses be chosen from "them that paint themselves" as this indicates a wanton pride which could be transmitted to the child. A nurse must be changed if she becomes sick or is given to drink "or anye other intolerable vice," for fear that the child would "sucke uppe sickness and wickednesse with milke." For the milk has the power to "chaunge and alter the disposition of the Infant."[90]

The behaviour of the nurse. The nurse must rule her passions. Jones makes the suggestion, for example, that should she become annoyed she can repress her anger by singing Psalms. Because the blood is corrupted by lechery the nurse should suppress her desires by taking lettuce, a conserve of water-lilies, pigeons, or by strewing her chamber with herbs. Regarding foods to be eaten, nurses must be careful to take only those which engender good blood. The foods should be medium in substance and of a mean temperature. Foods advocated include: Flesh

— mutton, young beef, kid, lamb, veal, pig, rabbit, capon, chicken, hen, turkey; Birds — all "cloven footed foules," except quails; Fishes — eighteeen kinds are listed, including both fresh and salt water. The only stipulation is that they shall be from good water; Wine — the nurse (because the climate is cold) may have a small draught of wine in the middle of dinner.[91]

Jones then discusses the "medicines" to be taken by a nurse and says they must be chosen with care. In fact, he gives a long list of foods which may be taken by the nurse "to keepe hir solible, or any others, and also to binde." These include broths made with flesh, and a wide variety of herbs and pulses, buttermilk, a variety of sweet fruits, meade, bread and butter. Instructions are also given as to what air, exercise, labour arts, and pastimes are suitable for a nurse. Finally, Jones emphasizes the importance of kindness and love in a nurse and the good relationship there should be between her, the baby, and the baby's mother.[92]

Breast feeding and weaning. Physicians advised against putting a child to its mother's breast at once; this should be delayed a day or two "because that the creme (as they cal it) straight after the byrth, the first day in all women doth thicken and congile."[93] No reference is made to any other suitable fluid that should be given to the child.

There seems to be no clear-cut idea of how often a child should be fed each day. Jones suggests that twice or three times a day is sufficient, but he points out that ancient authors warned against overfeeding. His own views tend the other way. He says:

> Yet for my parte, if an errour shall happen in the quantitie of the foode and propertie, as I confesse it will be harde for anye to desine the juste quantitie and qualitie as I had rather it should be a little to plentifull for yonglings, than anye thing to scant.[94]

The age at which weaning was advocated varied widely according to both ancient and contemporary advice, ranging from one to four years, or until the teeth appeared. Jones says the custom is one year, but adds that he knows of cases where children were weaned at less than one year old. He himself was not weaned until after he was big enough to bring his nurse her stool.[95] However, some general rules are given regarding the comparative duration of breast feeding: the child of an old woman should be fed longer than that of a young woman; the weak should be fed longer than the strong; twins longer than a single child; males longer than females, and nobles longer than "unnoble."[96]

No weaning should be done suddenly. This follows Hippocratic advice that "those that eat solid food while being suckled bear weaning more easily."[97] A recommended "pappe" was: one pint new milk; enough flour when boiled to make it thick; a lump the size of a chestnut of almond butter or sweet butter; and one ounce of sugar. This mixture is said to be better than that made of milk and flour alone, which was a pap in general use.[98] Paps should be taken until the teeth come through, at which time some tender flesh of good "temperature and juice," finely minced or bruised, can be given to the child.

Childhood. No clear picture emerges of the diet to be given after weaning. Advice about the care required is given in general terms in Hake's book about the training and education of children. The appropriate verse is

> . . . their childe they never feede
> With all that comes to hande, but they
>   observe with carefull heede
> Both what to give and how to give:
>   what quantity to use:
> And eke to feede it leisurely:
>   for if they should infuse
> And pour it in with reckless handes
>   they know they either should
> Their baby choke, or at the least
>   his clothes would be foul'd.[99]

Glimpses of children's meals are given in the books on instruction in the French language, by Hollyband.[100] It was accepted that children had considerable innate heat, a condition requiring plenty of nourishment, and that children (like old people) should eat little and often. Jones gives some of the advice provided for the children of the French king. They should have: Suppings made with fine wheatflour, fine starch, almonds, barley or wheat, rye, "peas and such like." Also, they should have soft bread steeped in the broth from the flesh of kids, calves and hens, and sometimes a capon wing or roasted pheasant's breast minced up finely. No drinks were listed, though wine was utterly prohibited.[101]

It would seem that this soft diet was intended for a period directly after weaning and would be changed gradually to an adult diet. The two elder sons of the fifth Earl of Northumberland, when about nine years old or less, took the same food as their parents, without the wine.[102] A

word of warning about child feeding is given by Elyot, who says that if
the child's belly is "fuller and greater than it was wont to be," then the
child is being given the wrong food.[103]

Section III
Diet in Old Age

Despite the great interest shown in the preservation of health and pro-
longation of life in sixteenth century England, it was not until 1586
that the first treatise appeared, in English, which was primarily concerned with diet in old age. This work was Thomas Newton's *The Olde
mans Dietarie*,[104] which he had translated from the Latin of an anonymous author. It is predominantly concerned with the proper food and
drink for old men. Supporting and supplementary information is also
given by Elyot, Cogan and Peter Lowe and Du Laurens.

Traditionally the time between birth and death was divided up into
set periods. In Hebrew, Greek and Roman literature the division is into
fourteen, ten or seven periods. Bartholomaeus Anglicus gives these
divisions: infancy, childhood, adolescence (giving seven years to each
period, making a total of twenty-one years). After this comes "Juven-
tus," which continues until middle age at about fifty years, and some
suppose that middle age lasts until seventy years.[105] In the sixteenth century the representation of the seven ages of man was a common theme
in art and literature.[106] However, all writers place great emphasis on the
fact that each individual varies. Newton explains the cause of this variety as being due to temperament, their divers trades and kinds of life,
and the constitution of the body.[107] Lowe says that age should be measured by the temperature of the body, not by its years, for "there be
many olde folkes of 40 yeares, and divers who may be thought young
of threescore." He also points out that women age sooner than men.[108]

Old age itself can be divided into three stages. Firstly, the "Greene
and lustie old age," which is the doorway to old age. In this period men
are still "lustie in bodie constant in minde and in strength serviceable
and active." Next comes "grave, reverent and honorable old age," with
the limbs weakening and a greater inclination to sleep and rest. The last
period is "Dotage," in which "being riveled and wrinkled . . . [they] are
not able any more for very feeblenes and impotencie to use any exercise."[109] The general picture of old age is of a thin, shrivelled, weak old
man who is costive and liable to gout and the stone. No reference is
made to fat old men.

The Old mans Dietarie quotes the works of Hippocrates, Celsus, Galen and Avicenna. Newton complains that Avicenna "confusedly, disorderly and unaptly" takes Galen's advice, which was intended for Antiochus, and "doth . . . jumble and shuffle [it] up in a heape or a generall rule for every olde man."[110] This is the sort of fault Newton inclines to himself. His advice for old men does not differentiate clearly between his three groups, and it is often presented in a somewhat confusing way. The basic fact to be considered was the change in temperament which occurred with ageing. Old men become cold and dry, changing from the hot:moist state of their young years. This is the Aristotelian and Galenic view of ageing, accepted by most English writers in the sixteenth century.[111] The reason for the change from hot:moist to cold:dry is explained as follows:

> For, the radicall humour and substantificall [sic] moysture beeing in tract of time by litle and litle wasted, which (like Dewe) is distributed, and interspersed in and among all the similare and principall partes of the bodie; together with the naturall heate likewise by litle and litle waning and drooping away: the whole bodie cannot choose but decay withall. . .[112]

Because of this the instrumental parts of the body become too dry and the whole body becomes weak and unable to function properly. Du Laurens points out that these changes take place at different rates, women growing old sooner than men (they are naturally more cold) and those of a sanguine complexion growing old very slowly, because "they have a great store of heate and moysture."[113]

It is emphasized that treatment must be gentle. A good diet for the old is

> in a maner like unto that renutritive and restorative diet that is prescribed unto pueling and still sickly persons: or to such as have beene lately recovered from their disease. . .[114]

Newton gives "Three ends to be observed in dyeting olde men," namely:

(1) Those places in the body which have become emptied should be filled with nourishing substances suitable to the part which has decayed.

(2) The distemper of the body, whether it is due to natural or accidental causes, should be qualified and altered by contraries.

(3) Superfluous excrements should be carefully purged from the body.

All these objectives can be achieved by using the right food and drink, by wholesome bathing, moderate exercise, and massage.[115]

In general, old people should eat foods which are "of good nourishment, and easie of digestion, abstaining from all grosse, viscous, windy, flegmaticke, and melancholique meates."[116]Newton is more specific and lists some foods which are "of ill juyce and give naughtie nourishment." These foods include frumentie (hulled wheat boiled in milk), cheese, roasted eggs, cockles, onions, scallions (spring onions), mushrooms, lentils and oysters.[117] The rejection of these foods is based on the fact that they yield "grosse clammy and tough nourishment and that they vary considerably in their qualities as well as the degree of these qualities. For example, scallions are hot (4th) and dry (3rd), while cheese is cold and moist, both in the second degree.[118] Some of these foods are listed again later (with some qualifying remarks) as suitable for old men.

Newton's advice about foods is summarized at the end of this section. Throughout the work it is reiterated that a man's normal custom should not necessarily be changed because he has grown old. In general the advice is fairly consistent, being based on the effect of the "juices" produced, as well as the qualities of the food. Newton explains in what measure and order it is most expedient for old men to take these foods. However, Lowe puts this out more clearly as eight "principall rules" to be observed, as follows:

1. To eat only when they have an appetite, for then the stomach is best able to deal with food.

2. Food should be well cooked and soft; otherwise it cannot be concocted in the stomach satisfactorily.

3. The stomach should never be overloaded, as this weakens the natural heat.

4. Only one sort of meat should be taken at one time, and never more than two. Foods which cause a thirst should be avoided, as drinking hinders digestion.

5. Foods which can be most easily digested should be taken first, including such things as soup and prunes, which loosen the belly. Heavy foods should be eaten last.

6. Eat more at supper than at midday (unless the individual suffers from catarrh). This is because there is a greater period of time between supper and dinner rather than the other way around. Also, sleeping between supper and dinner aids digestion.

7. Eat foods of good nourishment and easy digestion.

8. Eat little and often. This applies to the young as well as the old.

These rules are, in fact, quite general and only a few apply specifically to the old.

Newton continues by referring to other things which are "outwardly incident to us" — namely, air, water, fire, oil, baths, sleep, and affections of the mind. In this section he follows the general pattern of sixteenth century authors on these subjects. He does stress that anxieties are more dangerous to a man as he gets older.[120] Lowe provides a section of remedies for the "sundry inconveniences and diseases" of old age, though he adds "They be so many in number, that it will be tedious to prescribe remedies for them all." The remedies given are mainly broths made with herbs of the same sort mentioned above, and intended for such conditions as constipation, wind, aching, pain when urinating, coughing and running eyes.[121]

The temperament of old men was considered to be like that of a man of melancholy complexion, both being cold:dry. The foods advocated or forbidden follow the same general pattern for both groups with, naturally, some slight variations due to the debilities of old age.

Following is a summary of the advice on foods given by Newton in *The Old Mans Dietarie:*

Foods forbidden

All food and drink: Of ill juice, tough or clammy.

Cereals: New bread, unleavened or ill baked or that made from the finest wheat flour or purest meal. Pastries and cakebread[a] that are made using paste, butter, milk, cheese, honey and sugar.

Flesh: Flesh from beasts that are very large, old, lean or hard. Birds which live in watery places.

Fish: Big fishes and those that are strong or rank in taste or smell. Oily, shiny, tough or clammy fish.

Dairy produce: Eggs fried hard or roasted. Milk generally is forbidden. It is likely to cause obstructions. Cheese, especially if it is old, hard or rotten.

Fruits: Spanish prunes, ripe or dry figs, dates, pine apples[b] cause gnawings in the stomach and may stop up the liver and spleen.

Pulses: All sorts of pulses.

*Ale, beer and water:** Ale, beer and water should all be avoided.

---

*Boorde (p. 253) says water is "colde slowe and slacke of digestion."

Foods recommended

All food and drink: Of easy concoction, quickly nourishing and soon alterable into a man's own substance without any excess excrements.

Cereals: Bread, well baked, thoroughly kneaded, properly leavened, salted, and made from reasonably fine flour. Bread made from Zea or Spelt Wheat.[c] Barley bread.

Flesh: Chickens or young pullets are best. Wild birds from the hills or mountains.

Fish: Fish that live in clear rocky waters and which are tossed by the movement of the water, which prevents them from "being filthy."

Dairy produce: Eggs lightly poached. In summer, new milk — direct from the beast — if taken alone.[d] Cheese made from sour milk (buttermilk) may be eaten with a little honey at the beginning of the meal. This loosens the belly.

Fruits: Ripe summer fruits may be eaten at the beginning of meals; for example, cherries, prunes, peaches, and ripe grapes which have hung a while before eating.

Pulses: A decoction or broth of beans, peas, or chick peas is permissible.

Herbs: (None forbidden). Recommended are: Lettuce, malowes, orage,[e] Blite, wild carrots, white beets, sorrell, borage, buglosse, leaks (in small amounts), cheville and parsley. To provoke urine — parsley seed and roots. For the stone — betonie. To purge phlegm — capers pickled in oil or honey and eaten with bread, mercurie,[f] mallowes, cabbages, a fig now and then with a little senna.

Wine: (None forbidden). All wine is good. The best is that which is thin and fine in substance and yellow or reddish in colour.[g]

Notes (a through g) to above summary (pp. 161-162)

[a]Cake bread is a finer and more dainty quality of bread *(OED)*.

[b]Spanish prunes are also called damaske and are a type of plum. Pine apples come from the pine tree and have no connection with the fruit now given that name.

[c]Zea is the obsolete Latin name for a grain called Spelt. Spelt is *Triticum Spelta*. Now Z. Mays refers to maize or Indian corn and is sometimes anglicized as Zea maize *(OED)*. Newton says in a marginal note (Sig. C3ᵛ), "This Zea or Spelta, is thought to be our Rye." B. Googe, in *Foure Bookes of Husbandry*, London, 1577 (Sig. D2ᵛ), refers to this confusion but separates wheat from rye. To determine exactly which plants he describes is beyond the scope of this work. Tusser lists a number of varieties of wheats and refers separately to rye (D. Hartley, *Thomas Tusser 1557*, 1931, p. 112). See also Chapter XI.

[d]The list of permitted foods varies slightly according to the time of year. The recommendation of new milk directly contradicts the advice to avoid milk generally. Newton gives no explanation, but states that "newe milke warme from the udder" may be taken by itself when the weather is extremely hot (Sig. C4[r]). Milk itself is moist in the second degree and temperately hot, which might be considered valuable for a cold:dry temperament. Presumably it is the avoidance of oppilations which is more important.

[e]Mountain spinach, *Atriplex hortensis.*

[f]Mercurie, *Mercurialis perennis.*

[g]Wine moistens and nourishes. It should be avoided by all those who are hot and moist in themselves, but is most valuable to those who are cold and dry. The degree of qualities of a wine depended mainly on its colour, country of origin, and age. The general consensus of opinion was that a clear white or yellow wine of medium age was the most beneficial. See also Chapter IX.

Section IV
Diets for Students

Two books on diet which, according to the title, or author's stated intentions, would seem to be directed towards students, are: *A Direction for the Health of Magistrates and Studentes* by G. Gratarolus, translated from the Latin by Thomas Newton (1574),[122] and *Haven of Health,* described as "chiefly gathered for the comfort of students and consequently of all those that have a care of their health. . ." by Thomas Cogan (1584).[123] In fact, neither of these books is directed specifically to students as we would now understand the word, but both are fairly comprehensive works on the general principles of diet necessary for good health. This apparent discrepancy is due to a different use of the word student from our present usage. Today a student may be described as someone following a course of study or instruction. In Elizabethan times the term embraced a much wider though ill-defined social group, the title being given both to those who used their minds (as opposed to their hands) and also to those who were able to order their own lives and were not at the beck and call of others. Gratarolus points out that as all individuals vary in their needs there is no point in trying to provide dietary advice for those who must attend on others (e.g. servants on their masters) and so are unable to choose and follow their own particular regimen or observe any precise diet. Therefore his advice is directed to those who "live of themselves freely and are not enthralled or mancipated to the inconveniences above said."[124]

Cogan has the same sort of attitude but puts more stress on the differences between different groups. He says "So I write not these precepts for labouring men, but for students, and such as though they bee no students, doe yet folowe the order and diet of students."[125] Cogan differentiates between labourers and learned men, and also between "gentlemen and learned men" and "craftsmen and husbandmen."[126] An example already cited says that beans "are meate for mowers, as the Proverbe is,[127] and for ploughmen but not for students." He also says "but what Rustickes doe or may doe without hindrance of their health is nothing to studentes."[128]

Unlike Sylvius' *Regimen for Poor Scholars Readily observed and wholesome,*[129] little of Cogan's advice is specifically for students. Occasionally he refers to conditions at Oxford during the time he was a student there and comments on the needs for exercise and the time and order of meals "in the Universities."[130] Here and there he advocates, or warns against, particular foods for students. The resulting picture we get of students, from these irregular references, is a poor one in the sense of physique. They are not necessarily the traditional "poor scholar" as regards worldly goods, though Cogan does refer to the fact that he is describing a recipe in detail "because all studentes bee not of habilitie to have a Cooke, or a Physician at their pleasure."[131] We learn that students are weaker than labourers: "prooved by experience in labourers, who for the more part be stronger than learned men."[132] They are shorter lived and have poorer health than husbandmen. "For husbandmen and craftsmen for the more parte doe live longer and in better health, than gentlemen and learned men and such as live in bodily rest."[133] It was also a general belief that countrymen were longer lived than town dwellers.[134] The shorter life and poor health of the man who used his brain was attributed in part to the anxiety and loss of tranquility caused by mental work. Students are also unfortunately "Oftimes troubled with scabbes," due to lack of exercise;[135] Affected by rheum "which is a common and a continuall adversarie to studentes";[136] "Commonly cumbred with diseases of the head";[137] afflicted "for the more part" with ill or weak stomachs.[138] This is emphasized a number of times and agrees with the view that was held from early times to Ramazzini in the eighteenth century, that learned men have weak stomachs.[139] In general, students are melancholy, like all learned men.[140] In his chapter on Borage, Cogan lists the five things which, according to classical tradition, are "enemies to study." These are phlegm, melancholy, venus, satiety, and morning-sleep.[141]

No clear diet is advocated for students suffering from any of these conditions, but reference is made to them under the headings of various foods. Coriander helps against rheum. Borage "putteth away melancholie and madness" because it causes joy and mirth. It also comforts the brain, increases the memory and wit, and engenders good blood; therefore it is to be recommended for students.[142] Great emphasis is put on sweet smells, which clear the head of phlegm; they also aid the sight, and stimulate the mind. Three examples out of many are: betayne (the smell of the leaves clears the head), camomile (whose smell comforts the brain), and rose water, which aids dim sight.[143] The problem of the celibate student is raised and the old English saying quoted: "He that will not a wife wedde, must eate a cold Apple when hee goeth to bed."[144] Also, purslane "represseth the rage of Venus: wherefore it is much to be used of students that will live honestly unmarried."[145] Advice on satiety and morning sleep are given in Cogan's sections related to the timing and sequence of exercise, meals and sleep.

These two sixteenth century treatises which one might expect to deal with diets for students, do not do this in any particular or logical fashion. If the characteristics of students given by Cogan are accepted, then additional specific advice is available from other sources which refer to these characteristics, such as Elyot's lists of foods which make the stomach strong, digestives of phlegm; foods good for a cold head, or foods to be avoided because they hurt the eyes. The advice for a melancholy man is also applicable. From all the material available it would be possible to build up a fairly comprehensive dietary plan suitable for the general group which could be called students.

Section V
Diets for all Manner of Men and Women

This heading, which is taken from Boorde's "Chapter XXXIX which treateth of a general dyate for all manner of men or women beynge sick or hole,"[147] is a much wider generalization for a chapter heading than is usual, despite the contemporary reluctance to be specific. Others confine themselves to entitling their chapters according to groups already referred to in the above sections, or to providing superficial information regarding diets for those "whyche be ready to fall into siknesse," or during sickness, or for "healthy men," or a "natural diet for all."[148]

Boorde's title is itself misleading. In fact, he merely generalizes briefly on some principles of behaviour required to maintain good health, with

an emphasis on the avoidance of anxiety. It would have been surprising
if Boorde had provided the information that the chapter title indicates,
because the emphasis in all contemporary dietary advice is on the needs
of the individual. The advice given on the four complexions, taken in
conjunction with advice related to their age and state of health, provided guidance for each person. However, it was recognized that within
these four groups, the variation among individuals was enormous. Physicians frequently stated that no diet should be prescribed without the
doctor having a full knowledge of the individual concerned. Boorde,
after being asked to attend the Duke of Norfolk, says that before he
can give advice he must first consult Dr. Buttes (the Duke's own physician) regarding the Duke's usual condition, "not onely your [Nor-
folk's] complexion and infyrmitie but also he [Buttes] dyd know the
usuage of your dyet, And the imibecyllyte and strength of your body
with other qualytes expedyent and necessary to be knowen."[149] It is
this need for the consideration of so many factors which resulted in this
comment:

> Now, whereas there is both diversitie in bodies and also diverse trades
> of living, it cannot be that any one absolute way should be appointed
> to serve everie nature in everie facultie generally.[150]

The usual way of life of the individual was one of the most important
factors to be considered. This refers both to the individual's status or
work in life and to his own particular habits.

It has been shown already that the type of foods advocated for
labourers and gentlemen were different. The humbler people could live
on the cruder, harsher foods because they were considered to have
stronger stomachs, to exercise more, and to be more healthy. Referring
to peas-bread, Cogan says, "But I leave it to Rustickes, who have stom-
ackes like Ostriges, that can digest hardy yron."[151] There was, of
course, a certain convenience in this, as the foods given to servants for
payment in kind could, in general and from this advice should be of the
poorer and probably cheaper quality.

In the Elizabethan period many men of humble origin rose to positions of high authority. There was therefore no general belief that the
cruder digestions of the inferior classes automatically indicated that
they were in other ways inferior human beings. Archbishop Cranmer,
himself of fairly humble origin, said: "Poor men's children are many
times endowed with more singular gifts of nature, sobriety and such like;
and also commonly more apt to apply their study than is the gentle-

man's son delicately educated."[152] Within any specific social position
the individual's own particular habits had to be considered. Cogan says
about custom, "Which is of such force in mans bodie both in sicknesse
and in health, that it countervaileth nature it selfe, and is therefore
called of *Galen* in sundrie places, *an other nature.*"[153] Familiar foods
may be better for the individual than those which are theoretically correct if they are unfamiliar:

> for those meates, to the whiche a man hathe bene of long tyme accus-
> tomed, though they be not of substaunce commendable, yet do they
> somtyme lasse harme than better meates, wherunto a man is not
> used.[154]

Cogan adds a corollary to this: "For what the stomacke liketh, it
greedily desireth ... which thing is the cause that meate and drinke
wherein wee have great delight, though it bee much worse than other,
yet it doth us more good."[155] This view, taken together with the emphasis on a moderate diet, might almost be summed up by Marie
Lloyd's phrase, "a little of what you fancy does you good." It was recognized that custom, in time, may alter nature. Cogan gives the story of
the old woman of Athens who accustomed herself to drinking hemlock
by gradually increasing the dose, for "custome in processe of time may
alter nature and make that harmelesse, which is otherwise hurtfull."[156]
Great changes in ways of life were often inevitable, in which case
"Chaunge is profitable, if it be rightly used, that is, if it be done in the
time of health, and at leisure and not upon the sudden."[157] Or, as Lemnius puts it, "Old rooted custome may not be hastely and sodenly
chaunged, but softly, leysurely and discretely. For sodaine alteration
and chaung bringeth the body into daunger, and is very prejudiciall to
health."[158] Nevertheless, Elizabethans believed that they should be prepared for change, "as Arnaldus teacheth" (says Cogan):

> Every man should so order his selfe, that he might be able to suffer
> heate and colde, and all motions, and meates necessarie, so as he
> might chaunge the houres of sleeping and waking, and his dwelling
> and lodging without harme: which thing may be done, if we be not
> too precise in keeping custome, but otherwise use things unwont-
> ed.[159]

Accepting the notion that only a slow change of habit was desirable
for health, one hesitates to dwell on the turmoil of the stomach of
someone like Sir Walter Raleigh, who was a country gentleman's son,
Oxford student, soldier, naval commander, American explorer, with

interludes of being a Queen's Favourite and, finally, a prisoner in the Tower. The stress placed by all authorities on the need for care in making any change of diet is echoed some three hundred years later by Dr. Edward Smith in 1862 when reporting on relief diets for the unemployed in the English "Cotton Famine." He said: "It is necessary that no material change be attempted in reference to the fixed habits and tastes of these populations and also that any improvements which may be advised be effected in a gradual and unobtrusive manner for otherwise the appetites of the people will be lessened and the food will cause disorder in the system."[160]

The attempt to provide dietary advice for "all manner of men and women" resulted in the production of a large number of books following the same general pattern. A wide range of information was given, but all lacked specificity because the writers subscribed to the belief summed up by Cogan, when he advised that "He that is sound and in good health, and at libertie, should bind himselfe to no rules of dyet . . . a moderate diet is alwaies good, but not a precise diet."[161] This is a view that persisted through the centuries, with the result that the ideas in this chapter regarding an individual's diet can be summed up equally well by a twentieth century writer. R. H. Chittenden said that "On matters of diet every man should be a law unto himself, using judgment and knowledge to the best of his ability reinforced by his own personal experiences."[163]

CHAPTER IX
QUANTITY, TIME AND ORDER

> Let meager appetite be reasons page,
> Let hunger act on diets golden stage:
> Let sparing bits go downe with meriment,
> Long live thou then in th' Eden of content.
>
> T. Walkington (1607)

SIX FACTORS WHICH require special consideration in relation to "Meates and Drinkes" are Substance, Quantity, Quality, Custom, Time, and Order.[1] Of this list, Substance, Quality, and Custom have already been referred to in detail. Of the three terms left all the sixteenth century authorities studied make some direct or indirect reference to them. For example, specific references to Quantity are given by Elyot, Cogan and Lowe,[2] but only indirect references are provided by Boorde, Langton, Bullein, Newton and Jones. Time is more generally referred to because the time of year and time of day played a significant part in the regimen. Order is important because good digestion requires that foods arrive in the stomach in the correct sequence for proper concoction.

Quantity

Empirical ration scales have been used from ancient times; early records of monasteries, hospitals, institutions for the poor, houses of correction, and the army and navy provide a variety of examples of such allowances. In general terms, the basis of these scales was traditional practice, religious rules, food and money available, and the apparent health of those eating the diet. Modern tables of Recommended Daily Intakes,[3] with their detailed suggestions of the quantity of nutrients appropriate for different groups of the population, are derived from foundations laid down in the mid-nineteenth century.[4]

Reference has already been made to a number of attempts to quantify the qualities, but writers in the sixteenth century were under the influence of Aristotelian logic with its emphasis on classification rather

---

N.B. Footnotes to this chapter appear on pages 328-333.

than having a Pythagorean attitude with the acceptance of the importance of numbers and measurement that this implies. It could not be
expected, therefore, that writers would refer to quantities of foods
using a specific manner of measurement comparable to what we would
use today, either for recommending food for the individual or for itemizing the quantities of foodstuffs used. The latter are most frequently
given as numbers of items, by volume or in monetary value. Cogan,
writing of dinner at Oxford University, says "the quantitie of Beefe was
in value an halfepenie for one man."[5] Sometimes directions regarding
precise quantities in recipes are given. M. S. Serjeantson, discussing earlier manuscripts, quotes such directions as "Take a quart of hony" and
"ij galouns of Wyne or Ale and a pound of Pepir," and (with fine abandon) "Take a thousand eggs."[6]

Printed sixteenth century cookery books use the following style:
"Take sixe yolkes of Egs, and a little peece of Butter as big as a Walnut,
one handful of verie fine flower."[7] No indication is given for how
many portions a given recipe is intended. This is not surprising, because
the number of portions a recipe should provide is not generally indicated until cookery books of the nineteenth century and is sometimes
omitted even in modern works. In the use of spices and wine the directions were frequently more precise, using ounces and pints, but the
only time weights of foods *per person* are clearly indicated, is in medicinal prescriptions and allowances in public institutions.

This does not mean that the amounts of foods provided in households
were not supervised. Both Queen Elizabeth (and her father before her)
showed considerable concern regarding the provisions and catering in
their establishments. The allocation of quantities of foods and suitable
menus for all levels of the household hierarchy were usually laid down
in the household regulations of big houses.[8] The object of these regulations was the control of expenditure rather than the achievement of a
good dietary pattern. The Queen had a *Book of diet* which described
specifically the daily menus for monarch, retainers and servants, and as
well a *bouche of court* book which gave the allowances of bread, wine,
fuel and light for all persons at court. These allowances were called the
"Livery."[9] Woodworth points out, in her study of Purveyance for the
Royal Household, that no copies of these books have come to light,
though indications as to their contents are available from various
reports and memoranda that have survived.[10] Examples from other
reigns are given in *A Collection of Ordinances and Regulations for the
government of the Royal Household...*[11]

It is known from Queen Elizabeth's household that "one mutton will make ten messes or services; one veal twelve; one pig thirteen; and one stork twenty-four."[12] In modern dictionaries (besides the usually accepted meaning used in the armed services) mess is defined as a "portion of food or course of dishes."[13] Halliwell says a party of four people dining together was called a mess.[14] This definition will probably have been derived from records of households such as the *Northumberland Household Book* which, in referring to the service of meat and drink served in Lent on "Scramlynge"* days, lays down that two gentlemen-ushers and two yeoman-ushers equal one mess, and that for the gentlemen and children of the Chapel four messes contain ten gentlemen and six children.[15]

Though it seems the general practice to have four to a mess, there are exceptions to this rule. In the *Northumberland Book* itself, in the allocation for the "Clerks in Household," ten clerks are said to constitute two messes. In the earlier *Book of Carving,* directions to the Marshall show that people of high rank may sit with two or three to a mess, but "all other states" may sit with three or four to a mess.[16] Thomas Whythorne, in his autobiography, describing his position as a friend (not a servant) in a gentleman's house, says "whereupon they did not only allow me to sit at their table but also at their own mess, as long as there were not any to occupy the room and place that were a great deal my betters."[17] This does indicate that a small group of people would be served together though seated at a large table, and that this division of people to be fed was followed in the smaller establishments of gentlemen as well as the great households.

Household regulations seem sometimes to have been more excellent in theory than in application. Emmison says that Queen Elizabeth was personally a most frugal and abstemious monarch.[18] However, Woodworth says that Burghley, when he took control of the Royal Household, found that by and large the rules were disregarded and that the "quantity of victual [is] more than before time hath been." Apparently no one, least of all the Queen and her principal household officers, paid attention to the "book of diet." The menu served to the queen was twice as large as that in the book. She substituted costly delicacies for simpler fare. Ignoring "fasting days" she ordered a full menu every day of the week.[19]

This example of court behaviour underlines the real need for the continuous advice against surfeit given by sixteenth century authorities on

---

*That is "Scrambling" days of makeshift meals.

diet. Even where clear records of the provisions used are available, the exact amount of food actually eaten by a given number of people is impossible to calculate. Some of the unknown factors are these: provisions were listed by number (one mutton), not by weight, the quantity of food which was certainly consigned, from the Queen's household to the private households of court officers, is not known. Equally unknown are the number of "strangers" fed and the quantity of alms (in the form of food) given to the poor.[20]

Advisers on regimen and dietaries to preserve health give no precise advice regarding the quantitites of food to be taken. Hippocrates, Galen and Avicenna all write in general terms about quantities of foods required. In *Regimen III* it is suggested that the amount of exercise taken should be exactly proportioned to the amount of food eaten, but no explanation is given as to a scale of measurement.[21] It is also said that it is important to harmonize the amount of food taken with the ability to digest it. Elyot says "the quantitie of meate muste be proportioned after the substance and qualite thereof and according to the complexion of hym that eateth."[22] Having regard to this advice, sixteenth century authorities in general suggest that control of the quantity taken should be governed by the appetite. Cogan says "wherefore the surest way in feeding is to leave with an appetite according to the olde saying, and to keepe a corner for a friende."[23] Even so, there are pitfalls in this sensible advice. Elyot points out

> And here it wolde be remembered that the choleryche stomake doth not desyre soo moche as he maye digest: the melancholye stomacke maye not dygeste soo moche as he desyreth.[24]

According to Cogan, "the greatest occasion why men passe the measuring in eating is varietie of meates at one meal." He explains that in England this is due to the traditions of hospitality which overcome even the strongest wills.[25] The attitude of writers to the subject of quantity of food in the diet can be summed up by another quotation from Cogan:

> Pone gulae metas, ut sit tibi longior aetas,
> Esse cupis sanus? sit tibi parca manus.

That is to say, "use a measure in eating that thou mayst live long and if thou wilt be in health, then hold thine handes."[26]

Time

To a modern way of thinking, the greatest significance time has in relation to food lies in the number and spacing of the times that food is taken. In the sixteenth century the influence of time on the dietary regimen was of greater importance, and was considered under the following headings: (i) Time of year, (ii) Time in the life of a person (age), and (iii) Times in the day of meals.[27]

(i) *Time of the year.* This can be considered in two sections, the first being related to the season of the year, the second to the position of the planets. The factors of the seasons that made them important in relation to diet are: climatic temperature,[28] degree of moisture in the atmosphere and the length of the nights, which influenced the amount of rest taken. The taking of meals had to be planned in relation to the individual's pattern of exercise and rest.

The following information, obtained mainly from Elyot and Cogan,[29] is roughly similar to Hippocratic advice.[30]

In Winter (8th November-8th February) the cold surroundings cool the body, causing the body's heat to be drawn inwards and thus providing a greater concentration of heat for concoction and digestion. Because of this, more food and food of gross substance can be taken in winter than at other times of the year. Due to the atmospheric moisture present there is likely to be an increase in phlegm which is also influenced by the long nights and extra rest taken. Drier roast foods are better at this time than boiled foods. Raw herbs and fruits (except roasted or baked quinces) should be avoided.

Spring (8th February-8th May) may be cold like winter or hot like summer, or a temperate period between these two extremes. Diet should be adapted to the cold, temperate, or hot conditions as the occasion warrants. Phlegm is still present at this time of year, but increases in temperature cause an increase in blood. Cold conditions favour phlegm: warmer conditions will increase the blood; still hotter conditions tend to produce more bile. Therefore in spring the quantity of food taken should be reduced and the amount drunk increased.

In Summer (8th May-8th August) the inward heat becomes less so that the stomach cannot digest the food as quickly or as well as in the winter. Eating little and often is advocated. Cogan quotes Galen when explaining this advice: "because we neede more often nourishing, being then the more consumed through opennesse of the poares and because our strength is more resolved."[31] For those of hot complexion a larger amount of drink is recommended, especially wine diluted with water. The dilution of wine with water was not a step taken without due consideration but was a matter of some importance. Fasting should be avoided, as this dries the body. A variety of foods may be taken at this

season, but not all at one meal (see below). Boiled foods and those with
a high water content and cold quality are specially recommended.

Autumn (8th August-8th November) is "variable" and the air change-
able. This makes autumn a season of sickness when the blood decreases
and melancholy abounds. All summer fruits should be avoided because
they make ill juice and cause wind. More food can be taken than in the
summer, but it should be of a drier sort. All bitter foods, sweet wines,
fat meat (and much exercise) should be avoided. Drink should be less in
quantity and less diluted with water.

In addition to giving this brief advice on diet for each season, authors
explain which season is most beneficial (or harmful) to various groups.
Winter is said to be the enemy of old men, while choleric persons and
young men are "best at ease." [32] Of spring Cogan says "for all seasons of
the yeere the spring time is most wholesome, as *Hipp.* teacheth." [33]
(Elyot makes no comment on this aspect.) Summer, because it is hot
and dry, is best suited to those "whiche be cold of nature and moyst,"
and worst for hot dry natures. At the beginning of summer children and
very young men "are holest, olde folke in the latter ende, and in harvest." [34] Autumn is a dangerous time "to all ages, all natures, and in all
countreys, but the natures hote and moyst be leste indamaged." [35]

Thomas Hill breaks this down further in his translation of the works
of the "lerned menne of the Universitie of Padua," called *A most profitable rule for the preservation of mans Health,* and lists foods suitable
for each calendar month. [36] Examples given are: "salates well prepared
with oyle and spices" are commended in January (sixteenth century
salads included a wider range of ingredients than are generally used
today and could include herbs, roots, flowers and fruits). February is
the time "to eat confections cauded [candied][37] with Honye." Most
authors go no further than advocating foods according to seasons of the
year.

For those who accepted the influence of "the stars" upon the collection, preparation and eating of foods, the time of year would have an
added significance due to the varying position of the moon and planets
at different seasons. [38] As already indicated, the influence of the astrological herbalists was not strong in England in the sixteenth century,
but two titles of books by Anthony Ascham suggest that they advocate
the benefits of planetary influences. The books are, *A little Herball of
all the properties of Herbes. . . declaring what Herbes hath influence of
certain sterres,* London, 1550, and *A little Treatise of Astronomy, very
necessary for physick and surgery,* London, 1552. [39] The herbal is

derived directly from Bankes[40] and in fact contains no astrological law at all. The *Treatise* is very rare and has not been examined. Also, Manning's *Complexion's Castle* deals with herbs and other foods and has a table at the end to aid physicians in their diagnosis through the position of the planets.[41] This type of table had been in common use in previous centuries, though writers on health do not place any particular importance on the position of the planets in relation to particular foods.

(ii) *Time of life* (see also Chapter VIII). In discussing the influence of the "Age of the partie" (as Cogan puts it) on diet, both he and other authors discuss what age is, and the differences apparent at various ages. All recognize that "the dyet of youth is not convenient for olde age nor contrarywise."[42] The needs of children and old men have already been referred to in detail. In general, both are said to require hot moist foods, the children for growth and maintenance, the old to counteract cold and dryness. Reference is made to the fact that young men can eat grosser foods and those foods which are colder and moister such as salads of cold herbs.

(iii) *Times of taking meals.* Ideas on the number and timing of meals in the sixteenth century must have evolved from rather contradictory traditions. Hippocratic teaching advises "First a man should have one meal a day only, unless he has a very dry belly; in that case let him take a light luncheon."[43] Celsus makes many references to meals, from which it can be inferred that one or two meals a day was the common practice. He says for example that hunger is more easily borne by "one accustomed to a single meal than by one used in addition to one at midday,"[44] but does not appear to advocate either one or two meals per day. The stress is on maintaining the habits of the individual. Some descriptions of great Roman banquets suggest that for the rich at least it might be said that two meals were taken at once.

Arabic authorities went to the other extreme and advised that a person should eat only when hungry and should satisfy his hunger before the feeling had passed.[45] A. S. Way, in his translation of a medieval tract on hygiene[46] refers to Rhazes as saying in Book X of *Almansor,*[47] that "food should be taken when the weight of the previous meal has descended to the lowest point and the nether portion of the intestines lightened." As to the frequency of meals, the following "good rule" is given — not more than two meals in twenty-four hours, but preferably only one. For some temperaments, taking refreshment twice in three days is best. This view is also said to have been suggested by Averroes (commenting on the poems of Avicenna), where it is stated that the third stage of digestion is completed in eighteen hours and therefore an equivalent space of eighteen hours is recommended between meals. Thus the most commendable hour for eating is when a person is invigorated by the completed digestion of the food last taken. However, these writers do suggest that the number of meals should be adapted to the frame of the person: fewer meals for those with big fat frames, and more for the thin wiry types. They also say that those who take a great deal of exercise and work hard require more ample nourishment.[48]

The abstemious habits advocated by the Arabs did not suit the English way of life. Apart from the tradition of hospitality which provided meals more frequently, Harrison and others explain that the cold climate in England necessitates the taking of more food than would be needed in hotter countries.[49] This, they say, is because the cold here keeps in the internal heat of the body, and the resulting hot stomach requires more food to act upon if it is not to produce harmful humours. In general therefore, Englishmen need to take more food more often than do those who live in hot climates. However, it is recognized that this taking of extra food can be overdone, and Harrison is critical of his predecessors for taking too many meals. He blames Canute for introducing four meals a day into England and complains that though the Normans claimed to be abstemious they eventually exceeded Canute's gluttony and took five or six meals a day.[50] Fortunately, in his own time (he says) men are more restrained in England and take just two meals a day, namely dinner and supper.

The pattern of meals in general seems to have varied as the sixteenth century progressed and does not, anyhow, seem to have been uniform at any time. It is known (despite Harrison's remarks) that some people "took food" four times a day (breakfast, dinner, supper, and livery) during this period. The apparent contradiction is probably due to different definitions of the word meal, as well as different habits. In his reference to the Norman's five or six meals a day, Harrison must surely have included meals which could be called breakfast and livery, yet in describing contemporary habits he ignores them. He is supported, in his reference to two meals a day, by account books of some noble houses which list only foods for dinner and supper, yet other records show conclusively that in the fifteenth and early sixteenth centuries more "meals" were provided.[51]

Livery was a snack taken when required. This would usually receive no special mention as a meal. "The Gent. Usher maye commaund all tymes of the daye bred, wyne, beare and ale, to the chambers as he shall thinke goode."[52] The term can also refer to regular allowances of such things as bread, beer, wine, fuel and candles, made to members of a household. The word livery is said to be derived from things "livered" or "delivered out."[53]

Sixteenth century writers on diet were faced with a problem regarding breakfast, because the ancient teachers, and especially Galen, had never referred to it. Cogan gives this as a reason for the Universities (i.e., Oxford) providing only dinner and supper.[54] On the other hand, the predominance of hot stomachs in England demanded a pattern of meals which would not leave the stomach for too long without food. The result was that advisers differed in their attitudes. Many make no mention of breakfast. Langton is one of these.[55] Elyot puts great stress on the importance of breakfast and bases his argument on the necessity of giving a hot stomach sufficient food to work on. He describes the conditions under which breakfast is advised, i.e., for a person who is "not old," who has a clean stomach after a good night's sleep, and also for those who feel themselves "lyght in the morninge and swete brethed, let them on goddis name breake their fast."[56]

Cogan, though he patterned his work on Elyot's, is not so emphatic. He says that for students, provided the stomach is clean, foods of light digestion such as milk, butter, and eggs are recommended, and if there is nothing else available a little "breade and drinke" should be taken to give the stomach something to work on.[57] Without a detailed examination of all the records available it is impossible to say how extensively breakfast was taken in England. The pattern seems variable even in households of the same social level.

The first quoted reference to breakfast in the *Oxford English Dictionary* is dated 1463.[58] The household ordinances of King Edward IV's mother illustrate the rules governing the meals of different levels of officers within the household.[59] Breakfast is referred to and is taken under varying circumstances by different officers. The *Northumberland Household Book* (1512-c.1525)[60] gives lists of the foods to be provided at breakfast, throughout the year, for various members of the household. Three examples for "flesh days" are given below. The terms requiring explanation in these examples are as follows: a trencher is a slice of bread used instead of a plate; a manchet is a small loaf made of the finest wheaten flour; chine is backbone; potell is a half gallon measure; dimid *(dimidium)* means halved, i.e. half a gallon in this case.

For my Lorde and my Lady
a loaf of bread in trenchers
two machents
one quart of beer
one quart of wine
half a chine of mutton or else a chine of boiled beef.

For my Lord Percy and Mr. Thomas Percy
half a loaf of household bread
a manchet
one potell of beer
a chicken or else three boiled mutton bones.[61]

These ordinances were laid down in 1511, at which time Lord Percy would have been about nine years old. It is uncertain how long these amounts would continue to apply to the children but they provide an interesting contrast with the adult allowances.

For two Meas [mess] of Gentilmen o'th'chapel
and a Meas of Chylderyn
three loaves of bread
a gallon dimid of beer
three pieces of boiled beef.

On fish days the meat would be replaced by a piece of salt fish or a dish of buttered eggs. The quantities supplied diminished with the lower ranks and some of the more elaborate dishes, such as buttered eggs, seem only to have been supplied to senior officers of the household.

Later (edited) account books of the Northumberland family (1564-1632)[62] refer only to items to be accounted for at dinner and supper. Similarly Emmison's excellent picture of life in the household of Sir Thomas Petre gives no lists of foods for breakfast in his household, but simply those for dinner and supper.[63] However, it is known that Queen Elizabeth frequently breakfasted on salt meat, bread and ale.[64] Also in the same period Thomas Tusser directed that farmworkers should be provided with breakfast, saying:

Give every one some
Let huswife be carver, let pottage be eate
a dishfull eche one with a morsel of meate[65]

Despite the evidence given above, it was Fynes Moryson's belief that the English only took dinner and supper and that the Italian writer Sansouine's statement that the English covered their tables four times a day was mistaken, though Moryson agrees that sickly men and travellers sometimes took a small breakfast. He explains that at some inns travellers sometimes "set up part of supper" for breakfast. [66] It is likely that those who could did eat or drink between the time of rising and the dinner meal, though perhaps without always describing this taking of food in terms of a meal called breakfast.

Of dinner, Harrison says that the nobility, gentry and students ordinarily ate it at eleven (a.m.). Out of term students dined at ten, while husbandmen and merchants more usually took their dinner at noon. [67] (A comment on the time meals should be taken is given after the section on content.)

Naturally, physicians cannot specify exactly what foods should be taken at dinner because the choice must be determined by the complexion and habits of the individual. Some examples of the foods that were to be provided for dinner in various circumstances are given below:

From the provision account books of the week commencing Sunday, December 20th 1551 in the household of Sir William Petre. [68]

Dinners

FOOD	DAY AND AMOUNT				
Flesh days	Sun.	Mon.	Tues.	Weds.	Fri.
Boiled beef	3 pieces	3 pieces	3 pieces	3 pieces	6 pieces
Roast beef	1	1	--	1	3
Neats [cattle] tongue	1	--	--	--	--
Baked mutton	1 leg	--	--	--	1 neck
Roast pork	--	--	--	--	1 loin
					1 breast
Cony	2	1	1	2	4
Partridge	1	1	--	--	--
Goose	--	--	--	--	1
Capon	--	--	--	--	1
Pies (unspecified)	--	--	--	--	8

Fish days	Thursday	Saturday
Ling [salted cod]	1	½
Haberden [cod] [69]	1	½
Whiting	5	12
Plaice	3	6
Mud-fish	--	3
Cakes of butter	5	1½ (dishes)
Warden [pear] pies	2	--
Eggs	6	16

Christmas day fell on a Friday, which was normally a fish day, and the fish day was moved to the Thursday of that week. [70]

The numbers catered for in the Petre household are not given in the
material quoted by Emmison, but notes about the number of strangers
present are inserted. These give a name, or a description, of the type,
e.g. "5 pore women and 4 strange felowes."[71]

Cogan describes the dinner provided for students at Oxford as
"boyled Beefe with pottage, bread and beere and no more." The
amount of meat was a half-penny's worth per man, but if hunger was
not satisfied by this the authorities would "double their commons."[72]

In 1588 the "Orders . . . for the House of Correction at Bury, Suffolk" listed the following portions of meat and drink which were to be
given to each person:

Flesh days
(dinner and supper)

Rye bread	8 oz. (troy weight)
Porridge	1 pint
Flesh (unspecified)	¼ lb.
Beer	1 pint (the quality of the beer was controlled by cost)

Fish days

Rye bread	8 oz. (troy weight)
Porridge made with milk or peas	1 pint
Cheese	1/3 lb. *or* 1 herring (*or* an alternative to be decided by the Keeper of the House)[73]

This was the maximum normal allowance, but for those who worked
hard, a little more (quantity not specified) bread and beer was allowed
between meals. Those who would not work received *only* bread and
beer. Tusser does not describe the dinners to be given to farm workers,
but he warns: "Give servants no dainties but give them enough."[74]

In Elizabethan England, as would be expected, the pattern of the dinner meal varied greatly between different levels of society, and also,
within each level, on ordinary days as compared with times of special
celebration.

Supper was usually taken between five and seven p.m., depending on
the time of dinner. Again no precise directions are given regarding what
should be taken at this meal. It was a matter of controversy as to
whether supper or dinner should be the larger meal. *Regimen Sanitatis*
advises taking a light supper,[75] but Lemnius, when writing about the
melancholy man, suggests: "let their Supper be larger and more in

quantitye then dinner."[76] Cogan puts both points of view in his discussion.[77] He acknowledges that the *Regimen Sanitatis* advocates a light supper, and shows that this view is supported by the Oxford authorities who followed any sumptuous dinner by providing a smaller supper for the students, but he says that Conciliator (Petrus de Albano)[78] advised a larger dinner than supper because "the heate of the day, joyned to the naturall heat of the body may digest more," and because during the night nature has enough work to do to digest the superfluities of the food eaten earlier without adding a great deal more to it at suppertime.

Leonardus Fuchsius (says Cogan) argues the opposite – i.e., that supper should be greater than dinner.[79] This is because the coldness of the night and sleep both conserve internal heat and aid concoction. Cogan reconciles these two points of view by advocating the larger supper for those that "be lustie and strong of nature, and travaile much," because in these people there is no need for the digestion of superfluities, but only the need to strengthen their bodies, and this (he says) is best done in the night when the senses are at rest.

Alternatively, those that are diseased, aged or troubled with rheumes, or who have a sedentary occupation, will have raw and superfluous humours the digestion of which must not be hindered in the night. Therefore, people in these groups should take a light supper. Cogan underlines the importance of a light supper for Englishmen by pointing out that

> the whole booke of *Schola Sal.* was written specially for englishmen [who are] . . . rheumaticke above other nations.

The prevalence of rheums in England is variously attributed to the damp air, excess beer drinking, and gluttony. Cogan favours damp air, mixing foods, and eating too much as the causes. He concludes that "it is more wholsome to take more at noone than at night. Great Suppers then and late Suppers must be banished from all healthfull houses." As this is advice directed mainly to "students," Cogan is particularly concerned with the effects of meals on the brain and eyes. These are damaged by repletion at supper.

It is not possible to determine which advice was followed in practice. A high proportion of the transcribed or edited records available refer to banquets and Court functions and describe these held at both dinner and supper times. General reading about the period and household accounts, such as those of the Howard and Petre families (quoted above), give the impression that on the whole, dinner was planned as

the larger meal. Though Tusser is no help in advising on the size of supper for farm workers, he does, however, stress the importance of good
cheer at suppertime. This is echoed by many authorities on diet who
advise a gentle walk[80] and cheerful company after supper.

The timing between meals was taken seriously by physicians. Langton
opens his chapter "of dyner or eatynge tyme" with the story of Diog-
enes who, when asked when was the right time for a man to eat, replied
"a rich man when he will, and a poor man when he may." This statement is frequently quoted both by sixteenth century writers and by
others in later centuries.[81] They usually disagree with the advice, as
does Langton, who says:

> I do well alowe that a poore manne shall not eate before he have
> meate, so I do utterly condemne that a ryche manne shall eate when
> he whyll. For meate taken eyther out of tyme or to much in quan-
> titye is cause of many evyls and maladies to the bodye.[82]

Food is taken "out of time" when the accustomed time of eating is
changed or when meals are taken at times "ordeyned for an other purpose,"[83] e.g. eating at night, which is the time for sleep.

The time to eat is when one is hungry, but even so one time is better
than another. The very best time is after exercise because then the body
is purged of excrements, natural heat is increased, and the body is
stronger. Being "purged of excrements" could be said to be similar to
the Arabic idea of digestion being completed and "the nether portion
of the intestines lightened." It is stressed that exercising the body or
mind should be avoided after taking food. The stomach must be kept
rested and quiet if good concoction is to take place. Movement or agita-
tion can have detrimental effects because the "over mouth" (or
entrance) of the stomach will be opened and natural heat will be lost;
also, the opening of the "nether mouth" will allow the content of the
stomach to move on before it is properly concocted.[84] Readers are
advised to follow the examples of "brute beasts" which rest quietly
after food.[85]

It is concern about the proper digestion of food which makes writers
advise on the *minimum* time that should be allowed between meals.
Elyot is quite precise about this. The time between breakfast and dinner should be at least four hours, while that between dinner and supper
should be not less than six hours.[86] Cogan says four to six hours
between dinner and supper. It is frequently stressed that whenever too
much has been eaten at a meal the next meal can be omitted without

harm. Authorities also point out that "children and suche as be not yet at theyr fulle groweth and olde men whyche be weake and feble" need to eat more often, but taking less at each time;[87] nevertheless they should still put at least four hours between each meal. Thus four hours was considered to be a reasonable time for a meal to be digested, the slightly longer time being required for a bigger meal. A space of two to four hours (depending on the size of the meal) should be allocated before sleeping after supper to allow "for the consuming of the vapours which ascent."[88]

Meals, exercise and sleep had all to be related to one another and fitted into the general pattern of the day. The length of the day for the nobility was long, for the Gentlemen Ushers had to be in attendance (in two shifts) from seven in the morning until nine at night.[89] Tusser's description for servants gives an even longer day:

> In Winter at nine and in Summer at ten
> to bed after supper both maidens and men.
> In Whinter at Five oclock servant arise
> In Summer at four is ever good guise.[90]

It is likely that merchants and craftsmen had a workday somewhere between these two, while the poor (who had little artificial illumination) were probably compelled to regulate their lives by the rising and setting of the sun.

Order

The order in which foods should be taken was an important part of a proper regimen. Under their chapter headings of "Order" authors use the word to refer either to the overall plan of the dietary or to the sequence in which foods should be taken. Both meanings are used in this section, but the greatest emphasis is on the sequence in which foods are taken. Cogan says that order is the first and last thing to be considered in relation to foods because order in eating can greatly help or hinder a man's health.[91] He gives Galen as the example of a man who (from the age of twenty-eight years) followed a correct order of diet and lived a healthy life until dying of old age at 140 (sic) years. He also recognized that sometimes people who ignored a proper diet remained stronger and healthier than some who "keepe a precise diet, and eate and drinke as it were by weight and measure." However, it was generally agreed that the effect of an "immoderate diet" was merely deferred and would eventually take its toll on even the soundest body and strongest nature.

Three general rules concerning the sequence of taking foods were stated clearly by sixteenth century writers.[92] These were frequently qualified in detail and appear to have been often contradicted in practice.

1. *Foods that are easy to digest should be taken before those that are more difficult to digest.* The basis for this advice is the belief that during the concoction of food in the stomach heat was applied in a way rather similar to that of a fire under a cooking pot. Therefore, if food which is difficult to digest entered the stomach first, the heat would take so long to work upon it that easily digested foods taken later might putrefy before the concocting heat could reach them. Alternatively, care had to be taken to see that "fine" (easily digested) foods were not left alone in a hot stomach because they might be burnt up too quickly and produce ill effects.

2. *Moist foods should be taken before dry.* The term moist referred not only to those foods which naturally had a greater degree of the moist quality but also to foods made more moist by the method of cooking. For example, boiled meats should be taken before roast or baked meat (of the same sort). Also, the timing and quantity of drink to be taken had to be considered. Drink was required for two purposes: (i) to conserve natural moisture, and (ii) to help the food down into the "places of digestion."[93]

Despite the advice to take moist things first, meals should never begin with a drink; the minimum of a morsel of bread should be taken first. When drink is taken it should be in "sundrye lyttell draughtes"[94] and not all at once at the end of a meal. Just enough should be taken to quench the thirst (which is "a desire of cold and moyst" caused by heat and dryness)[95] and to moisten the food. Too much liquid taken at once "drowns" the food and causes it to pass onwards too soon.

3. *Foods which are "leuse and slipperie" should be eaten before those which are hard and binding.* Slippery foods taken after hard foods may cause the hard foods to move on too soon, before proper concoction has taken place, concoction taking longer for a hard food than for a soft one. Boorde explains why slippery things such as butter should be eaten first in the morning before other foods.[96] He says that anything unctious "that it is to say butteryshe oyle, grease, or fat doth swymme above" in the stomach in the same way that fat remains at the top of a boiling pot. Also, if too much butter is taken it will putrefy on top of the stomach contents, causing harm. The old English proverb says that butter is gold in the morning, silver at noon, and lead at night.[97]

The analogy of the stomach with a cooking pot comes over clearly in sixteenth century writings. It seems to be a pot which is never really stirred because the advice given indicates that the contents of the stomach were expected to remain in the same sequence as they had entered, until they were properly concocted and passed on to the gut. The terms "laboured and concocted" are used to describe the action of the stomach on food, but there is no clear reference to any churning or mixing movement. Sixteenth century anatomists recognized (as had Galen) that the stomach could expand or contract. Bannister describes it as the stomach being "made therfore to dilate and readely gather together agayn."[98] But Galen had not referred to a mixing movement in the stomach when he described his experiment on dividing the peritoneum of a living animal. Here he found

> all the intestines contracting peri-staltically on their contents while the stomach on the other hand is not displaying such a simple activity, for it is observed to be embracing the contents tightly, above, below, and on every side, and further it is seen to be motionless so that it would appear to be in intimate union with the food.[99]

The three groups of fibres in the wall of the stomach (which enable the stomach to mix up its contents) were known to anatomists in the sixteenth century. Bannister refers to them and attributes to them the virtues of attraction, retention, and expulsion. The straight fibres are said to have the attractive power, while the transverse fibres have the expulsive virtue. He is not clear regarding oblique fibres. In one place he rejects the idea of their being present, saying they would cause the stomach contents to be retained too long.[100] Elsewhere he refers to oblique fibres with their "needful vertue of retention."[101] The immobility of the stomach seems to have been accepted generally, but the part played by the actual movement of fibres and their virtues of attraction, retention, or expulsion in the action of the gut was a matter of controversy which is discussed at length by Helkiah Crooke in his *Microcosmographia,* a description of the body of man.[102]

Besides these three general rules, some other more detailed advice regarding groups of foodstuffs, is given:

Flesh and fish ought not to be eaten together at one meal, according to most sixteenth century books on diet. This division had not been adhered to so precisely in earlier centuries in either England or Europe. Examples of mixtures can be found in English Court records of the fourteenth century and are illustrated clearly in *Le Ménager de Paris* (c.1393).[103] The Elizabethan practice of having "meat" and "fish" days would seem to provide for a clear separation of the two kinds of foods.

Regarding fruits and herbs, those which "do mollifie and louse the belye" should be eaten before any other foods. Fruits which are binding should be taken at the end of a meal.[104] Langton underlines this by saying "for it is a preposterous ordar, to beginne with quynces or orynges and ende with sallades, made of herbes and oyle."[105] Fruit sweetmeats, especially those made with honey, should not be taken with other sorts of foods.[106]

Fat and lean meat should be eaten at the same time. Boorde explains: "The fatness of flesshe is not so moche nutrytyve as the leenes of flesshe; it is best whan leene and fat is myxte one with another."[107] Harrison records that the order of eating in England was at variance with accepted rules. Here "we commonlie begin with the most grosse food and end with the most delicate."[108] Others describe the order in which types of foods are commonly taken in England. Below, Cogan's list is compared with examples of the instructions for dishes suitable for various courses, as given in contemporary cookery books.[109]

Cogan's general sequence[110]

Potages or broths
boiled meats
roasted or baked meats
cheese or fruits

Meat days[111]	*Fish days*[112]
DINNER	
First Course	
Potage or stewed broth	Butter
Boiled or stewed meat	A salad with hard [cooked] eggs
Baked chickens	Pottage of eels and lamphreys
Salted beef	Red [smoked] herring freshly boiled
Pies	White [fresh] herring
Goose	Haberdine [large cod]
Pig	Salted salmon (minced)*
Roast beef	Salted tunges [conger eel]
Roast veel	Shad
Custard	Mackerel*

Whiting*
Plaice*
Thornback [skate] *
Fresh cod*
Dace [Leuciscus vulgaris]
Mullet
Eels upon soppes[113]
Roach upon soppes
Perch
Pike*
Trout upon soppes
Tench in jelly
Custard

Second Course

Roast lamb
Roast capons
Roast rabbit
Chickens
Pea hens
Baked venison tart

Flounders*
Fresh salmon
Fresh conger eel
Brette [brill or turbot]
Turbot
Halibut*
Bream upon soppes
Carp upon soppes
soles (or any other fish) fried
Roast eel*
Roast lamphreys
Roast porpoise
Fresh sturgeon*
Crevis [crayfish]
Crab
Shrimps*
Baked lamphreys
Tart
Figs
Apples
Blanched almonds
Cheese
Raisins
Pears

*Note. The appropriate sauces to go with the dishes are mentioned but are too complicated to be included in this outline. The most usual sauce was mustard with vinegar of "vergious" (i.e. verjuice, an acid juice from sour fruit). Others include herbs and spices. Two references are made to "liver and mustard" and refer to the liver of the fish, e.g., "Whiting. Sauce with the liver, and mustard." [114]

Besides lists of dishes suggested for different meals, books on instruction on the serving of foods advise on a long list of items which should be available at all seasons.[115] These include butter, cheese, a variety of fruits and herbs, as well as a number of spices and "sauces." The spices include such things as saffron, nutmeg and sugar.[116] Examples of "sauces" are mustard, salt and vinegar.[117]

Cogan was certainly not exaggerating when he said "we feed on divers sortes of meates [foods] at one meale."[118] England was well known for the plentiful variety of dishes served.[119] As indicated by the range of dishes mentioned, advice from cookery books is on a grand scale. Certainly noble households would be served with a great variety of dishes each meal and these would be increased when guests were present. The gentry and merchants would probably provide four to six dishes when guests were present, and have between one and three choices when alone.[120] A similar pattern was still found in England towards the end of the eighteenth century. Parson Woodforde, writing in 1783, describes a dinner at which he was a guest as being of two courses besides dessert, and says: "Each Course nine Dishes, but most of the things spoiled by being so frenchified in dressing."[121]

Regarding the order in which foods were served, the lists of foods per course (as exemplified by those given above) do, in general, follow the pattern described by Cogan, and the instruction for not mixing flesh and fish does seem to have been observed,[122] though (as already pointed out) in previous centuries fish and flesh dishes were served in the same meals.[123] How closely the three general rules of order were followed by the general population is impossible to estimate. This is partly because different habits were followed in different parts of the country: for example, milk (which, according to its characteristics, might be taken first) was said to be taken last in Lancashire.[124] Nor do records give a clear description what number of dishes (of the many likely to be available) an individual would actually eat. It is known that the most senior person present would be expected to taste every dish. After this tasting, it is likely that an individual would make the choice of a particular dish or dishes which then constituted the main part of the food eaten.[125] The selection would be based on an individual's preference and his ideas of his needs according to his constitution.

Harrison points out that a large supply of foods was required in noble households because, besides all the guests and members of the family who partook of these dishes, enough had still to be provided for the large number of servants, with some left over for the poor.[126] The fact that in England gross foods were eaten before the fine was a matter for discussion, the question being as to whether this was a good thing. The argument against this English order was a practical rather than a dietetic one. At present, it was said, people fill themselves up so much with the gross foods that even if they have the will to eat the delicate foods they no longer have the appetite. This was considered rather wasteful as the leftover fine foods will then go to the servants, whereas eaten the other way round the appetite will be good for the delicate foods and any leftover food will be of a grosser sort. However, this type of argument is overwhelmed by the weight of belief that the hot choleric stomachs of England needed to be fed gross meats first. While it is recognized that cold stomachs should start with the finer foods it is perfectly acceptable to the writers on diet that the English custom is right for Englishmen, and order must be adapted to the needs and desires of those eating. The conclusion, as put by Cogan, is "that almost a man may say: as divers men desire divers meates, so use they divers orders in eating."

PART II

CHAPTER X
INTRODUCTION TO FOODS

> The soil is fruitful and abounds with cattle, which inclines the inhabitants rather to feeding than ploughing.
>
> Paul Hentzer (1598)

CAMEL'S MILK AND pomegranates seem unlikely foods to find in England, yet both are referred to by sixteenth century writers on diet.[1] The reason, of course, is that some of the advice about foods was taken uncritically from earlier writers who had a Mediterranean background. Nevertheless the variety of foods available in England was large. Cogan, for all his occasional references to unusual items, gives over 200 chapter headings for different foods and Langham, in his *The Garden of Health*,[2] gives information about 693 simples.

Modern historians point out that this period was one of generally favourable economic conditions for farming and quote, as evidence, the comprehensive schemes for improvement in farming, formulated at this time.[3]

> Men were imbued with the conviction that everything could and should be employed and improved. With economy and ingenuity every living thing, where possible, was pressed into the service of man — wild fruits, wild animals, weeds wildflowers, insects all found a use in agriculture or as medicine to promote the health of men and stock.[4]

Both contemporary works and modern historical studies imply that the range of foods available to all classes in sixteenth century England was not limited to the comparatively small group of familiar foods which are in daily use now. The following brief indication of the food supplies available in the Elizabethan period is derived from recent studies in the history of agriculture and of London markets. The type of cereal grown varied in different parts of the country, depending on conditions there. The many varieties of common arable crops, both cereal

---

N.B. Footnotes to this chapter appear on pages 333-334.

and legume, show that attention was paid to the quality of different varieties and that people were on the lookout for new strains which would give better yields, be more resistant to disease, and be easier to harvest.[5]

Great attention was paid to stock development and much care and effort expended to overcome the problem of inadequate pasture land,[6] by such methods as reclamation of marshes, and by increasing yields of hay by "floating" meadows. This meant the flooding of land under carefully controlled conditions. The water protected the land from severe frosts and gave early grass crops, by which method a number of crops of hay would be provided in the year. Many areas formerly grazed by deer had been turned over to cattle in the last part of the sixteenth century.

The number of sheep in the country was increasing because of the growing importance of the wool industry. Pig-keeping was regarded as one of the peasant's stand-bys, though the demand for pork and bacon in the towns was met by the larger farmer, or the dairyman who had whey available to feed his pigs.

At the end of the century poultry keeping was an industry in Norfolk. Poulterers in London bought supplies from Bedfordshire and Northampton.[7] At least a few hens would be kept by most households for their own use.

Goats were kept in mountain areas such as Northumberland, and in Wales. Their value was for milk and their skins, though young goat was considered tender and acceptable as food.

Rabbits were not considered a pest, and could provide additional income for those who built warrens or were prepared to risk being caught poaching.

A number of the wide variety of fish and birds available are given by Emmison in his records of the Petre household.[8] Besides sea and river fish, another source of supply was from locally built fish or "stew" ponds.[9] Salted and cured fish was also used and some shellfish are mentioned. The names of birds recorded include what are now called game birds, as well as domesticated flying birds (e.g. doves) and what might be called wild-country birds (e.g. larks and rooks), and wild coastal or marshland birds.

Areas devoted to root crops were being extended. Carrots were grown quite extensively in East Anglia, and a principal occupation at Fulham, near London, was market gardening with carrots, parsnips, turnips and other vegetables grown in the common fields.[10]

Fruit growing had received royal encouragement. Richard Harris, gardener to Henry VIII, is said to have been the first to import grafts of French cherries, pears and apples.[11] In counties where fruit could be grown, orchards were developed and fruit growing became a profitable enterprise.

Besides the cultivated herb gardens, innumerable useful plants grew wild throughout the countryside.[12]

Wine was an important import,[13] but for the country folk and those who could not afford wine, beer, ale, cider and perry were local products.

Much advice is available on the care and preservation of foods to be stored so that they could be safely transported.

In addition to those produced at home, a number of imported foods were available. These can be divided into two groups: the "familiar," and the new foods from the New World. The familiar imports ranged from exotic spices and citrus fruits to more prosaic items such as cod and carrots. New foods, like potatoes, maize and oil seeds, were on their way (via Europe), but did not become established until later. Tobacco had arrived and was cultivated in England about 1571.

A large part of home produced food was consumed within the household of the grower whether on big estates or small farms, but towards the end of the sixteenth and early part of the seventeenth centuries, there was an insistent demand for food in all parts of the country, brought on by the rise in population and growth of towns and villages.

One of the most important factors in determining which foods an individual is actually able to have is the cost of the food in relation to wages. Accurate prices of foodstuffs are notoriously difficult to find, partly because prices fluctuated from place to place and time to time. In the last century, figures for prices and wages through the centuries were collected by J. E. Thorold Rogers.[14] A recent price index from the thirteenth to twentieth centuries indicates a marked fall in the relation of wage rates to consumables during the sixteenth century, the lowest ratio being that of 1597. Information available now is in the archives of noble households and the records of some merchant families.[15] The most detailed data are in the Ordinances of the Royal Households, but these prices give a distorted reflection of general prices because of the system of purveyance used. Purveyors most usually paid less than the market price. The experience of a poor Hertfordshire woman is said to be typical: taking six chickens to market, "she had intended to ask 5d. or 6d. apiece for them but the purveyors forced her to part with them for a penny each."[16]

The examples of prices given in the following chapters are taken from various accounts where the year is specified. Otherwise only an indication of the probable sort of price is given.

Reference has already been made to the foods provided for noble-men, merchants, students, farmers and farm workers, house servants, and the inmates of a house of correction. The range and contrast between the richest banquets and the poor of Suffolk is naturally very great, and though many records are available of the richer households, no clear picture emerges of the dietary condition of the poorer groups of the population. A number of efforts have been made to calculate the nutritional value, in modern terms, of diets based on information from old records. The results have been inconclusive because of the number of assumptions that have to be made.[17] The poor groups most acutely felt the effects of the comparatively frequent shortages, but the country as a whole was rich in produce and it is likely that, except in times of dearth or local crises, all except the incapable poor fared reasonably well.

CHAPTER XI
BREAD AND CEREALS

Fiat panim
Motto of the United Nations'
Food and Agriculture Organization

THE IMPORTANCE, through the centuries, of bread and cereals in English life is illustrated by the following three references to the statute books. The earliest authoritative *Assize (or Assay) of Bread* was passed in the statutes of the realm assigned to 1267,[1] though this form of control of the sale of bread is believed to have dated from Anglo-Saxon times.[2] The Assize remained in amended forms until it was abolished in 1815. Secondly, the Corn Laws and their repeal in 1856 were of immense political significance.[3] It is notable that in modern times, following the Second World War, the British government's control of bread was not lifted for eleven years (until 1956).

The object of the *Assize of Bread* was to lay down the weight of various sorts of loaves (for sale) in relation to the changing prices of a quarter of wheat.[4] Sir William Ashley has shown that the rules of Assize originally referred to breads made from any grains,[5] but that by the sixteenth century wheat was used as the standard.[6] Moreover, Gras[7] suggests that the proportion of wheat used in England had always been large enough to warrant it being used as a basis for historical comparisons of prices. Sixteenth century writers stress the benefits of wheaten bread but do also refer to breads of other grains made in different parts of the country.[8]

The *Assize of Bread* was intended to give the baker a proper return for his labours and to enable the consumer to "be secured from fraud and imposition."[9]

Below are given two examples of the regulations from the *Assize of Bread*, [1580] and 1600,[10] as published in pamphlet form by J. Powell.

N.B. Footnotes to this chapter appear on pages 334-337.

1580   *1600*

Types of loaves
  a farthing wastell
  a farthing symnell
  a farthing whyte lofe
  a half-penny whyte lofe
  a half-penny wheaten lofe
  a penny wheaten lofe
  a half-penny household lofe

    a half-penny white lofe drawn
from the fine cocket [11]
    a penny etc. etc.
    a half-penny white lofe drawn
from the corse cocket
    a penny etc. etc.
    a half-penny wheaten lofe
drawn from the corse cocket
    a penny etc. etc.
    a penny householde lofe
drawn from the corse cocket

Weights
are given per quarter of wheat, giving forty different prices from 12d. to 20s. 6d. An extra 2s. per quarter must be allowed to the baker for baking.

Weights
per quarter of wheat giving one hundred and twenty different prices from 12d. to 60s. 6d. Powell suggests that the allowance for baking should be raised to 6s. per quarter. [12]

"Wastell" and "symnell" breads were both made from a fine flour but the latter was originally a boiled bread.

    Basically, the three types of bread covered by these regulations are white, wheaten, and household.[13] Unfortunately, the various terms used by writers in the sixteenth century to describe different types of bread, vary considerably and are frequently impossible to identify exactly. An attempt to correlate some of the terms used then is given below. Confusion is not restricted to the sixteenth century.[14] A study of modern authorities on the subject has not completely clarified the position, and this classification is recognized as being very rough. It needs to be remembered that in the sixteenth century, milling would be by stone grinding,[15] which at best could give the following separation:

Flour	79% [16]
Middlings	11%
Bran	10%

Modern fine white flour (or 72% extraction rate [17] or less) is only obtained through sophisticated techniques using steel rollers. In the sixteenth century the ground meal would be bolted [18] (more than once) through fine cloth (usually linen) or through a "temse" or sieve. [19]

Breads were prepared from the individual parts, or mixture of parts, of whole-wheat meal. Besides wheaten bread, loaves were made from other cereals, including rye, barley, oats, peas and beans, and mixtures of these grains.

The rough groupings of types of bread given below are based on Harrison's[20] description of the breads used in England, together with examples from the *Assize of Bread*,[21] Andrew Boorde's description,[22] and the account of breads used in the Petre household.[23] The grouping goes from A to D, where A is of the finest quality, and D of the coarsest.

	A	B	C	D
Harrison	manchet	cheat or wheaten	revelled (cheat)	brown (2 sorts) miscelin
Assize of Bread	wastell symnel white loaf	wheaten	household	
Boorde	manchet			mestlyng
Petre household 1548	manchet		ravel	tems
" " 1552	manchet		yeomans	carters

Group A. Manchet is the term used in Tudor times for small fine white loaves. These had previously been called "pandemayn" (with a variety of spellings) in Plantagenet times.[24] In the Petre household two manchets were equal to one loaf. The size of a manchet can be estimated from the instructions given in *The Booke of Carving and Sewing*,[25] for laying the table at mealtimes:

> lay the one side of the Towell uppon the left arm . . . and lay on thine arme seven loves of breade with three or fower trencher loves with the end of the towell in the left hande.

Trencher loaves were made from whole-meal flour and used with the upper crusts "chipped" off as plates. By Tudor times bread trenchers were being replaced by wooden ones.

Group B. Cheat or wheaten bread was made from flour with the coarser bran removed. More than one quality of cheat is referred to. Harrison describes it as yellow or gray in colour. The part removed was called the "gurgeons" or "pollard."[27]

Group C. Ravelled, household or yeoman's bread retained more of the whole grain with only the coarsest bran removed. (This description could sometimes also be applied to breads in Group B.) Residues from the manchet flour were sometimes added to the coarser flour before baking.

Group D. Brown bread was made of a variety of ingredients. Harrison describes two sorts. One is whole wheat flour "as it cometh from the mill, so that neither the bran nor the flour are any whit diminished." The other sort of "brown" has "little or no flour left therein." This is very dry and brittle and is often made up with rye flour to form "miscelin." This mixture of flours is spelt in a large number of ways. Boorde says "mestlyng" can be half wheat and half rye or half rye and half barley, and some "evil" people put wheat and barley together.[28] This mixture was usually made by the mixing of meals after milling, but in some parts of the country two grains (wheat and rye) were actually grown together. This was not easy to do, as the grains grow and ripen at different rates. Nevertheless, it was a practice followed by some farmers for centuries. Dr. Edward Smith, writing in the mid-nineteenth century,[29] advises against growing two grains together and refers to the mixed product (two to three parts wheat: one part rye) grown in Yorkshire at that time.

Other mixtures could include meals from oats, peas or beans. The coarse bread from peas and beans was intended for feeding horses. In times of famine the poor have to eat what is usually given to the horses, hence the proverb already referred to: "Hunger setteth his foot first into the horse manger."[30]

In London the "dark" breads could only be made by members of the Brown Bakers Company.[31] These restrictions applied only in London or big cities. The division of the bakers into "white" or "brown" was intended to "safeguard the diet of the poor and to ensure that the brown bread they ate contained the whole wheat grain. In 1645 the two groups, in London, joined to form one bakers' guild. This underlines the effects of rising standards of living in London and southern England generally, with the trend going away from dark wheaten and rye bread towards a paler wheaten bread.

Generally speaking, in sixteenth century England bread was made of "such grain as the soil yieldeth."[32] The nobility and gentry commonly ate wheaten bread made from the finest or a good quality flour. The relationship between social position and the type of bread eaten followed the general rule that the higher the position the greater the choice of fine-flour breads.[33] Those lower on the social scale would eat darker bread, and Harrison describes how, in some parts of the country, sometimes even in the households of the gentry, they were forced to eat rye or barley bread. While the poor in times of dearth ate pea, bean, oaten bread, or even bread from acorns.[34]

Not all those who ate bread made from grains other than wheat did so because of shortages. Jones gives this incomplete summary of areas where different breads were used. Bread from "clean wheat" was used in Kent, Somerset, Lincolnshire, and Nottinghamshire; in parts of Leicestershire and Nottinghamshire beans and peas were used; rye in Urchenfield and Staffordshire; miscelin in Worcestershire and Shropshire; oaten bread was found in Lancashire, Cumberland, Westmoreland, and Cornwall, while some use lentils, vetches, and buckwheat for their bread.[35] This information includes only the names of breads most commonly used and omits altogether any reference to the local terms used in various parts of the country.

Dietary Value of Breads and Cereals

The advice of sixteenth century authors on the dietary value of breads often appears confused. This is because advice from the ancients (which is not always consistent) is frequently mixed up with contemporary views which may often differ in some respects.

In general the points to be considered in assessing the dietary value of bread are:

(i) *Type of grain used.* The grains selected for discussion below, include only those generally referred to by writers on diet or husbandry. Following sixteenth century practice, beans and peas are included here.[36]

(ii) *Fineness of flour or quantity of bran.*

(iii) *Degree of leavening.*

(iv) *Degree of salting.*

(v) *Method of baking.*

(vi) *Degree of staleness.*

(i) *Type of grain.*

Wheat. By general consent, the best bread is made from fine wheat flour.[37] The wheat should have been grown on "wholesome" soil and the flour should be clean. Unfortunately Buttes, who itemizes the characteristics of his "dry" foods, giving the qualities and degrees of each, does not include wheat or bread. Neither does Cogan give the qualities and degrees of wheaten bread taken as food; but he says, obviously referring to a type of bread poultice: "Wheate in nature is manifestly hotte, and being laide to outwardly in a medicine, is hotte in the first degree without any manifest moysture,"[38] while Gerard, in his *Herball* describes wheat as "according to their natural qualities."[39] Boorde refers to Avicenna as saying that wheaten bread makes a man fat. He adds that fine wheaten bread (without leaven) is slow of digestion and nourishes well, and manchet breat is good for all ages. [40]

The types of wheat mentioned by sixteenth century writers on diet or husbandry include: white, red, yellow, gray, and hard wheats. Also listed are a few certain "straunge grayne," not much used in England, two of which are:

(1) Turkey or Purkey wheat, i.e. maize. The name "turkey wheat" for maize was derived from the belief (held for a short time) that the plant had originated in Asia.[41] This was considered to be less nourishing than wheat, rye, barley, or oats. Gerard points out that the "barbarous Indians which know no better, . . . thinke it a good food."

(2) French or Bucke or Branke wheat, i.e. buckwheat. This was used mixed together with barley meal in parts of Lancashire and Cheshire to make household bread during the winter.[42]

Naturally, a number of dishes were made with wheat. The main dish is "frumenty," which is made with hulled wheat boiled in milk and seasoned with cinnamon or sugar or some appropriate spice.[43] It was considered to be a wholesome and nourishing food rather like boiled wheat, which is described as heavy and difficult to digest, but strengthening when digested.

Bread crumbs were frequently used in dishes such as "good white puddings" (this included liver and lights), "spinage fritters," "puddings from grated bread," and in a number of sauces.[44] Flour seems to have been used less than bread crumbs but was necessary for items like pancakes and shortcakes and some types of fritters. Cogan explains that dishes made from flour and "simnels," "Cracknels," "Bunnes" and "Wafers" should (according to Galen) be rejected, because wheat meal is only easily digested if it has been leavened, salted, thoroughly kneaded, and baked.[45] However, experience in England had shown that unleavened manchets were satisfactory, so this remained a point for controversy.

Rye. Cogan says "secale commonly called Rye, a Grayne much used in Breade, almoste throughout this Realme."[46] The proportions cultivated in England at different periods are discussed by Ashley[47] and by Gras.[48] Rye bread is not as wholesome as wheaten bread. It is heavier and harder to digest and is considered "windy and hurtful to manie." Exceptions are labourers, those who work hard and those with a strong stomach. These people find rye bread beneficial.[49] As a medicine, rye is hotter than wheat.[50] Used externally it is considered to be hot and dry in the second degree and is said to be "meane between Wheate and Barlie."[51] Rye flour was specifically indicated in some recipes, e.g., for "blewe manger." This includes rye flour, flesh from a capon, milk, cream, sugar, and rose water.[52]

Barley. Here again reference is made to Cogan, as his information on foods is more comprehensive than that of other writers.[53] Barley does not nourish as much as wheat; it troubles the stomach, makes cold and tough juice, though "some affirme that it is good for such as have the gowte." Barley itself is cold and dry in the first degree, but when made into bread is of a "cooling nature," makes thin juice, and is "somewhat cleansing." In general it is thought better to "drink" barley in the form of ale or beer than to eat it as bread. However, the comment is added that though "barlie be colde, yet it maketh such hotte drinke, that it setteth men oftimes in a furie." It is of note that both the Hippocratic *Regimen II,*[54] and Gerard advocate the benefits of barley water[55] as opposed to malted barley drinks) with and without additional ingredients. The administration of barley water and barley gruel should be done with great care, according to Hippocratic teachings.

Oats. It was of course well known that oats were widely used in Scotland. But in England in general oats were more commonly thought of as food for animals. Hence the later and much quoted definition from Dr. Johnson's *Dictionary,* "*Oats,* a grain, which in England is generally given to horses, but in Scotland supports the people." Cogan, like Jones, points out that in a number of northern counties of England and in Cornwall, oats, besides being used in the form of malt for ale (as elsewhere), are also used as oat bread or groats for man.[56] In Cogan's experience oats are somewhat similar to barley, being fairly cold and binding. Because of this last characteristic he found them helpful in cases of the laske (diarrhoea). Gerard describes oats as "dry and somewhat cold of temperature as Galen saith."[57]

Bread is made from oats both in thin and thick cakes and in "broade loaves, whiche they call Janockes." Oaten bread is light of digestion but "somewhat windie." It becomes stale quickly and is not considered very appetising by those who are not used to it. "Greates or grotes" are made by drying the grain lightly and shelling it. From groats a pottage is made, named according to the fluid used, e.g. water pottage, whey pottage, or ale pottage. These dishes are very wholesome, temperate, and easy to digest. If you want to taste such a pottage Cogan's advice is to ask a Lancashire woman.[58]

Besides being used in pottages, "oatmeal grotes" were used in other dishes, such as puddings. For example, "Ising pudding" contained: groats soaked in cream for four hours, eggs, beef suet, salt, saffron, cloves, and mace.[59] (According to the *OED* the meaning of "ising" is obscure, but is related to stuffed forcemeat and sausages.)

Beans and peas. Gerard classes these items under pulses[60] and includes beans, peas, and tares (vetches) in the classification. He subdivides the group to include both wild and "tame" (garden) varieties. Some examples under "beans" are the great garden bean, the kidney bean, and lupins. As for peas, Gerard comments that wild peas grow in divers places, especially about the fields belonging to Bishop's Hatfielde, in Hertfordshire. He also describes a number of varieties of chick peas and refers to such things as lentils, vetches, "the oylie pulse called Sesamum"[61] and the "Pease Earth nut" *[Lathyrus montanus]*.[62] The number of pulses (both wild and garden) available is large, but sixteenth century writers on diet usually refer rather generally to beans and peas without providing the details of varieties found in herbals. Some general subdivisions are given, such as those of "green" and "dry" beans, and the grouping of peas in "garden," "grey," and "green" peas, the last two being field peas. Cogan dismisses such things as vetches and tares as being only food for animals.[63]

The striking fact about beans and peas is that they are universally recognized (then as now) as being "windy."[64] Beans produce more "ventosyte" than peas and both are more windy if taken unshucked. Pythagoras is said to have advised against beans.[65] Hippocratic teaching had said "beans afford an astrigent and flatulent nourishment."[66] The Ancients pointed out that no matter how beans were prepared, or how long cooked,[67] they remained windy and hard to digest.

Sixteenth century advice classed beans as cold in the first degree and dry in the second.[68] Though before green beans were ripe they were considered cold and moist, and when dried they had the power to "binde and restraine." Their benefits are that they "Cause sleepe, restraine Migrain, fat the bodie." Unfortunately, besides causing wind they dull the senses and cause terrible dreams. They are best eaten in cold weather by "gross and homely" feeders. Beans were considered more suitable for those with strong stomachs and for those people accustomed to eating them.[69] Both green and dry beans can be eaten boiled. Green beans are eaten with butter, the dry are eaten with salt unbuttered. Care must be taken not to eat unripe green beans, as these will give "very moyste nourishment to the bodie" and produce much excrement all over the body, not just in the bowel.[70]

Peas were considered cold in the first degree, and temperately moist.[71] They are pleasant to the taste (the taste of a food was considered to make a greater contribution to its value than is accepted today). Peas "mundifie the brest," cure coughs, and give singularly good nourishment. Compared with beans, they are not so windy nor so cleansing, i.e. they pass more slowly along the alimentary tract. They are said by some to "hurt evil teeth." Again, peas are better eaten when the husks are removed. The proper method of preparation is considered: Buttes advises "Dresse them [peas] well with salt, oile, pepper and the juice of sower hearbes."[72] Cogan refers to peas pottage, saying that for the best pottage, peas should be sieved after boiling.[73]

It is clear that on the whole pulses were considered mainly a food for animals, and the use of beans and peas was not very common in the diet of the well-to-do who could anyhow afford a good variety of foods. Cogan points out that "pease pottage" was, in England, most commonly eaten in Lent and on other fasting days, when "gross and oppilative" foods were taken. He notes with what seems like surprise that people in Leicestershire use bread from beans for feeding their families[74] and again explains this behaviour by the fact that their stomachs are stronger. The poor in rural England undoubtedly ate (and digested) many of the wild and cultivated pulses which have been mentioned. These, it can be assumed, would be an important protein supplement to a diet in which the amount of meat, milk and cheese would be extremely variable.

Rice. Descriptions of the value of rice appear in most books which describe the value of foods. Gerard says that he grew (or rather, unsuccessfully attempted to grow) rice in his garden in 1596; rice, he explains, is "brought unto us [in England] purged and prepared" from Spain and other places.[75]

According to Rhazes and Avicenna (says Buttes)[76] rice is hot in the first degree and dry in the second. Bullein says there are many opinions about the virtues of rice, but he too accepts the views of Avicenna.[77] Rice stops and binds the belly and nourishes well if it is boiled in milk (Bullein notes that rice should be steeped in water overnight before cooking). Besides being boiled in milk, rice pottage should be flavoured with such things as almonds, sugar, cinnamon, rosewater, and if intended primarily to stop the flux oak bark should be added. As rice was imported it could only be eaten by those who could afford it, but it was obviously well liked, for "many other good kinds of foode [besides pottage] is made with this graine [rice], as those that are skilful in cookerie can tell."[78]

(ii) *Fineness of flour or quantity of bran used.* As indicated above, the best bread is made from "fine wheate flower cleane boulted from all branne and other baggage."[79] Bread from the "coarsest wheat," with a large proportion of bran, passes through the stomach quickly and fills the belly with excrements. Flours of higher extraction rate were only suitable for those who were physically active – that is, for members of the lower social orders (such as carters and "rustics") who had strong stomachs. It was recognized that brown bread and butter could act as a laxative for those who were constipated and who normally ate fine bread.[80] Bread containing bran could be used to make one "leaner," because the bran nourishes only a little and loosens the belly. From the advice given it becomes clear that the outside parts of any grains were considered less valuable (or even harmful) compared with the material obtained from the parts closer to the centre of the grain.

(iii) *Degree of leavening of the loaf.* The advice regarding the leavening of bread is confusing for two reasons. Firstly, what was actually done in England conflicted with the advice of the ancients (which in itself was not always consistent), and secondly, this led to apparent contradictions in the advice given by the English writers.

Galen advocated leavened bread;[81] Celsus had previously accepted unleavened;[82] Boorde (1542) explained that bread made from fine flour without leaven is slowly digested but is nourishing, providing the loaf is well made. He reminds his readers that, according to the ancients, when bread is leavened it is more quickly digested. However, English stomachs find leaven "hevy and ponderous" and are better suited by unleavened bread.[83] Cogan (1589) quotes Galen as saying that bread "must be wel leavened, *for breade without leaven is good for no man,*" and adds (speaking for himself), "Howbeit in England our finest manchet is made without leaven."[84]

In general, this was the form in which writers in the sixteenth century presented this information – i.e., by quoting Galen as advocating leavened bread, and then observing that leaven does not suit English stomachs and that the finest bread used in England is unleavened. In contrast to this, recipes for manchet bread[85] and for "leavened bread" describe how to use yeast for breadmaking. Furthermore, in describing the best and proper loaf one of the factors included is that it should be "lightly leavened," with the additional advice that "the lighter the bread is, and the more full of holes, it is the wholesomer."[86]

The dilemma of the sixteenth century authorities, in trying to reconcile English practice (which was related to the best quality bread) with the weight of Galen's advice, can be appreciated. In practice it was probably the size of loaf and type of flour used which influenced the baker to add or omit yeast. Manchets were small loaves made from fine flour and even without leaven should never turn out like hard little stones, while the larger loaves made of coarser flour are difficult to keep light without a leavening agent.

(iv) *Degree of salting of bread.* Following an ancient tradition, the necessity of adding salt to bread was generally recognized. "Moderately salted" is the term most commonly used. The manchet recipe "after my Ladie Graies way" describes the amount of salt required. It is "as much white salt as will [go] into an Egshell" for two pecks of flour.[87] Bread "oversweete" (i.e. under-salted) is a "stopper" and over-salted a "dryer," according to the *Regimen Sanitatis Salerni.*[88] No mention has been found of the improvement in the *taste* of a bread which is correctly salted.

(v) *Method of baking.*[89] It will be appreciated that the method of baking a loaf will affect the moistness or dryness and the type of crust a finished loaf will have. These characteristics were a matter of concern when advising on diet. The most influential factors in the baking were the heat of the oven and the size of the loaf.

The type of oven illustrated in both versions of the *Assize of Bread,* referred to above, is a peel oven — that is, one that is heated either by coals inside (which are then removed), or less usually from the outside, and then the loaves being placed within, using a peel or bakehouse bat. This method should give a good all-round heat. It is pointed out that breads not baked in ovens, "but upon yrons or hotte stones, or upon the earth, or under hotte ashes, are unwholesome because they are not equally baked, but burned without and rawe within."[90] The heat of the oven was important and it was obviously part of the bakers' craft to be able to estimate it correctly. The advice given is that the oven should be of medium heat, "not extremely hot ... nor less than meane hote."[91]

The size of the loaf mattered, in that large loaves were more difficult to cook through properly, but they were considered to be the most nourishing if properly cooked, because "the fire hath not consumed the moysture of them." But, Cogan concludes:

But whether Breade be made in forme of Manchet, as is used of the gentilitie, or in great Loaves, as it is used among the Yeomanrie, or betweene both, as with the frankelinges, it maketh no matter, so it bee well baked.[92]

Readers are warned that burnt bread and hard crusts "aduste," and engender choler and cause melancholy humours. For this reason it is commonly advised that the upper crusts should be removed from the loaf before it is served. Bullein comments: "Therefore in great mens houses the bread is chipped and largelye pared," and he infers that these crusts, which would help to feed a great number of poor people, are fed to the dogs. Bullein adds dryly that "many be more affectionate to dogges than men."[93]

(vi) *Degree of staleness required in bread*. There is very wide general agreement about how old bread should be before it is eaten and also at what age it should not be eaten. Tradition differentiates between new bread for the sovereign, one-day bread for others, three-day bread for the "house," and four-day bread for trenchers.[94]

Hot bread should never be eaten; it is bad for everyone. It lies in the stomach "lyke a sponge," hastening the production of unconcocted humours because of its vapourous moisture. However, the smell of hot bread is not harmful but is comforting to the head and heart.

Bread should not be eaten when it is less than twenty-four hours old, nor after more than four to five days old. Too new bread causes "drinesse, thirst and smoking into the head, troubling the braines and eies through the heat thereof."[95] Old bread dries the body and causes damage to the memory and engenders melancholy humours.[96]

The best bread is that which is well cooked and one day old. It must not be mouldy or musty.

Bread and cereals played an important part in the diet of English people in the sixteenth century, and the ideas about their value in the diet were inherited from the traditional views of the ancients with some slight adaptation to conditions in England. The general description of a good loaf is one made from good quality wheat, with little bran, lightly leavened, moderately salted, well moulded, and baked at a suitable oven temperature. This is to be eaten when one day old, with any hard crusts removed.

Bread of good quality was considered a suitable food for most people most of the time, but it was not advocated in quantity during sickness because it could only be digested slowly.[97]

A small point of interest is Boorde's reference to "rascally bakers."[98] Distrust of millers and bakers is a long standing one. With millers it is understandable, for a client never seems to get back all the grain he gave to be milled and yet he has to pay for the service. With bakers the position is slightly different. In the sixteenth century, bread could have been obtained either by baking it at home, by giving the baker the materials to bake, or by buying the finished loaves. It is in the bought loaves that adulteration could readily be practiced. It was there in later centuries, when the sale of bread became more widespread, that its adulteration became a matter of serious public concern.

CHAPTER XII
WATER, WINE AND OTHER DRINKS

Ale for an Englysshe man is a natural drynke.

A. Boorde (1542)

THE SEVEN COMMON drinks listed by sixteenth century authors are: wine, ale, beer, cider, whey,* metheglyn or mead. Water was not considered to be a drink. Boorde states quite dogmatically that "water is not holesome sole by it selfe, for an Englysshe man."[1] Despite this antipathy, water was obviously included in many drinks and was necessary for cooking. Its importance for the life of all living things was full recognized, being

sary for cooking. Its importance for the life of all living things was fully recognized, being

> the cheepest of all liquors not onely because it is one of the four Elementes, but also for that it was the verie naturall and first drinke appoynted by God to all manner of creatures.[2]

Classing various sorts of water in order of merit, the best was considered to be clean, pure, rainwater; next, the water that runs through rocky places (preferably from the east). Running water from "pure ground" is better than either river, pond, flood, or sea water. Ice and water from snow are dangerous for man and beast,[3] but of all the ordinary waters available, the worst is standing water.

Characteristics of a good water include the speed with which it can be heated (or will cool down); also, the lighter the better. Cogan notes that "a pinte of that [good] water is lighter than a pinte of standing water of wells or pooles."

Good water should have no "froth" on it when boiled. It can be tested by dipping a linen cloth into the water and then drying the cloth; there should be no sediment left when this is done. A way suggested by Vaughan to "revive" water which has begun to "putrifie" is to add a

---

*Whey is considered in Chapter XIV.

N.B. Footnotes to this chapter appear on pages 337-339.

little oil of sulphur or aqua vitae.[4] Boiled water should be used for the dilution or preparation of other drinks, and running water is advocated for all cookery. Water may be drunk more safely "and without hurt of the inner parts" if barley is boiled in it until the grains break.[5] This might be thought to give an indication as to the length of time water must be boiled to make it safe, but the advice is followed directly by suggestions that boiling prunes, sugar or liquorice in the water will make it harmless without any clue to the time required.

Water in itself is not nourishing;[6] it is "colde slowe and slacke of digestion."[7] Nevertheless, those who are accustomed to drinking "rawe" water from childhood are not harmed by it. Cogan gives proof of this:

> As in Cornewal although that the countrie be in a very cold quarter, yet many of the poorer sort, which never or very seldome drink another drink than pure water, be notwithstanding strong of bodie and live and like wel until they be of great age.[8]

Drinking water with food cools the stomach too much and prevents proper digestion. The same effect results from drinking water after meals except in cases where too much food or wine has been taken. A good drink of cold water after drinking too much wine may give a good night's sleep; it will also "clense the stomacke, and represse the vapours and fumes, and dispose it to retaine new sustenance."

Great care should be taken when thirsty, for "though small drinke or [of] colde water seeme to quench thirst better than wine," the water can cause too great an alteration by suddenly changing the body heat to cold, and this may be dangerous. Wine diluted by water is advised.

Wine

Contemporary writings suggest that little wine was drunk in comparison to ale, beer and cider. Coke, rather boastfully praising England to a Frenchman, says:

> Item for your wyne, we have good-ale here [in England] metheghelen, sydre and pirry, beyng more holesome beverages for us then your wynes, which maketh your people dronken, also prone and apte to all fylthy pleasures and lustes.[9]

Nevertheless, about twenty years later (1568), William Turner, in the preface to his *A new Boke of the natures and properties of all wines. . .*, says he is writing the book because he sees there was "so much use of wine in all countries of England."[10] Though country folk and the poor were still satisfied with ale, those who had money were fast developing a taste for sweet wines. In the reign of Edward VI "An Acte to avoyde Excesse of Wynes" attempted (rather ineffectually) to limit and control the sale of wines.[11] Henderson says "The English, however, were now too much accustomed to wine to be restrained by such enactments from indulging in their taste for that luxury."[12] In the early part of the sixteenth century the Earl of Northumberland's household (which was regulated with the utmost economy) allowed forty-two hogsheads of wine per year.[13]

Sixteenth century books giving dietary advice usually devoted comparatively long chapters to wines. This is likely due to the much greater amount of information available from ancient texts about wine, rather than to a comparatively greater importance in the English dietary. It is suggested that viniculture had made some progress in England by the beginning of the eighth century.[14] But the climate and soil are not really favourable here and by the sixteenth century Tusser commented:

> For as much as the nature, temperature and clymate, of our soyle is not so truely proper and agreeing with the Vine as that of France . . . thus we have it more for delight, pleasure and prospect, than for any peculyar profit.[15]

Of the wines imported into England, Boorde lists Gascony, French and Raynysshe (Rhenish) wines.[16] He describes the characteristics of good wines as follows:

> All manner of wynes be made of grapes, excepte respyse [raspberry wine], the which is made of a bery. Chose your wyne after this sorte: it muste be fyne, fayre, and clere to the eye; it must be fragraunt and redolent, havynge a good odour and flavour in the nose; it must spryncle [sparkle] in the cup whan it is drawne. . .; it must be cold and pleasaunt in the mouth; and it must be strong and subtyll of substaunce.[17]

Writers acknowledge the importance of wine in the regimen. Cogan compares the vine with life and says:

> so that the vine may seeme as it were life: because it greatelie preserveth life. An no marvaile, considering that life, as *Aristotle* affirmeth, standeth chiefly in *heate and moysture.* Which two qualities are the very nature of wine.[18]

Here it is implied that wine has the predominant qualities of hot and moist, which is the more generally accepted view. However,

Hippocrates had said that wine was hot, dry and purgative,[19] and Cogan, when discussing Galen's view that wine was hot in the second degree, and adds that "it is drie according to the proportion of heate."[20] Galen's statement about wine being hot in the second degree is widely discussed and criticised by sixteenth century authorities. In fact, Galen's much quoted statement seems to have been lifted out of context because in *De simplicium medicamentorum temperamentis ac facultatibus* he expounds at length on the characteristics of wines of different ages, colours, sweetness or sourness and country of origin and, like his critics of the sixteenth century, he acknowledges that the degree of heat in a wine will vary but in general will increase with age.

Great emphasis had always been put on the medicinal virtues of wines. The Hippocratic teaching on the subject is to be found in *Regimen in acute disease* and *Regimen II*, and Galen provides more information about wines in his *De simplicium* than in *De Alimentorum facultatibus*. William Turner's book, the most authoritative of its time, takes a predominantly medical viewpoint throughout because one of his objects in writing the book was to show that Rhine wines are not responsible for the formation of kidney and bladder stones.[21]

Turner's classification of wines follows earlier authorities.[22] He divides them by country, colour, age, taste, and smell, referring to some twenty wines by name. Those most commonly used in England were: Sack, Malmsey, Muscadel, Claret, French, Gascony, and Rhenish. Because of the varieties of wines and the number of factors to be considered, the advice sometimes seems somewhat confused. However, three points are clear. All wines must be avoided by those who are hot and moist in themselves — e.g., children and those of an excessively sanguine complexion; young men up to the age of twenty-two years should take only a little wine; lastly, wine is most valuable to the old who are cold and dry.

Country and Colour. While it is agreed by writers that, other things being equal, yellow and red wines were hotter than white wines, most emphasise that a direct comparison can only be made between wines of the same country. Cogan says "the Red wines of Fraunce are not so hoat nor so strong as the white wines of some other Countreys."[23] When describing dietary values, authors sometimes give information as to the country of origin of named wines, but on the whole they refer to the colour rather than the name. Colour was classified as white, claret, and red, these terms having a slightly different meaning from the mod-

ern interpretation. White referred to the same type of wine as would be
called white today. Claret then meant a yellowish or light red coloured
wine.[24] Red wines referred to deep red or "black" wines.

Age. Turner describes two sorts of new wine: one that is called Must*
and the other which is wine proper, but newly made. Galen had said
new wine was up to five years old. Others decided age by taste, calling
it new while the sweetness lasted, — that is, until the sharpness came.
There was a divergence of opinion on this matter; in France some of the
most notable wines were termed old before they were fully one year
old. This variation is understandable in view of the fact that the time of
maturation of a wine depends a great deal on the type of grapes used.
New wine, by whatever criterion it was measured, was hot in the first
degree; wine of "middle age" — that is, between five and ten years old
— was hot in the second degree; old wine (more than ten years) was hot
in the third degree.

Taste. Turner is much concerned over an exact translation for Greek
or Latin terms regarding the taste of wines. The English words used are,
he says, crude compared with the finer differentiations of the older
languages. Basing his ideas on the works of ancient authors, Turner concludes (not very precisely) that:
Sweet tasting wines are hot and gross. They cause wind and trouble
the stomach, they are "suitable" for the kidneys and bladder, and they
are less apt to cause drunkenness.
Sour-binding wines (no elemental quality is mentioned) can hurt the
head, but they will not do so if "waterish." They strengthen the stomach but are not good for those in a swoon.
Rough and binding wines are cold and dry. They stop vomiting and
"flowings" of the belly and have a cooling and drying effect.
Cogan follows the *Regimen Sanitatis* and classifies the tastes of wines
as sweet, sour, rough, and lyth. He also refers to the need for wine to
have a fragrant smell, and he describes the substance of wine as thick,
thin, clear, or muddy.[25]
Despite the various natural classifications of wines and the different
approaches in presentation, the following ideas emerge clearly. All
stress the value of wine taken in moderation and support their views by

*"Must" is the juice of the grape either unfermented or before fermen-
tation is complete *(OED)*.

Biblical quotations. An excess of wine is said to be useful on occasions, but drunkenness is generally deplored. Wine must always be drunk moderately "and bycause wyne is full of fumosyte, it is good, therefore to alaye it with water."[26] Also, because of the contemporary aversion to water, wine was often recommended as the vehicle for herbs and medicines. A comparison between Boorde's *Breviary of Helth* (1552) and the recipes in various works by John Jones in the period 1572-79 suggests that the number of times wine was chosen as a vehicle seems to increase toward the end of the century.

Effects of wine

Beneficial

A quickening of man's wits and quickening of the heart;

"It easily conveyeth thy meate that it is mingled with, to all the members of the bodie."

It rejoices all the powers of man and nourishes them.

It engenders good blood. It purges the watery part from the blood because of its diuretic action.

It helps digestion and resolves phlegm.

It expels melancholy.

Because wines are high and hot in operation they comfort old men and women.

Harmful

Troubling the belly and causing wind. Wine is however recommended in cases of long continued wind and the hiccups.

It is unsuitable for children and nurses and should be taken sparingly up to the age of 22 years.

It is bad for those with a hot complexion, or with a great rheum or gout or any signs of the palsy.

Strong wines inflame the liver and breed choler.

On the whole, wine is beneficial. The best wine is a clear white or yellow one, not too old or too new, though some say thick red wines are the most nourishing. It is agreed that all sweet and gross wines make men fat.[27]

Ale and Beer

Beer is now the generic term for malt liquors including ale and porter. In the sixteenth century, theoretically, ale was made with malt and water, and beer had added hops. Despite the familiar rhyme

> Turkeys, Heresies, Hops and Beer,
> All came to England in one year.

which is said by some to refer to the year 1520,[28] Bickerdyke puts the
introduction of hops into England at a little before the middle of the
fifteenth century.[29] The growing of hops received an impetus from a
number of Flemish immigrants who settled in Kent in 1524 and cultivated hop gardens. From this the county became famous for its hops.
It is evident that the use of beer had spread quite widely by the time
Boorde was writing, for he says "And nowe of late dayes it [beer] is
moche used in England. . . ."[30]

Drummond and Wilbraham say villagers brewed a crude ale in their
homes and that the manors brewed "prodigious quantities" to be used
both for their own use and sometimes to supply the village ale house.[31]
Harrison's account tells of brewing done once a month to produce the
best part of three hogsheads.[32]

Cogan believed that ale was the more usual drink in Great Britain.
This was true, he says, particularly in the north where, except in the
cities and "worshippes houses" they had not yet learnt how to brew
beer.[33] But Paul Hentzer, travelling in England in 1598, commented:
"The general drink is beer, which is prepared from barley and is excellently well tasted but strong and what soon fuddles."[34]

Drummond suggests that beer eventually ousted ale because of the
preservative quality of the hops.[35] Thomas Tusser also supports the value of hops as a preservative. In praise of hops he says "It strengtheneth
drink and it favoureth malt:

> And being well brewed
> Long kept it will last.[36]

Elyot and Paynell do not always make a clear differentiation between
ale and beer, but often refer to them together. Boorde has strong views
on this matter and disapproves of beer; he explains that it is now much
in use in England, to the detriment of Englishmen. Beer, he says, kills
those suffering from colic, the stone and "the strangulation."[37] This is
because beer has the elemental quality of being a cold drink. Beer
makes men fat and inflates their bellies (the example of "Dutche men"
is quoted).[38] However, if the beer is of good quality and not new it
qualifies the heat of the liver.

Cogan makes a comparison between ale and beer. Ale generally (that is, small ale) is better. It is beneficial in sickness and in health.[39] Desirable characteristics in ale are summed up by Boorde: "it must be fresshe and cleare, it muste not be ropy nor smoky, nor it must have no weft nor tayle."[40] All stress the importance of using clean, wholesome water and good "corne" to start with. New ale is bad. It should not be drunk until it is at least five or six days old. This was the generally accepted period. About 1547, complaints had been made about brewers delivering their ale too soon after brewing. An ordinance was made that the finished liquor should not be delivered for eight hours in the summer or six hours in the winter. Sour or flat ale and any "which doth stande a tylt," that is, which has not been properly cared for is no good for anyone.

The widespread acceptance of ale and the quantities consumed in England indicate that ale was in general considered to be beneficial. Elyot (classing ale and beer together) calls them "a necessary and convenient drynk, as well in syknes as in helth."[41] Unlike attempts to give specific advice on wine, descriptions of the advantages and disadvantages of ale are given in fairly general terms. This may be partly due to a lack of background guidance from ancient writers, for Cogan points out that neither ale nor beer are mentioned by Hippocrates or Galen.[42]

The value of an ale was derived from the barley it was made from. Other names for ale include "barley-broth" or "oyle of barley." Sometimes ales were made from wheat or oats or mixtures of grains. In times of scarcity the use of wheat for malting was sometimes forbidden. Using wheat for this purpose was considered to increase the price of bread.

Eight properties of ale and beer.
1. *Engenders gross humours.* The grosser the substance of the corn used, the grosser the humours produced.
2. *Augments the strength.* The better the preparation and the grain used, the greater the value for nourishing and strengthening.
3. *It increases flesh* because of its powers of nourishment.
4. *"Breeds" blood.*
5. *Provokes urine.*
6. *Causes* looseness of the bowel (laske).
7. *Inflates the belly.* Holland beer is referred to. This inflates and stops, and therefore "fatteth ryghte moche."[43]
8. *Cools moderately.* The amount of cooling produced depends on the type of malt used.

The value of ales made from various grains. It is pointed out in *Regimen Sanitatis* that "as the grayne is altered so is the complexion of the ale."

Barley produces a colder ale, for barley is cold.

Barley and oats. This ale stops less, engenders less wind and is less nourishing.

Wheat. Ale from wheat is hotter and nourishes more and stops more.

The grosser the ale the worse it is, the subtler the better. The grossness depends on the substance of the materials from which the ale is made.

Ale made of things that make one drunk (such as darnell) is worst.[44] This grain causes headaches and hurts the sinews.

The two names for the malted liquors (ale without hops, beer with) were retained into the seventeenth century. However, the division between the two drinks did not remain clearcut. Sir Kenelm Digby (1603-1665), in his collection of recipes, prepared towards the middle of the seventeenth century, gives one for "A Small Ale for the Stone:"[45] This was a mixture he frequently used himself. Hops are used for this "small ale," so turning it into a "small beer," according to Boorde's criterion. Despite Boorde's strong views we now have a small beer which is good against the stone.

Throughout the centuries there has always been in England a desire to believe that beer was a beneficial drink,[46] culminating perhaps in the familiar slogan, "Guinness is good for you." This statement was, happily, proved to be true when Guinness' contribution of B vitamins was estimated.[47]

Cider and Perry

The modern differentiation is that cider is made from the juice of apples and perry from pears. Boorde does not mention perry as such, but Cogan refers to that "Cider which is made of pure Peares, commonly colled Pery."[48]

Cider, when first made in England (about 1284), was called wine.[49] In the late sixteenth century Cogan tells how a certain Mistress G. tried to pass off perry as Rhenish wine when he was a student.[50] This was not at all appreciated, as cider was not praised, the reason being that as cider is made from fruit it cannot (under any condition) be very wholesome, for fruits engender ill humours. Those who regularly take cider are said to have pale wrinkled skin when they are young. Cider will also hurt the stomach and digestion. The few benefits from cider seem to be for those with hot stomachs and hot livers, but only under certain circumstances. If moderately used by those who have the red choler it will mitigate excess heat. The cooling effect is caused by the fact that cider is cold in operation. However, for those who are used to cider, it may be drunk at harvest time with little harm. If taken at all it is best after Christmas and about the time of Lent.

Cogan reports that cider is made extensively in Worcestershire and Gloucestershire (no mention is made of Somerset),

> where fruites doe most abound . . . And if a man travaile through that countrey, when they [apples and pears] be ripe, he shall see as manie lie under his Horse feete, as would in some places of England be gladlie gathered up, and layed in store under lock and keye.[51]

Mead and Metheglyn[52]

Before the Norman Conquest mead was also called metheglyn, but by the sixteenth century they were recognized as separate entities. Both were made with honey and water, but metheglyn had a more elaborate process of preparation, was more concentrated, and contained herb juices. The name is of Welsh origin and Cogan says (in the first edition of his work): "it is marvellous to see how Welshmen will lie sucking at this drink." This statement was omitted in later editions because of complaints.[53]

Instructions for preparing metheglyn are:

> Take a handful or two of all sorts of garden herbs and boil them in twice as much water as the final quantity of metheglyn required. When the quantity of water is reduced to half by boiling, cool and strain off the herbs, add honey in the proportions (by volume) of 2 parts water to 1 part honey. Boil it well removing the scum and place it in a vessel with some barme letting it stand for three or four days. Cleanse the liquor in the same way as beer or ale is cleansed and put in a barrel. After three or four months "drawe it and drinke it at your pleasure."[54]

If it is well made metheglyn is a very good winter drink, especially for the phlegmatic, those with cold stomachs or troubled by a cough. It is best taken in the morning well spiced with ginger.

Meade or meath is made of one part honey to four parts of pure water and boiled until no scum remains. This had been much recommended by Galen, to be drunk in the summer time. If well made mead cleansed the lungs making it easier to spit, it was a diuretic and acted as a moderate purge.

In the next century there were many variations on these two drinks, which were not clearly differentiated. Sir Kenelm Digby gives 106 recipes for metheglyn and meath, most of which were the favorites of his noble friends.[55]

The seven common drinks are described by Cogan as

simple drinkes, for of these, sundrie others are as it were compounded or made for our necessities but yet are rather used as medicines than with meates. . .[56]

Examples are: Aqua vitae, Aqua composita, Rosa Solis, Dr. Steven's water, Cinnamon water, Hippocras, Bragget, Buttered Beere, and such like. Cogan describes these "for the behalfe of students who neede now and then such comfortable drinkes."[57] These comfortable drinks were either prepared by distillation or made with a basis of wine, ale or beer. To make Aqua vitae, liquorice and aniseed are added to strong ale or strong wine and steeped together for twelve hours, then distilled with a Limbecke (i.e., Alembic) or serpentine. For every gallon of original liquid a quart of "reasonable good *Aqua vitae*" can be produced. Cogan stressed the importance of having a temperate fire, keeping the head of the Limbecke cool with fresh water and the bottom "fast luted [i.e., stopped up, as with the use of clay] with Rye dough, that no ayre issue out." [58]

The preparation of spiritous drinks might generally be termed "medicinal" in the sixteenth century, wine and ale or beer being the general drink. Inventories of contemporary household equipment show that some households did their own distilling. The Irish are said to have introduced their national beverage, usquebaugh (later called whiskey) when they settled in Pembrokeshire in the Tudor period, and this became increasingly popular. Permission to distil brandy commercially was given in the next century after the Revolution.[59] Distilleries multiplied and by the end of the first quarter of the eighteenth century spirits became sufficiently cheap for the mass of the population to be affected by the drinking of gin.

> . . . .no man of honour or worshippe, can be saide to have good pro-
> vision for hospitalitie, unlesse there be good store of Biefe in
> readinesse.
>
> T. Cogan (1589)

> Good Ploughman looke wekely of custome and right
> for rostmeat on Sundaies and Thursdaies at night:
>
> T. Tusser (1571)

AMONG ALL THE records of the social habits in the many countries
he visited, Fynes Morison's "England's fertility, traffick and diete"
shows a country plentifully supplied with natural resources and particularly abundant in flesh, fowl and fish. He notes that "In generall the
Art of Cookery is much esteemed in *England*, . . . the English Cookes in
comparison with other Nations, are most commended for roasted
meats."[1] The tables were so plentifully furnished that "other Nationes
esteeme us gluttons and devourers of flesh."

As has already been indicated the maintenance of the country's herds
of cattle was a matter of governmental concern. Cogan says "Biefe of
all flesh is most usual among Englishmen,"[2] and much of this beef
came from Wales. The practice was continued in the sixteenth century
of sending cattle from Wales to the great households and rich feeding-
grounds in England.[3] Kentish farmers bought lean cattle and fattened
them up for the nearby London markets. Butchers were not allowed to
do this by the Act of 1550, which forbade any butcher to buy cattle or
sheep and resell them alive. The demand for beef was such that Mc-
Grath suggests a yearly figure of 67,000 beeves killed by freeman
butchers.[4]

Stone has indicated the proportionate costs of foods spent in some
noble households, and he gives the following percentages for meat out
of a total food and wines bill: the Early of Derby, in 1561, 23% on
meat; Lord Lumley, in 1588-89, 45%.[5] Those who were employed in
households where meat was freely available, or those whose wages included rations would be likely to have eaten meat more or less regularly, but the increasing price of foods, especially in the middle and
towards the end of the sixteenth century,[6] would have put meat out of
the reach of the poor. An alternative source of flesh for them was the
"unlawful hunting" of game with which the country abounded. Cogan
refers to the risks in stealing venison,[7] and the Statutes against it were

---

N.B. Footnotes to this chapter appear on pages 339-341.

quite severe. However, Emmison, in his study of poaching, as recorded in the Essex Quarter Sessions and Assizes, gives a picture of surprising moderation in the punishments of those who were caught. He points out that Elizabethans

> . . .were relatively lucky in the mildness of the Tudor game laws, bearing in mind the ferocity of the old Forest Law and the heavy punishments inflicted in the eighteenth and nineteenth centuries.[8]

This suggests that the Elizabethan deterrents to poaching were not too fearful, and to judge by the number of gentry who indulged in it, there was less general disapproval of it than in later centuries. From the point of view of possible dietary supplements from poaching (unfortunately for the records) the greater proportion is likely to have been consumed by unknown poachers who were never caught.

The addition of Queen Elizabeth's so-called "political Lent" to the traditional two fish days per week, taken together with the dietary advice that flesh and fish should never be eaten together, give fish an important place in the diet. According to Boorde,

> Of all nacyons and countres, England is best served of Fysshe, not onely of al manner of see-fysshe, but also of fresshe-water fysshe, and of all maner of sortes of salte-fysshe.[9]

In the country the rivers, natural ponds, and artificial "stew" ponds provided a variety of fishes. The population of London had fish in the Thames and in ponds and ditches nearby, with additional supplies brought from country fish-ponds at distances of some twenty to fifty miles away.[10]

Sixteenth century books on diet give a mass of detailed information about meat and fish which, of necessity, has been drastically condensed in this chapter. The basic framework is taken from the chapter headings given by Cogan, with additional notes from *Regimen Sanitatis,* Gratarolus, Bullein and Buttes.[11]

Two important general points to be considered are the effect of the age of the animal on its value and the effect of different methods of cookery. Age was divided into four parts: suckling, youth, middle age, and old age. On the whole, animals in the second period were best. Suckling animals were considered too moist and old animals too dry. The effects of cooking were judged by the observed results. "Rosted meats or fried meates give dry nourishment to the body: but boyled meats are more moyste."[12] The theme of the suitability, in various circumstances, of boiled, broiled, baked, roast or fried foods runs through all advice on diet.

Flesh

Animals. (The letters H, D, C and M indicate the quality; the number the degree of the quality, e.g. $C^2 D^1$ is cold in the second degree and dry in the first.)

Beef[13]($C^2 D^1$):

Biefe of all flesh is most usual among English men, . . . I neede not to show how plentifull it is through-out this land, before all other countries, and how necessarie both by sea, for the victualling of Shippes, and by land for good house-keeping. . . . And how well it doeth agree with the nature of English men, the common consent of all our nation doth sufficiency prove.

Beef gives stronger nourishment than other meats. This can be plainly seen by comparing those that "feede of Biefe and them that are fedde with other fine meates." It is recognized that Galen, Isaac Judaeus and the School of Salerno all say that beef breeds melancholy, but in Cogan's opinion these authors have erred because they have classed all beef as the same.

For hadde they eaten of the Biefe of England, or if they had dwelt in this our climate, which through coldnesse *(Ex antiperistasi)* doeth fortifie digestion, and therefore requireth stronger nourishment, I suppose they woulde have judged otherwise.

Cogan makes further excuses for the ancients, saying they must have meant old beef or very fat beef, for there is a great difference in beef at different ages. Young beef is best, ox (under four years old) is better than bull and young cow is the best of all. Veal is approved of; the English habit is to kill calves at three weeks or a month old. At this time the flesh is full of "superfluous moysture," which is improved by roasting. "Therefore veale is better rosted than sodden."

Fortunately, in view of the need for the preservation of meat, "light powdered" – i.e., lightly salted beef – is considered more wholesome than fresh beef, "Because by the salt it is purified and made more savourie." Beef is better for hot stomachs, such as are common in England, than finer meats. Cogan ends his chapter on beef with this comment, "The good ordering of biefe and other victualles I refer to good cookes."

Mutton[14] (H.M.). Some authors give separate headings for lamb and mutton. The animal should be at least a year old before being eaten, but even so "the disposician and temperature of the country must be respected." Avicenna is referred to as saying that lamb and mutton can be eaten in the eastern and southern parts of the world, but it is not always expedient "in our moyst countrey, and in moyst bodies."[15]

It is noted that the sheep which give the finest wool do not give the sweetest meat. Gelded or young animals are best. "Wherfore [Cogan says] Rammes muttom I leave to those that would be rammish, and old mutton to butchers that want teeth." Mutton should (unlike veal) be rather under roasted than overdone, for one seldom saw a man who had suffered from eating raw mutton, because it is so light and easy to digest.

Pork[16] (H^2M^2) or swine flesh. This is generally commended, on the basis of its resemblance to human flesh. "Moreover the flesh of swine hath such likenes unto mans flesh, both in savour and tast, that some hath eaten mans flesh in steed of porke." The blood of man and pig appeared so similar that it was difficult to differentiate between them. The inner parts of the pig ("as is proved by Anatomie") are also very like man's.

Pork was said to give good nourishment, being especially recommended for strengthening wrestlers, but it was considered unsuitable for students or those that had weak stomachs.

The flesh of wild swine is better than that of the tame animal. Brawne, "which is of a boare long fedde in a stie," cannot be wholesome meat. This is the reason that brawn is taken at the beginning of meals, particularly in cold weather, because then it will lie longest in the hottest part of the stomach.[18]

Goat[19] (H.M.). Authors note that goat's flesh (of both male and female) "is dispraised of Galen." This is because besides producing bad blood it is tart. Yet Galen commends kid's flesh as next in merit to pork. Avicenna and the "secte of the Arabians" had (according to Cogan) placed kid's flesh above all other flesh, because it was halfway between hot and cold and subtle and gross and therefore did not cause either inflammation or repletion. It was good for those with a weak stomach or for those who took little exercise, but not for labourers, "because great labors woulde soone resolve the juice engendred thereof."

Hare[20] (H^2D^2). This animal and its parts were said to be the most useful in physick. They are recommended principally for the treatment of conditions of the liver, kidneys and bladder, for the stone, and for the flux (diarrhoea). Examples are: the whole animal should be baked (skin and all) in a tightly closed vessel, then made into a powder which, if taken in wine, was good for the stone, kidneys and bladder. Hare's blood taken immediately after the hare's death, boiled with barley meal and then eaten, will help the flux. The gall mixed with sugar "doth take away flewmes of the eyes, and helpeth dimnesse of sight." Besides these parts Cogan also refers to the liver, kidney, testicles, hair, the ankle bone, and hare's dung. Rhazes is said to have recommended the roast flesh, but in England it was usual to roast the hind parts, boil the front parts, or bake the whole.

Cogan points out that the old idea that every hare is both male and female is untrue.

Rabbits[21] (C^1D^2) or Conie (considered to be a kind of hare). The flesh was considered to be "of verie good nourishment: consumes all corrupt humours." Though rabbits were very plentiful in England, writers encourage the keeping of warrens, and advice is given on the preparation and care of warrens and the feeding of the rabbits. Special care is required in feeding, as the flesh can become tainted and take on the smell of a substance eaten.[22]

Venison[23] (H^2D^2) is given under the two headings of Red Deer and Fallow Deer. The flesh of both these animals should be avoided. Cogan suggests that there was more virtue in stag's horns than in the flesh. Horn burnt and powdered can be given with great success in the treatment of all kinds of lasks (fluxes) and the spitting of blood and jaundice. The flesh engenders melancholy; he comments:

> A wonder it is to see howe much this unwholesome flesh is desired by all folkes. In so much that many men rashly will venture their credite, yea and sometimes their lives too, to steale venison when they cannot otherwise come by it.

He adds a point which a number of other authors also make:

> And I coulde wish (saving the pleasure of honourable and worshipfull men) that there were no Parkes nor Forestes in England. For a great parte of the best pasture in this Realme is consumed with Deere, which might other-wise be better employed for a commonwealth.

This situation was changing, as Thirsk has shown.[24]

Strange beasts used for meats.[25] It is noted that Galen had referred to the use of asses, lions, dogs, wolves, bears, and snails as food. Cogan adds fried frogs, rooks, and hedgehogs, with a passing reference to "The Canibals who feede on mans flesh, as sometime the Scots did," referring to an old tale of cannibalism which was said to have taken place in France.

Parts of animals.[26] "Some say that everie part doth best nourish his like," but Cogan disagrees with this view, giving as his reason: "I knowe that the flesh of heades is very hurtfull to them that have the falling sicknesse, which is a disease of the head." The parts referred to by our authors are: brains, tongue, ears, eyes, heart, lungs, stomach, liver, spleen, "inwards of beasts" (these may be made into puddings), kidneys, testicles, udders, bone marrow, fat, and feet.

The parts recommended are tongue, eyes, testicles, udders, and feet, and also puddings made from hogs. Fat should only be eaten together with the lean of the meat.

Birds.   Comparing the flesh of animals and birds, Cogan says:

> And if the comparison bee made betwene both generally, whether is lighter of digestion, I say that the flesh of Byrdes is much lighter than the flesh of beastes, and againe that the flesh of those foules which trust most to their wings, and doe breede in high countries is lighter than the flesh of such as seldome or never flye, and be bred at home.

It was generally accepted that domesticated varieties were less good for food than the untamed.

In the *Regimen Sanitatis* birds are divided into "wylde foule [which] are moste holesome to eat," namely:

Hen	Pheasant
Capon	Woodcock
Turtle [pigeon]	Partridge
Stare [starling]	Ruddocke [robin redbreast]
Dove	Oser [pheasant hen?]
Quail	Tremulus [wagtail]
Osell [blackbird]	Amarellus [probably a moorhen]

Unwholesome birds are listed as: geese, peacocks, mallards, and all fowl that have long necks, long bills, or live upon the water. It is noted that sparrows are bad because they cause lust.[28]

There are differences in detail over the value of different birds in the advice given by Greek, Arab and sixteenth century authors. In general the pattern follows *Regimen Sanitatis*. Cogan's list, with some notes, is given below as being representative of English advice. More information about the large number of birds available is given by Emmison when referring to the birds of Essex, near Ingatstone.[29]

Chickens[30] (temperate). The flesh of a young capon is the best: "it is easily digested, for it maketh little ordure, and much good nourishment." The flesh is most tender after it has been kept a day or two. In winter hens are almost as good as capon. The flesh is soon turned into blood and has the "marveilous propertie to temper a mans complexion and humours." The broth is good for lepers. Young hen's flesh (particularly before they start laying) also helps understanding, clears the voice, and increases the seed of generation. In summer, chickens are best taken by the weak; the healthy are advised to take grosser meats. Cock's flesh is hard to digest, but a good (and rather elaborate) broth can be made from it which is good for the sick.

Pheasant[31] (temperate). This "exceedith all foules in sweetenesse and wholesomenesse" and is as nourishing as capon. Cogan says that pheasant is a food for princes "and for poore scholers when they can get it."

Partridge[32] (H^1D^2). Cogan comments on the pleasures of hawking, saying "the flesh of these birds is very precious, and every morsell worth golde."

Woodcocks[33] (temperate). The flesh is wholesome. The birds come to England "at the fall of the leaf" and go again in the spring. No one knows where they come from, but Cogan speculates: swallows come from hot Africa and return there when England gets cold; conversely, woodcocks, because they come for the winter, are likely to come from cold countries such as Denmark or Norway.

Pigeon[34] (H^2M^2). Being very hot and moist this flesh is not so good except for those which are "flewmaticke and pure melancholie, they [pigeons] are very wholsome, and be easily digested." The birds should be killed when ready to fly, and should be well bled. They are best baked with some grapes. In the sixteenth century pigeon lofts were kept for food, not for racing.

Quail (H^1M^2). Cogan does not commit himself as to value but refers to the Biblical story of the quails raining from heaven to feed the Israelites. He adds, "But God gave them a sower sauce to their meate," meaning the plague that then struck the people. "Gode defende [he says] this land from such a sauce."

Blackbirds[36] (H^1D^1). These are greatly commended for lightness of digestion and are classed with starlings, robins, moorhens and wagtails.

Other birds[37]. Cogan makes brief references to them in this order:

Larks	Lapwing
Sparrows	Teal
Geese	Peacock
Duck	Turkey
Mallards	Crane
Swan	Bustard
Plover	Heron
	Bittern

Other foules also are used to be eaten, which I omit, because I find little written of them.

Boorde gives a warning note about small birds, like the titmouse and wren, "the whiche doth eat spyders and poyson be not commendable."[38]

Parts of birds.[39] The wings and necks of geese, capons, hens, pheasant, partridge, and fat small birds are better than the legs. In wildfowl and pigeons the legs are better than wings. The fattened stomachs and liver of capons, hens and geese make good juice and are easily digested.

Fish.[40] Generally speaking, fish is less nourishing than flesh because it is "full of flewmatike superfluities, cold and moist." Sea fish is better than freshwater fish, though freshwater fish is sooner digested and so is better for sick people.[41] The place of origin of fish, whether the water was turbulent, clear and running, or still and muddy, was important.[42]

An English proverb, quoted by a number of writers, states: "young flesh and olde fish doeth men best feed." In fact, the best age at which a fish should be eaten varied according to type. Bullein says, "If the fish be soft, the eldest fish is best; if fish be hard the yongest is best, for it is either soft or hard."[43]

Ten Fishes recommended.[44] The list includes both salt and freshwater fish:

Pike	Gunard
Perch	Plaice
Sole	Carp
Whiting	Gugeon
Tench[45]	Trout

Cogan makes two comments about the trout. He quotes the saying
"hee is as sound as a Troute," meaning he is a good sound man. He then
points out that the trout is easily flattered; it "will suffer itself to be
rubbed and clawed," and so be caught — an example, he says, "I would
wish no maydes to follow."

Other Fishes "verie wholesome."[46] Cogan lists fish familiar today:

Breame	Haddock
Bret [brill]	Tunny
Turbot	Mullet
Halibut	Mackerel
Cod	Shad [herring or catfish]

Many scales and finnes betoken the purenesse of the fishes substance.

Two comments by Cogan are entertaining rather than instructive. The
mullet acts like an ostrich and believes its whole body is hidden if it
hides its head. Mackerel are difficult to catch except in tempest or
when it thunders and lightnings.

Eels[47] (C^1M^1). Pleasant to taste but not wholesome, they are slimy,
clammie, and "greatlie stopping"; this makes them bad for the voice.
Slimyness can have a congealing effect, therefore eels should be avoided
by those with the stone.

Lampreys[48] (H.M^1). Lampreys are partly of the nature of eels, but
they are "more wholsomer and less jeopardous." Some people believe
they are venonous. After this food, wine is recommended, as the
French proverb says: *"Poisson sans vin est poison."*

Conger[49] is of hard substance and therefore hard to digest.

Salmon.[50] A sweet pleasant fish, but not as wholesome as many already mentioned. The proof of this is "that it is not used to be eaten
hoat, or immediately after it is boyled." Cogan does not explain the full
significance of this remark.

Thornback,[51] or ray. The flesh is soft and full of bones. If eaten hot it
disposes toward the falling evil. The spines on the back can be dried,
powdered and then drunk (while fasting) with white wine, as a medicine to "avoyde the gravell and to breake the stone."

Porpoise and Sturgeon.[52] Cogan classes these as "not much better
than Bacon and brawne," despite the value placed upon them due to
their scarcity.

Herring and Pilchards.[53] "Herring is a fish most common and best
cheape." Yet it is not wholesome, as has been shown by those who

became feverish after eating fresh herring. Nevertheless, they are still important to the poor. Pilchards are similar to herrings; red herrings and spratts are summarily dismissed as unwholesome.

Shellfish.[54] These include mussels, oysters, cockles, crabs, and shrimps. The general characteristic of shellfish is that they make "a salte juice which louseth the belly." Oysters are eaten raw, in broths, or roasted upon coals. They are good in that they do not "lightly corrupt in the stomacke," but they should be followed by wine. Mussels and cockles are best boiled or roasted. Cogan tells of the pearls found in a kind of mussel around England's coast which were said to have adorned Julius Caesar's breastplate.

Cogan ends his section on fish with "Of the Puffin." The reason for classing this bird as a fish is because it "liveth altogether in the water." Puffins are eaten fresh or salted. Their "in-between" position is illustrated by the fact that "A Carthusian [monk] may eate them and never breake his order."[55]

The Preservation[56] of Meat and Fish

The word preserving in the sixteenth century, commonly referred to preserving with sugar. The main methods of preservation of meat and fish were by salting or curing. The salting could be done by immersion in brine of the whole or parts of an animal, or by the use of dry salt. The term "powedered" is used to describe foods preserved by salt, though it can also mean the addition of other spices.

A salt beef "much used in some places of England is 'martilman' beef." This name refers to the time of year the beast is killed. After salting, it can be "kept in brine or hanged up in the smoke."[57] Either way it is an unwholesome food. Boorde puts it more graphically:

> If a man have a peace [of martilmas beef] hangynge by his syde, and another in his bely, that whiche doth hange by the syde shall do hym more good, yf a showre of rayne to chaunse, than that the which is in his bely, the appetyde of man's sensualyte notwithstandynge.[58]

Lightly powdered meat has been referred to above as being acceptable.

Maison Rustique directs the reader to kill animals for salting only in the new moon or the first quarter. If the animal is killed during the waning of the moon it will require more attention in the salting and there will be a greater loss when the meat is boiled.[59] Animals should not be allowed to eat or drink the day before slaughter so that the flesh will be improved and drier. The animal should be boned immediately after death and can be salted in layers of salt in tubs or have the salt beaten into each half of a pig's carcass "with a rowling pinne: and this thing is not done at one time, or in one day, but at two or three times and in two or three daies space."[60] The parts can then be hung up in the roof where they will keep for more than a year.

The wet salt pickle is the old "sea pickle" of Elizabethan sailors. Dorothy Hartley describes a number of ways of pickling flesh, some of which are still used today.[61] One interesting method is the "Potting and Preserving Poultry" which is a sixteenth century recipe for shipload storage. Drawn ducks or mallards are laid in salt, with pepper, for twenty-four hours. They are then roasted. The birds are then covered in a vessel with salted and spiced melted fat (fat from the roasting and added butter), after which "Lay a Trencher on them to keep them down till cold."[62]

No reference has been found to a "biltong" type of dried meat in the sixteenth century books studied. It would certainly have been used on long journeys.

Both Thirsk (in her discussion of agricultural records) and Emmison (referring to the records at Ingatstone Hall) conclude that the use of salted meat in the winter in England was not nearly so widespread as had been thought by earlier historians.[63] Certainly sixteenth century dietary and agricultural advice puts little emphasis on salted meats. It is likely that the amount of salted meat kept by substantial farmers was limited, though in poorer households a higher proportion of beasts may have had to be killed in the autumn.

The salting and curing of fish was important, and many references are made to fish treated in these ways. The terminology is confusing: from various contexts halberine can mean cod or salted cod, while stock-fish can indicate that the fish was salted or salted and cured. Tusser describes the care with which salt-fish should be chosen at market and advises that it should be packed in clean place-straw directly it is brought home.[64] Cogan says that salmon, conger, cod, eels, herrings, "and such like," are eaten fresh or salted.[65] Fresh fish is considered to be the better, except for those people who need a "drying" food. Stock-fish is "brought to us dryed from Iseland and other countries Northward."[66] The fish itself does not seem to have been very highly thought of as to nourishment or taste. However, Cogan has had a tasty pie made of stock-fish; the good taste he puts down to the cook, for it is said "a good Cooke can make you good meate of a Whetstone."

Despite the wide variety of foods referred to above, the tables of seasonal foods in "A Breviate touching the order and Government of a
Nobleman's House etc." (1605) includes even more items.[67] It is impossible to relate prices to all the foods listed. The short list below of
the prices of flesh foods is made up from different parts of the country.
The prices of meat and fish are obviously of great importance to the
diet of most people. Detailed prices are difficult to find. The following
have been selected from the accounts of St. Margaret's Westminster and
Eden's "Table of Prices" derived from many sources.[68]

1550	one day's work for a carpenter	8d
1554	4 green geese	2/4
	1 dozen rabbits	2/8
	1 dozen pigeons	2/6
	1 sirloin of beef	6/8
1572	Best capon in the market	1/—
	1 best green goose	9d
	1 dozen pigeons	1/2
	A fat rabbit	4d
1573	5 herrings	2d
	A stone of beef	1/10

In 1587 two days threshing earned 1/4 while the year before the Westminster accounts give another perspective, with the entry "Paid for the
ringing at the beheading of Queen of Scotts, one shilling."

CHAPTER XIV
WHITE MEATS

Why, sir alasse my Cow is a commonwealth to mee, for first sir, she
allowes me, my wife and sonne, for to banket our selves withall,
butter, cheese, whay, curds, creame, sod [boiled] milke, raw-milke,
sower-milke, sweete-milke, and butter-milke.

T. Lodge and R. Greene (1594)

WHITE MEATS are those foods which we would now class as dairy produce. Cogan places them clearly in the category of "meats," saying
"There remaineth yet a third kind of meates which is neither fishe nor
flesh commonly called white meats."[1] With minor variations the grouping of white meats in the sixteenth century was:

(i) Eggs	(v) Whey
(ii) Milk	(vi) Curds
(iii) Butter	(vii) Cheese[2]
(iv) Cream	

Some authors put eggs under "flesh," and whey is frequently discussed
with other drinks. The classification of dairy produce remained difficult
for it was, as Cullen said of milk in the eighteenth century, "commonly
and justly held to be of an intermediate nature between entirely vegetable and entirely animal aliments."[3] Harrison, in his description of
contemporary England, says that white meats, which had previously
been "woont to be accounted of as one of the chiefe staies throughout
the Iland, are now reputed as food appertinent onlie to the inferiour
sort"; the wealthy were said to prefer flesh and fish.[4] Modern studies of
agriculture in the sixteenth and seventeenth centuries show that the
dairy was frequently a significant part of the farm and that dairy produce was being sent to an ever increasing number of markets and fairs.[5]
Records and recipes indicate that milk, cream, eggs and cheese were still
in use in wealthy households.

N.B. Footnotes to this chapter appear on pages 341-343.

Eggs

> The egg is good and for delight:
> Thats long and new and white in sight.[6]

Though modern market research shows that consumers now believe that brown-shelled are best, the tradition that long white eggs are more nutritive than round eggs is an old one and can be traced, according to Cogan, from Horace through the *Regimen Sanitatis*. Of the varieties available hen's eggs are best, pheasant and partridge acceptable, but the eggs of ducks, geese, turkeys and other fowl should be avoided. Boorde says that "in England there is no egges used to be eaten but hen-egges."[7]

The particular value of the egg lay in the speed with which it moved down into the stomach, was digested, and provided nourishment. "They [eggs] have all the properties that belongeth to good nourishment, and are soon transmuted into the bloud, and leave small superfluities."[8] This general statement about eggs has to be considered in relation to three facts: the part of the egg used, the age of the egg, and the method of cooking.

The whole egg is considered to be temperate, but the parts differ. The yolk is temperately hot and the white cold and clammy, less easily digested, and only capable of making poor blood. There is a difference of opinion as to whether the chicken is engendered in the white and nourished by the yolk as Cogan believes.[9] This view is also held by Aristotle and Albertus Magnus, though other authorities believed the contrary.

The emphasis throughout is on the use of new eggs. Books on poultry-keeping give advice on how to keep hens laying all through the winter. This is done mainly by special diets, which may include toast soaked in wine and good supplies of earthworms.[10] The *Book of Thrifte* gives suitable yields to be aimed for, which are small by modern standards. It is suggested that one hen in one year should lay 150 eggs and breed seven chickens.[11] Instructions are also given on how to gather and keep eggs. Views differ, but packing eggs in straw, bran, or bean meal, and treating with dry salt or brine are all suggested.[12]

Because of the drying or moistening effect that methods of cooking could have on foods, it was always a matter for consideration when advising on the value of a food. There is general agreement on the effects of different methods of cooking on eggs and the methods of boiling, roasting and frying are described.

Boiling. This is called poached when out of the shell, and seethed when in the shell. Poaching is the best method, seething the next best. The moistness of the water tempers the heat and prevents drying up.

Roasting. Roasted eggs provide ill nourishment: "[they are] heavie to digest causing stinking fumes in the stomach."[13]

Frying. This is the worst method of cooking, producing the same effects as roasting, in an exaggerated form. Cogan comments, "wherefore collops and Egges which is an usual dish toward shrovetide, can in no wise bee wholsome meate."[14]

It was recognized that in all cases a lightly cooked egg was better than one overcooked. Eggs were used in a wide variety of recipes, both with flesh and in sweet dishes. They were considered especially beneficial taken in wine or in pottages.[15] On the whole, yolks seem to have been used more than whites for cooking. Reference is made to other uses of eggs. The white and shell could be used for a cement to mend glass; also "an egge spred upon wood or any kinde of garment doth keepe the same from the burning of the fire."[16]

The detailed advice on poultry raising and egg production, available in English in the sixteenth century, had been developed from ancient authors, frequently translated from collections of information prepared on the Continent. Most of the information used by a number of contemporary authors can be found in *Maison Rustique or the Countrie Farme.* Here advice is given on the care and feeding of the flock in health and sickness, the hatching of eggs (the author notes that a tiresome hindrance to hatching is impatient women who will not let the eggs rest, but must keep looking at them), and the storage and preserving of eggs. The aim of the advice is to provide eggs for home and market. The considerable variation in the price of eggs is illustrated by the following figures:

1552	693 eggs for 15/7
1567-68	100 eggs for 4/– to 6/–
1590	100 eggs for 8/– to 12/–
1594-96	One dozen for about 3½d (in town).[17]

The amount of information given about egg production indicates that they were an important market commodity; in addition to this, the egg was often discussed in a philosophical context. The shape of the egg and the fact that a whole chicken could emerge from it had caught the imagination of writers from ancient times. Cogan quotes Aphrodissaeus as saying: "A man may say that the type of the whol world is shewed in an Egge: for it is made of the fowre Elements, and is rounde like a Sphere, and hath life in it." The shell is likened in qualities to the earth, the white to water, the foam or froth of the white to air, and the yolk to fire. This makes the egg "a little world."[18] The vexing question of which came first the chicken or the egg is raised but neatly side-stepped, one author referring the reader to earlier writers, saying: "I doe not intend here to make any discourse, which of the two was the first made, the egg or the hen. Looke for the deciding of this curious question in. . . ."[19] and he continues with references to Plutarch, Aristotle, Pliny and Hippocrates.

Milk, Butter, and Cream

Milk. Sixteenth century writers accepted the traditional view that "milk is made of bloud twise concocted."[20] Opinions differed as to the order of merit for different milks. All place women's milk first, usually followed by that of cows, sheep, and goats. Some authors put goat milk before cows', and some include comments on camels' and asses' milk.[21]

Besides the variations according to the type of animal, it was clearly recognized that the characteristics of a milk were also influenced by the diet taken, the time of year, and the circumstances of milking. Here the discussion is limited to cows' milk, unless otherwise stated. The milk varied according to whether the cow was on good or bad pasture, eating unsuitable herbs or a diet of dry food, such as barley or straw. It was clearly understood that cows fed on the best pasture gave the best milk, and that the quality of the milk deteriorated if the diet of the animal was poor. All milk produced in the springtime "is waterisher than the milke of sommer."[22] Autumn milk is best according to the old saying

> when Fearne waxeth redde,[23]
> then milk is good with bread.

Many writers give clear instructions about the location and cleanliness of the dairy and its staff.

The milk produced directly after the birth of a calf should be rejected.[24] The best milk is that taken freshly from the cow and not kept for long; in the summer it should be used in a day, but in the winter, when yields are small, several milkings can be put together and made into butter and cheese.[25]

In describing the proper care of milk the term thicken has to be differentiated from souring; to thicken milk it should be set in a warm

place, "inasmuch as heate doth saveguard and thicken the milk, as cold
doth sowre it and make it turne by and by"; the danger of souring can
be avoided by boiling the milk.[26] That heating would delay or prevent
souring was accepted, but the amount of heating required to destroy
the bacteria which cause souring could not, of course, be understood.

The general view of the value of milk was that "All milke is of good
juice, it nourisheth the bodie, it looseth the bellie, yet it filleth the
stomacke and belly with winde."[27] This unfortunate wind-producing
characteristic could be lessened by boiling the milk or by adding spices
to it. Whole milk was considered to be moist in the second degree and
temperately hot.[28] However, the three different parts of milk had their
own characteristics. The parts are:

(i) Whitish, cold and moist, nitrous and powerful to make the belly
soluble." [Whey]
(ii) Fat and oyly, of temperate qualitie, of which butter is made.
(iii) Grosse, clammy and flegmaticke, whereof cheese is made.[29]

Readers are warned not to take more milk than they can digest. It
should be avoided by the choleric, by those suffering from the stone,
and in cases of headache and ague. In some situations milk had a loosening action and in others a binding.[30] In bodies that are distempered
milk becomes corrupted in the stomach and produces choleric fumes.

Occasionally milk is prescribed for a particular illness, such as goat
milk for consumption.[31] Milk is advocated for all melancholy people.
Students, who are particularly liable to melancholy, should drink milk
in the morning before other foods.[32] Milk boiled with a little sugar is
good for children and old men and for all those who are accustomed to
taking milk. References to drinking milk alone are rare; it was more
commonly used in cooking and in posset drinks. A posset may be made
with a variety of milks (whole, skimmed, sweet or sour) mixed with ale
or wine.[33]

Prices of milk are not often recorded because it was mainly used by
the family or sold in the form of butter or cheese. A figure for 1594-96
in London is 6d per gallon.[34]

Butter. Books on husbandry give quite detailed advice on procedures
for making butter. The yield expected was 2½ lb. of butter from 10 lb.
of milk.[35]

Three main types of butter were in use: fresh butter, which was for
immediate use: salted butter, which was pressed into earthenware pots

or barrels for storage, and clarified butter, usually for kitchen use, but which could also be potted and stored.[36] Butter could be clarified by standing it in shallow dishes in the sunshine for twelve to fourteen days; Cogan adds, rather sensibly, in view of the English climate, "if there bee faire sunne shining."[37]

Butter was used chiefly in made-up dishes, in pastry, and for frying. It was the cheapest fat available for the latter.[38] Frying butter is sometimes called "pound" butter. Prices for butter are:

    1552   7d per dish or 5d per dish in the spring.
    1589   5d per pound.
    1594-96 4½d per pound in London and 3d per pound in Gloster.[39]

From a dietary point of view new fresh butter was considered very wholesome, especially if eaten in the morning. Because of its slippery characteristics, butter "mollifieth and moysteneth and looseth the belly," and is therefore good for costive (constipated) people.[40] Taken in moderation with other foods, butter is good and can be further improved if sugar or honey are added to it. Butter should be avoided by those with fevers or with liver trouble. Cogan stresses that May butter is best and says, "such as have children to bring up would not be without May Butter in their houses."[41] Modern theory accepts that summer butter contains significantly more vitamin A than butter produced in the winter, but this is not Cogan's context; here May butter is linked with clarification and is also advised for external application.

Cream. This is best taken from slightly cooled fresh milk and is called "the very head or heart of milke."[42] Cream was used in two forms: (i) raw cream, taken from unheated milk, and (ii) clowted or clotted cream prepared from milk which has been gently heated. Raw and clotted cream taken together are "more for sensuall appetyde than for any good nowrysshement."[43] Both types of cream were frequently used in the summer with sugar and fruits such as strawberries or bilberries. However good this may taste, readers are warned against cream. It is hot and moist in the first degree,[44] but its fatyness loosens the stomach and cream "swimmeth above all other meate, it rejecteth the nourishment and maketh grosse bloud."[45] Therefore, says Cogan, those who go all the way from London to Islington to eat cream have a useless journey.[46] However, it was accepted that cream boiled with sugar was nourishing for weak students. It is doubtful if their Lordships of the Privy Council took cream because of their weakness, even though cream was supplied to them daily, winter and summer, usually at a gallon a day. Rising prices are illustrated by the changing cost:

1567   per gallon 12d, 16d or 20d.
1568   per gallon 18d.
1590   per gallon 2/−, 2/4, 3/− and 3/4.[47]

Cream was used in a number of dishes and is sometimes designated "cream for custard" and "cream for tarts." The word cream (with various spellings) in recipes refers not only to fat from the top of the milk, but also to other soft mixtures which would now be called custards or fools.[48]

Whey, Curds, and Cheese

Both whey and curds are produced in the making of cheese. The separation of the curd can occur due to souring by the action of lactic acid which forms an acid curd, or by the action of rennet. Acid curd is the basic curd for a group of soft and semi-soft cheeses, but it does not ripen on storage and so has to be eaten fresh. Rennet curd makes true cheese, being gradually ripened by enzymes present. In both cases whey is a by-product.[49]

Whey. Advice of French origin suggests that whey can be used to feed hogs and dogs except in times of dearth when the family will eat it.[50] In England, though it was fed to pigs in some parts, it was drunk more often, rather as a medicine than a food being used as a mild laxative. In the spring it was commonly drunk with an infusion of herbs, being considered good against skin troubles and as a purge of choler and melancholy.[51] Whey was sufficiently important for a recipe for its clarification to be included in a cookery book.[52] No prices are available in the records consulted, as it would have been used by members of the household or farm workers.

Curds as such are not often referred to. Buttes does describe them as cold and dry in the first degree and says they annoy a cold stomach and the sinews, are slowly digested, and make a person drowsy.[53] They were most usually made into cheese.

Cheese. The making of cheese was a woman's work, and sixteenth century writers stress the importance of clean healthy dairymaids. Thomas Tusser, describing the duties of Cisley the dairymaid, writes at length about the difficulties and pitfalls to be avoided when making cheese.[54] In some parts, sheep were still used as milk producers, five ewes being considered equivalent to one cow. Tusser gives this figure in "Mary's husbandry," and it is quoted elsewhere. Walter of Henley referred to ten milking sheep as being equivalent to one cow.[55]

The best cheese was made from full cream milk, but most were made from skimmed milk because the full cream cheese was too expensive for tenant farmers or labourers.[56] Gorge points out that skimmed milk produces a hard cheese which will not keep well. Just how hard the cheese could be is illustrated by one of the many doggerel verses written about cheeses:

> Those that made me were uncivil
> They made me harder than the devil.
> Knives won't cut me, fire won't sweat me;
> Dogs bark at me, but can't eat me.[57]

whereas full cream milk makes a cheese which "wyll very long endure, and long continueth in his fatnesse and softnesse."[58] The best cheese was carefully curdled with rennet or the juice of certain plants, and was not just allowed to form an acid curd.[59]

Boorde separates cheeses into five generally accepted sorts:[60]

(a) *"Grene chese."* This does not refer to colour, but means a new cheese. Its qualities are cold and moist.

(b) *"Softe chese."* This is best not too new or too old. Its qualities are hot and moist.

(c) *"Harde chese."* This is hot and dry and difficult to digest.

(d) *"Spermyse."* This is made with curds and the juices of herbs. Its nutritional value will depend upon the mixture of herbs added.

(e) *"Rewene"* cheese. This was considered to excel the rest. The meaning of rewene is obscure.[61]

Good cheese should not be too hard or too soft, not tough or brittle, neither sweet nor sour, not tart, not too salt nor too fresh. It should not have eyes, mites, or maggots. Not everyone disliked maggots in their cheeses, for in Hygh Almen (Germany) it is reported "they will eate the great magotes as fast as we doe eate comfetes."[62] Authors are much given to using Biblical descriptions for the characteristics of a good cheese; these were taken, for the most part, from old Latin verses, "nor full of Whey or weaping as Marie Magdalem was, nor rough as Esau was, nor ful of spots as Lazarus."[63]

Dietetically speaking, cheese was considered to be cold and dry in the second degree,[64] and to be unwholesome because it "annoyed" the stomach, engendered ill humours, caused the colic and the stone, and in general made gross blood. Cheese should be avoided by students and those with weak stomachs, though Cogan says, "I knowe that labouring men eating it daily, feel no inconvenience thereby."[65] Those who wish to eat cheese should eat it in small amounts after other foods, for it was recognized to be a "digestive." Roast cheese was despised as being (according to Cogan) "more meate to baite a trap, to catche a mouse or a ratte than to be received into the bodie."[66] In his first edition Cogan also refers in the same general context to Welshmen liking cheese. This point is diplomatically omitted in later editions.

References in contemporary accounts to the cost of cheese give the price per cheese without indicating quantity or quality. The mildest, lightest and most easily digested cheese was, according to Googe,[67] made from goat milk, but the type of cheese was hardly ever referred to, the distinction being by place of origin. The best cheeses were Parmesian, made in the valley of the River Po; then came Dutch and Normandy cheeses. Of English cheeses the saying goes,

> I never sawe Banbury cheese thicke yenough,
> But I have seen Essex cheese quicke yenough.

Between the Banbury and Essex came Cheshire, Shropshire and Suffolk in that order of preference, "and the very worst [is] the Kentish cheese."

The references to white meats in doggerel verse and everyday speech, the records of shipments of butter and cheese from Suffolk to London,[68] and the quotation at the head of this chapter, all indicate that both urban and rural dwellers used and enjoyed dairy produce when they could get it. Tusser advises it as a standby for poorer farming households when other foods are scarce:

> Where fish is scant and fruit of trees,
> Supply that want with butter and cheese.[69]

Contemporary dietary advice did not put the same emphasis on the benefits of milk, butter, eggs and cheese that we do today, though it was recognized by Platt in his advice in times of famine that "A man may live with milke only and it will serve instead of meat, drinke and medicine."[70]

CHAPTER XV
HERBS, VEGETABLES, FRUITS AND NUTS

> There is no Herbe, nor weede but God have gyven vertue to them, to help man.
>
> A. Boorde (1542)

THE IMPRESSION THAT in the sixteenth century the English lacked vegetables has been fostered by the repetition of two familiar statements about salads and cabbages. John Evelyn, in his *Acetaria: a Discourse of Sallets,* had said that

> 'Tis scarce 100 years [i.e., about 1599] since we had Cabbages out of Holland, Sir Arthur Ashley, of Wilburg St. Giles, in Dorsetshire, being the first who planted them in England.[1]

and is quoted by Dorothy Hartley in her *Food in England* (1954).[2] John Simon, Medical Officer of Health to the Privy Council, writing in 1863 about the incidence of scurvy at that time, suggested that the English were not great vegetable growers, referring to the fact "that in Tudor times Queen Catherine of Aragon could not procure a salad till a gardner came from the Netherlands to raise it for her."[3]

Both these statements are misleading when taken out of context. While it is obviously impossible to estimate what quantity of fruit and vegetables were actually eaten in England towards the end of the sixteenth century, contemporary references and the practical advice given on a wide range of fruit and vegetables, suggest that many varieties were available. The number of references is so great that only a few have been arbitrarily selected for comment here.

The sixteenth century herbal was derived from early writings on materia medica which had included items related to animals and minerals as well as plants.[4] In Dioscorides' work on materia medica Alston counted more than 90 minerals, 168 animal substances, and 700 plants.[5] Two English herbals were written by William Turner and John

---

N.B. Footnotes to this chapter appear on pages 343-345.

Gerard;[6] Turner's illustrated edition of 1568 contains about 500 wood-cuts and figures, while Gerard describes some 2,850 species. Johnson, in his later edition of Gerard's herbal (1633), added 800 more.[7] These works include a large number of plants which could be grown only in foreign countries. Though Timothy Bright wrote a treatise (1580) declaring "the sufficiencie of English medicines,"[8] English herbals continued to include a number of plants which could not be grown in the English climate. However, Bright's approach does reflect the increased interest in agriculture, horticulture and kitchen gardens which developed in England in the latter part of the sixteenth century.

Amherst, in *A History of Gardening in England*,[9] describes the changes in English gardens which came with the early Tudors, based on the fact that gardens had no longer to be confined within castle walls. This encouraged the development of elaborate flower gardens, and though changes in the kitchen or "cooks-gardens" were not so marked, more emphasis was placed on the growing of vegetables than had previously been the case. Harrison, writing in 1577, says "And even as it fareth with our gardens, so dooth it with our orchards, which were never furnished with so good fruit, nor with such varietie as at this present."[10] However, the growing importance of gardening at this period is indicated by the granting of a Royal Charter to the gardener's Company of London in 1606.[11] The first English book on gardening had appeared in 1603.[12] Amherst suggests that contemporary writers tend to exaggerate the progress made in fruit and vegetable growing during Elizabeth's reign and that this change was not as sudden as they imply.

Originally the word "herb" applied to all plants, excluding only shrubs and trees. Therefore no clear distinction was made between herbs, vegetables, and fruits in the way that is done now. Under his heading of herbs, Buttes gives the following:[13]

Sage	Burnet (*Sanguisorba officinalis*)
Fennel	Parsley
Asparagus	Tarragon
Spinach	Radish
Artichokes [globe variety]	Carrot or red parsnip
Lettuce	Onions
Endive	Garlic
Borage	Scallion or little onions
Succory	Leeks
Hops	Colewort (*Brassica oleracea*)
Mint	Sorrel

Cogan, in his much more detailed work, describes nearly 100 herbs and vegetables.[14]

To Buttes, "fruites" meant literally the fruit of the plant, and he includes nuts and some plants that we now call vegetables. Cogan, writing before Buttes, makes some distinction between fruits and herbs, putting his information about gourds, melons, and cucumbers directly after herbs because "though they bee fruites, yet because they are commonly set in gardens [they will] be here specified."[15]

Nuts are usually discussed towards the end of the section on "fruits," directly before spices. The latter are frequently "annexed" to fruits, "because they are for the more part fruites of certayne trees growing out of this Realme."[16] Some spices are occasionally to be found under the heading of sauces.

The importance of herbs and vegetables is indicated by the mass of advice and information given about them, though much of this is medicinal rather than strictly dietary. Langham's books of receipts for alleviating symptoms runs to some 702 pages and gives a large number of uses or recipes under each plant.[17] The dietary value placed upon a herb or vegetable does not seem to be related directly to the presence of any particular quality. Cogan divides his list of herbs into "hot" and "cold," saying "And of herbes I shall declare first such as be hotte and after those that be colde."[18] Of the plants he lists, about two-thirds are hot:dry (in the second or third degree), six are hot:moist, seven cold: dry, one temperate, and four not clearly described.

The value of most popular herbs is far-reaching. Two examples described here are sage and daisies, being the first and last items given by Cogan.

Sage. "Of all garden herbes, none is of greater vertue than sage."[19] Its virtue is so great that if it were possible it would make man immortal.[20] It is hot and dry in the third degree and has important properties: "sage comforteth the sinewes: it taketh away shaking of the hands: it resisteth sharpe Agues." Because it is also good for the brain it is valuable for students who are "commonly cumbred [sic] with diseases of the head." Sage was taken in many forms, e.g. with bread and butter, and in sauces and drinks. A drink containing sage and rue was recommended against infection.

Daisy. All daisies are cold:moist.[21] They are used in potions for fractures of the skull or deep chest wounds. The juice from the leaves and roots clears the brain when put up the nostrils. Daisies are good in pottage, in salads, or boiled with fat flesh, when they act as a laxative.

Vegetables are listed within the group of herbs. Parsnips, carrots and leeks have been chosen as examples.

Parsnips and Carrots. The reference here is specifically to the roots,[22] but the greenery can also be eaten. Both roots are hot and dry, they "breake winde and expell urine," and they are aphrodisiacs and restorative. Taken in excess they make poor juice but can be good for the colic and the stone, and help the weak and those "in a consumption"; carrots are considered to be better than parsnips.

Leeks.[23] Leeks are hot:dry in the third degree and "their nourishment is naught." They can, in fact, they do, cause much damage by hurting the eyes, sinews and teeth, engendering black melancholy, and causing terrible dreams. They should not be eaten raw by choleric or melancholic individuals. Boiling with honey or in a pottage can make them acceptable; they will then help to get rid of phlegm. Boiled leeks can also aid those suffering from colic, the stone, and toothache. For those of an appropriate complexion, they may be eaten raw, boiled, or dried and powdered.

Fruits are not thought to be as valuable as herbs. Galen recommended that some be avoided,[24] but on the other hand herbs and fruit were the first food "that ever was appointed to man, as appeareth by the commandment of God given to Adam."[25] Cogan then explains that from Adam's time until after "Noahs floud," man was vegetarian and did not eat flesh or drink wine.

> But now by the chaunge of dyet of our progenitors, there is caused in our bodies such alteration from the nature which was in man at the beginning that now all herbs and fruits generally are noyfull to man, and do engender ill humours, and be oft times the cause of putrified fevers, if they be continually eaten.

To judge from the large number of references to fruits, and their inclusion in many recipes found in sixteenth century cookery books, the attraction of fruit overcame these dietary considerations. From the practical point of view John Taverner, writing in 1600, says

> If the benefit arising unto the commonwealth through the abundance of fruite were well weighed and pondered, there would be lawes established for the increase and maintenance therof throughout this Realme.[26]

The examples chosen are apples and oranges — that is, one home-grown and one imported fruit.

Apples[27] are cold:moist in the first degree, but there can be a great difference between varieties, depending on taste. Some of "of a mixt temperature both sweete and soure these incline to heat." In general, apples are "unwholesome in the regiment of health"; they hurt the sinews, cause wind, and in the "seconde digestion" can make ill and corrupt blood. Nevertheless, they are included in a large number of recipes, some of which dishes are mentioned as being beneficial. The bad characteristics of apples were exaggerated if they were eaten raw, though (as Cogan acknowledges) "unruly people through wanton appetite will not refraine [from] them." He adds: "I have knowen in my daies many a shrewde boye for the desire of Apples, to have broken into other folkes Orchardes."

Oranges. Not all parts of the orange have the same qualities. The rind is hot in the first degree and dry in the second; the juice is cold in the second degree and dry in the first, and they are colder or hotter according to their sourness or sweetness. The rinds were used preserved in sugar, as were orange flowers. Either of these preserves would "comfort a feeble stomacke." The "substance" of the orange was eaten raw or used in sauces taken with roasted flesh. The juice was used with added sugar, or sugar and spices, and was considered good for the stomach, and caused an appetite.

Nuts[29] are placed amongst other fruits. They may be hot:moist or hot:dry, but are all considered rather indigestible but nourishing. According to Galen (says Cogan) chestnuts are the most nourishing of the wild fruits, but then (also according to Cogan) Galen contradicts himself and says that whether chestnuts be "rosted, fryed or boyled they be hurtfull: but much more if they be eaten raw."[30] The nut most frequently referred to is the almond.[31] Bitter almonds should be avoided; sweet almonds are hot and moist in the first degree and are recommended because "They do not extenuate and clense without binding. Wherefore they purge the brest and lunges." Almonds were used in a number of prepared dishes but also in the form of almond butter, cawdles and milks. Almond butter is good "for a stuffed brest." Almond cawdles are made with blanched, pounded almonds, ale and spices; these cawdles are "comfortable to the principall partes of the bodie," and are soporifics. Almond milk is the most widely used of the three. Cogan's recipe says: take a pottel of fair water, add two handfuls of violet or strawberry leaves (or other cooling herbs), add an ounce of licorish cut into thin slices, boil gently until the quantity is reduced by half, strain and cool. Then mix in a quarter of a pound of blanched, ground almonds, strain and press almond mixture through the sieve, add sugar, and bring slowly to the boil. The result is described as a "verie temperate meate in hoat diseases."

These brief references to the dietary value of these selected examples give an indication of the complexity of determining the nutritive value of herbs, vegetables and fruits. As has already been indicated, historians have commented on the scarcity of vegetables in the sixteenth century English diet. It is true that the main emphasis was on meat at that period, but a large number of leafy and root plants, both wild and cultivated, must have been available in normal times. The idea of a shortage would seem to be based on a lack of records in household accounts and menus. The difficulty of interpreting a lack of reference is obvious. Homegrown materials are frequently omitted from accounts and menu details available often make no reference to such things as bread and salt, which are known to have been used. It is possible, therefore, that some vegetables were used but not listed. Whatever the actual situation was in this respect, the list of vegetables referred to by sixteenth century writers which could be used today, is not insignificant. Included are:

Asparagus	Leeks
Artichokes (globe)	Lettuce
Beans	Marrow[32]
Beets (white and red)	Onions (including spring onions)
Cabbages	Parsnips
Carrots	Peas
Chicory	Turnips
Cucumbers	Radishes
Endive	Spinach
	Watercress

Asparagus, cabbage, and carrots are considered briefly from the point of view of cultivation.

Asparagus is also called "sperage," and is divided into garden and wild varieties. The roots as well as the "first sprouts or naked tender shoots"[33] were eaten.

The reference to cabbages being brought from Holland by Sir Arthur Ashley has already been given. He must have brought a special kind of cabbage for, as De Candolle points out, cabbages or coleworts are native to England.[34] Originally the cabbage was the compact heart or head of the plant, the whole being called cabbage-cole or colewort. Gradually the term came to refer to the whole species or genus, whether with a heart or not.[35] Buttes refers to the fact that Gerard lists eighteen different sorts of coleworts. One of these is called Cole Florie or Colieflorie[36] and is the cauliflower of today. Also familiar were the red cabbage and the savoy cabbage.

The demand for cabbages is illustrated by Gardiner's reference to those who devour them:

> but of al wormes or caterpillars knaves, which are the greatest devourers of cabadges and doe consume many of them at one time: those catterpillars doe never repent, until they come to Tyburne or the gallowes.[37]

It is of note that it was generally believed that cabbage seed more than three years old produced radishes. The old proverb is quoted: "sow coleworts and there will grow up radishes."[38]

Descriptions of carrots are often closely allied with parsnips. Buttes gives the heading "Carot, or red Parsnip." [39] Gerard describes three types — yellow, red, and wild.[40] He also refers to "candie carrots" and "stinking and deadly carrots." Here candie refers to the place of origin; the stinking and deadly types were not as fearful as they sound, and were used in medicine by French physicians.[41]

Gardiner, writing from the practical gardener's point of view, describes three sorts — the great long yellow carrot, the great short carrot, and the pale yellow common or wild carrot, which is small and long. He says the first two types can be profitable but the last sort "yeeld small profit, neither are they so good meate as the other two kinds by much."[42] The stated object of Gardiner's book is the "helpe and comforte of poor people"; besides giving directions for cooking carrots, Gardiner makes an impassioned plea for the growing of more carrots in England. His words have a faintly familiar ring.

> It is not unknowne to the Citty of London, . . . what great aboundance of carrets are brought by foraine nations to this land, whereby they have received yeerely great summes of money and commodities out of this land, and all by carelesnes of the people of this realme of England, which do not endevor themselves for their owne profits therein. . .[43]

John Coke, describing England in the middle of the sixteenth century, tells of many fruits such as "wardeines, quynces, peches, medlers, chestnottes and other delycious fruites serving for all seasons of the year,"[44] and refers especially to the plentifulness of pears and apples in the west of England and Sussex. The following list of fruits and nuts is divided into "local" and "imported" and refers to varieties familiar to-day.

Most of the fruits could be found in abundance in suitable parts of the country.

Many countries [sic] as Glocester-shire, Hereford-shire, Worcester-shire, great part of Kent and Sussex are so replenished with fruite, that it serveth the poorer sort not onely for foode a great part of the yeare, but also for drinke the most part of the yeare.[45]

Examples of local fruits and nuts mentioned are:

Apples	Pears
Apricots	Plums
Blackcurrants	Quinces
Cherries	Raspberries
Damsons	Rhubarb
Gooseberries	Strawberries
Hurtle or whortleberries	Almonds
Mulberries	Chestnuts
Medlers	Hazel-nuts
Peaches	Walnuts

Imported fruits and nuts mentioned are:

Capers[46]	Olives
Currants	Oranges
Dates	Raisins
Figs	Pomegranates
Grapes	Prunes
Lemons	Pistachio nuts

Imported fruits would have had a much more restricted market, but by the sixteenth century would be familiar in England. Oranges, for example, though a luxury until the end of the next century, had been known in England since the thirteenth century. Eleanor de Montfort, the Countess of Leicester, does not include them in her household accounts for 1265[47] but it is said that Edward I's queen bought seven oranges from a consignment of Spanish fruit landed at Portsmouth.[48]

By the sixteenth century oranges appear in the menus of noble houses and well-to-do merchants.[49]

Fresh fruits were rarely eaten, though occasionally used in salads. Fruits were used mainly in the making of drinks, syrups and conserves. They were also used in cooked dishes such as tarts and fritters.

The story of Catherine of Aragon needing a Dutch gardener to provide her with a salad has been used as an illustration of the lack of salads in England. Certainly the interest shown in salads by writers in the second half of the sixteenth century fell far short of that shown by writers in the next century, but salads are mentioned albeit without great enthusiasm. Langton places salads in the lowest of the three orders of foods.[50] Elyot recommends them for young men[51] and Hill describes the proper way to gather leaves for salads.[52] The type of "herbs and roots for sallads and sauce" are listed by Tusser:[53]

Alexander *[horse parsley]*	Rampions
Artichokes *[globe variety]*	Rocket
Blessed thistle	Sage
Cucumbers	Sorrell
Cresses	Spinage
Endive	Sea-holye
Mustard seed	Sperage
Musk-myllions *[Cucumis Melo]*	Skirrets
Mints	Suckery [Chicory]
Purslane	Tarragon
Radish	Violets

and he adds:

> These buy with the penny
> or look not for any

Capers	Oranges
Lemons	Rice
Olives	Samphire *[Crithmum maritimum]*

Other records show that carrots and onions were used as well as flowers. In fact, a wide variety of plants were advocated for use in salads. Of the ten salads for fish days in *The Good Huswifes Jewell*, three examples are given. Most salads were served with oil and vinegar:

(i) Olives and capers in one dish with vinegar and oil.

(ii) Minced (sic) carrot roots put in the dish with a proportion of "Flower de luce" (iris). Lay shrimps on it, with oil and vinegar.

(iii) Salmon, cut long ways, with slices of onion, "cast on violets," with oil and vinegar.[54]

How often, or how much, salads were taken is difficult to determine. André L. Simon points out[55] that the use of salads may be indicated by the reference to "herbs" and to salad oil, rather than to salads as such. Salad oil appears regularly in most household accounts.

The two modern vegetables conspicuous by their absence are potatoes and tomatoes, both of which had their origin in the New World. The first English printed description of a potato is given by Gerard, who caused some confusion between the sweet potato, the potato, and the so-called Jerusalem artichoke,[56] thus confusing chroniclers as to the date that *Solanum tuberosum* was introduced into England.[57] It is now believed that the potato came from America to Spain between 1564 and 1570. It may have been carried to Ireland by the ill-fated ships of the Armada, from where it was eventually carried back to Virginia as the "Irish potato." English sixteenth century writers on diet make no mention of the potato, for though it was established in Ireland it was not until the end of the eighteenth century that it became integrated into English farming.

The tomato is native to tropical America. The first reference in the *Oxford English Dictionary* is dated 1572, but tomatoes are not generally referred to by sixteenth century writers. Under the name "love apples" they were unpopular for centuries because of their supposedly aphrodisiacal or even poisonous characteristics. Although in the nineteenth century Mrs. Beeton gives a recipe for "Baked Tomatoes (Excellent),"[58] and Sir Henry Thompson writes favourably about them,[59] it is only in the present century that they have become so universally acceptable and generally available.

Other foods from the New World are: maize, buckwheat, and cacao. Coffee and tea were also new to England, originating in Ethiopia and China respectively. The last three (cacao, coffee, and tea) were introduced into England in the seventeenth century. Some tea came into the London market from a Dutch consignment in 1609[60] but remained exorbitantly expensive until it was sold to the general public by Thomas Garway in 1657.[61] The first English Coffee House was opened in Oxford in 1650 and the first in London in 1652. The first Chocolate House was opened in London in 1657.

Another important plant to arrive from America was tobacco. This was quickly accepted in England and so many people wished "to drink tobacco" (to use the contemporary expression) that King James I wrote disapprovingly about it being smoked or sniffed up,[62] but made good money from the taxes on it. Buttes, writing at the end of the sixteenth century, had advocated tobacco to counter excess in eating. Cogan does not refer to it at all.

Practical advice about the transport of fruits is given in *The Husbandman's fruitfull orchard*[63] written at the beginning of the seventeenth century. Here advice is given on the carriage of soft and hard fruits. Firstly, care must always be taken in the gathering of the fruit and all damage, bruising, and rough treatment must be avoided. Cherries can be carried on the head, in sieves reinforced underneath with lathes to prevent the head making a dent in the pile of fruit. When carried by ship or cart, cherries should be put into baskets, leaving a space at the top so that the basket above will not damage them. For short distances and small quantities the fruit can be taken on horseback in panniers lined with fern.

Pears should be gathered before they are fully ripe and packed in fern, the hard coarse stalks of the fern being kept outside the baskets. The pears will ripen on the journey but should be unpacked before quite ripe and laid on clean straw in a well aired, moderately cool place.

Apples can be wrapped in straw in layers and placed in maunds [wicker or woven baskets] directly they are picked, even if they are not dispatched directly. This will avoid double handling. Some suggest wrapping each apple separately in fern. Frosty weather or in March, "if the winde blow sharp" are "unfit times to remove or carry fruite by land or water."

The transport of herbs and leafy vegetables is not described. Root vegetables can be moved packed in a suitable dry material such as sand. To be stored, they should be chosen with care and have "all the branches" cut away. They can be packed unwashed in dry sand towards the end of December. When the roots start growing they should be taken out and the top cut off. They can then be repacked in sand and should last until Easter.

Detailed advice is given about the storage of apples, pears and nuts. Proper varieties must be chosen for storage, and the place where they are to be put chosen with care. The heaps must be watched and rotten fruit at the top and sides removed. Apparently rotten fruit in the middle or underneath was an expected loss. Handling of the fruit should be avoided where possible; nevertheless, it should be turned. The first time for turning is before Christmas, the second about Shrovetide, i.e, the beginning of April; thereafter it should be done at regular intervals, once a month, then once a fortnight. Pippins, considered a good fruit for storage, were expected to become wrinkled by the middle of May.

Methods by which plant foods can be preserved are: the removal of water, exclusion of air, preserving in acid, preserving in salt, preserving in sugar. All these methods were used to a greater or lesser degree in sixteenth century households. Herbs for drying should be gathered when properly grown, of a medium size, and in the right weather. This is on a dry day, preferably after rain. The leaves should be plucked off carefully and dried in the shade, away from dust and smoke. They should then be put in specially made boxes of leather or wood. Herbs treated in this way should keep a year.

Fruits can be dried whole or sliced either in the sun or a cool oven. Whole apples, for example, were peeled, cored with a bone corer, and strung up from the ceiling in long lines.[64]

The most usual way of excluding air was to use clarified fat or wax to stop up the opening of the vessels used. This was usually done in conjunction with pickling or the addition of sugar. Platt describes an elaborate method in which cherries or flowers can be preserved whole. The method requires special vessels with hooks inside, from which the cherry stalks can be hung over some "fayre" water. A tight lid is put on the vessel and this in turn is put within other suitable containers. It is claimed that fruit and flowers can be kept in good condition for two months.

References to pickled vegetables and fruit are not common, though it was recognized that fruits can "be long maintaind in vinegar."[65] A way which might be called partial pickling was to keep walnuts green and moist for two or three months by packing them in the "stampings of crab after verjuice is expressed."[66] This acid residue from crab apples preserved the nuts.

From English cookery books and household accounts it seems as if brine was used mostly for preserving animal materials, but such things as capers, peppers, and samphire are reported as being imported in brine.

The most common way of preserving vegetables, fruits, and flowers with sugar was in conserves or syrups, or by candying. Quince marmalade is mentioned by Buttes[67] and advocated to be eaten in the last course of the meal. Cogan gives instructions on the making of quince, pear, apple, medlar, cherry, strawberry, prune, damson ("or other plummes"), and marmalades.[68] The method is similar to that used to-day, but the proportions of the ingredients are not given.

Preserving fruit in a syrup was done in the following manner:[69]

> Take a pint of faire running water, halfe a pint of rose water, halfe a pounde of sugar, seethe all together upon a soft fire of coales, till the one halfe be consumed. . .

The mixture should then be taken from the fire and, when slightly cooled, cherries and plums shoud be added, of the same weight as the sugar used. This should be put on the fire again and cooked gently until the fruit is soft, "the space of an houre if neede bee." When it is cold, add some bruised cloves and "keepe it in a glasse or gallipote [glazed earthenware pot], the stronger the syrupe is with sugar the better it will continue." Other spices can be added, but there is a word of caution: "Seethe them not hastily for feare of much breaking."

Candied means "preserved or incrusted with sugar," a method commonly used at that time. The imaginative Sir Hugh Platt even prepared "candied" flowers on the plant by shaking a concentrated syrup upon the flowers in the sunlight.[70]

According to modern nutritional theory the importance of fruit and vegetables in the diet is due mainly to their contribution of the precursor of vitamin A (carotene) and to their vitamin C (ascorbic acid) content. Also in modern refined diets their contribution of roughage is important, a consideration which would not be of much significance with the less refined foods of the sixteenth century. The questions arise as to what, if any, was likely to be the incidence of deficiency diseases caused by lack of vitamins A and C during normal times in the sixteenth century.

The need for carotene is particularly important where the intake of dairy produce is restricted and liver is not eaten regularly, as these foods supply vitamin A.[71] Carotene is present in most red, yellow, and dark green leafy vegetables, and it appears that most groups of the English population would regularly include herbs and perhaps vegetables of this type in their dishes. Because carotene is stable in normal cooking procedures (damage is done by higher temperatures rather than longer cooking times), it is likely to have remained available even with the prolonged methods of cooking of the period. Therefore, under normal conditions gross deficiencies of vitamin A were likely to be unusual.

The matter of vitamin C is different. This vitamin is required at regular intervals (preferably daily) as it cannot be stored in the body in the way that vitamin A can be stored for later use. It is extremely unstable, being affected by heat and storage, though this occurs to a lesser degree in an acid medium (as in acid fruits). The amounts of the vitamin believed to be required daily are still unsettled.[72] Furthermore, although a deficiency of each of the vitamins produces individually characteristic symptoms, in poor diets these can often overlap and confuse the diagnosis. Also, in the early stages of a vitamin deficiency it is not always easy to distinguish deficiency symptoms from those of other common complaints. This modern viewpoint has been put at some length to help illustrate the difficulties of trying to estimate any incidence of scurvy in Elizabethan times. Lind, in the "Bibliotheca scorbutica," *A Treatise of the Scurvy* (1753), indicated that a number of Latin works by continental writers on scurvy were published in the sixteenth century.[73] However, English writers on the preservation of health make only passing references to scurvy, usually in company with other conditions which present some similar symptoms. Towards the end of the century the disease and its symptoms were known in England. Gerard gives a clear description[75] of the

> disease which the Germaines call Scorbuck and Scorbuyt: in Latin *Scorbutus*: which we in England call the Scurvie and Scurby, and upon the Seas the Skyrby . . .[75]

Of the variety of remedies suggested, many include plants which we know today to contain ascorbic acid and which would have been available in England at that period. Gerard, for example, emphasizes the benefits of cresses,[76] but a large number of anti-scorbutic herbs and vegetables would have been available.[77] The position regarding fruit is best described by the author of the *Fruitful Orchard,* who says:

> Now, therefore, since it hath pleased Almighty God, to give encrease & plenty of fruite in this land, and that divers have taken paines in the maintenance thereof, of all degrees: (the better sort for their pleasure, & in that they doe delight to see the worke of their owne handes prosper, as also to eate the fruite thereof; the common sort, for profit, and for the better reliefe of their family) In regard, I say, of the great paines that have been taken, in planting, setting, grafting, & proyning, whereby a great deale of ground hath been taken up, which might serve for other good purposes; I thought good to shew what course might bee taken, that mens Labours be not lost, nor such great quantity of ground, wherein fruite doth growe, lye in waste (as it were) and become unprofitable, through ignorance of well handling the fruite, after God hath given it.[78]

That the Elizabethans neither lacked or ignored fruits and vegetables is apparent from both the mass of material written and the practical advice given for their use. How frequently, or in what quantities they were used, by the average person at various levels of society, is impossible to decide, but it does seem likely that in normal times and conditions the plant foods available were sufficient to prevent any marked incidence of scurvy.

CHAPTER XVI
SPICES, SAUCES AND SWEET THINGS

... hunger and thirst are the best Sawces for meate and drinke. . .but there bee other sawces which bee artificiall of which I will set down those that bee most usual.

T. Cogan (1584)

And this precious iewel hony, hath beene evermore praysed above sugar, for it will conserve and keepe any frute, herb, rote, or any other thing that is put into it an exceeding long time.

William Bullein (1595)

THE WIDESPREAD REFERENCES to spices and sweet things in early English cookery recipes are well known. Numerous examples of their use can be found in the *Forme of Cury,* in fifteenth century cookery manuscripts and the printed cookery books of the sixteenth century.[1]

For a long period the pattern of the spice trade exerted a profound influence on European politics, and for centuries England obtained imports of spices from Asia via Europe, where trade was under the control of Mediterranean powers such as Genoa and Venice. The discovery of the Cape of Good Hope (1486), and the development of new routes, drastically altered the balance of monopolies. By the Treaty of Tordesillas (1494) the Pope divided the world into two spheres of influence, the dominating forces being Spain and Portugal. However, this dictum was ignored by many and towards the end of the sixteenth century the Dutch had made a powerful entry into the field of the spice trade through their carefully designed and strictly controlled monopoly of trade with the Spice Islands. So far England had been only on the outskirts of the competition, but the foundation of what was to be centuries of profitable trade was laid by the incorporation under royal charter (in 1600) of "The Governors and Company of Merchants of London trading into the East Indies." Voyages to the Far East started in 1601 and in time reached as far as Japan. Eventually competition

N.B. Footnotes to this chapter appear on pages 346-351.

between the English and Dutch came to a crisis (in the so-called "Massacre of Amboina" in 1623), after which England withdrew her operations to the area of India and adjoining countries.

From the pattern of monopolies it was inevitable that most spices should be quite costly in England, and records show that these valuable commodities were kept carefully under lock and key in a spice box or cupboard. Because these items were frequently stored together they were also often grouped into one item in the household accounts against one overall price. Current retail prices for individual spices are therefore often difficult to find. The figures given here are intended as an indication of prices in the year quoted and are taken from domestic accounts and commercial records.[2]

The grouping of spices and sauces given below is based on that used generally by sixteenth century writers on diet — that is, the classification into "spices" and "sauces or condiments." The designation of sugar and salt as "sauces" may seem odd to modern eyes, but it is understandable when dictionary definitions are examined. According to the *OED* "sauce" is described as any preparation, usually liquid or soft, and often consisting of several ingredients, intended to be eaten as an appetizing accompaniment to some article of food, and formerly occasionally applied to a condiment of any kind. A "condiment" is anything of pronounced flavour used to season or give relish to a food or to stimulate appetite.

The table below includes those items emphasized by a representative selection of writers. It omits a number of plants used for flavourings, which authors class under the heading of herbs. A large proportion of the spices and sauces were imported. The material presented in the table is not arranged chronologically but in the form best suited to the table and its contemporary groupings.

	Cogan	*Buttes*	*Bullein*	*Boorde*	*Gratarolus*[3] (Newton)
	(1589)	(1599)	(1595)	(1542)	(1574)
	pepper	pepper	cloves	ginger	not
S	cloves	cinnamon	galingale	pepper	classified
P	mace	cloves	pepper	cloves	
I	nutmegs	ginger	ginger	mace	
C	ginger	nutmeg	cinnamon	cardamoms	
E	galingale[4]	saffron	saffron	saffron	
S	cinnamon			nutmeg	
	saffron[4]			cinnamon	
	(sugar)			liquorice	

S	salt	sugar	salt	not	salt
A	vinegar	honey	vinegar	listed	oils
U	mustard	salt	mustard		honey
C	common	vinegar	honey		sugar
E	sauce	mustard	treacle[5]		vinegar
S		green sauce	methridatum		(cinnamon)

Of the five authors listed, Cogan and Buttes classify items under spices and sauces; the other authors group together the appropriate items, but do not call them spices or sauces. Reference is also made to the *Regimen Sanitatis* (1528), though it lacks any classification of spices or sauces. In it the various items are put (seemingly) anywhere — e.g., nutmeg is placed after eggs and before the advice about drinking wine and eating pears.

The spices discussed include: pepper, cinnamon, cloves, ginger and galingale, mace and nutmeg, saffron, cardamon, and liquorice.

Spices

Pepper. Pepper is one of the commodities which had a marked effect on the pattern of commerce for many centuries. It formed one of the earliest staple commodities in Indo-European trade. Sanskrit writers frequently mentioned it. Theophrastus referred to black and long peppers,[6] and Dioscorides to white pepper.[7] It was considered a valuable commodity in Rome and was awarded as booty to victorious Genoese soldiers in Caesarea in A.D.1101.[8] Clair also suggests that the earliest reference to the pepper trade in England is in the statutes of Ethelred (978-1016). During feudal times the payment of "pepper rents" (usually about one pound by weight of pepper) for land held in "socage"* was exceedingly common and indicates the value of the commodity. The cost of pepper in the mid-thirteenth century fluctuated around 10d. per pound. This can be compared with the price of fresh pigs at 3/6 each quoted for the same period.[9]

In the sixteenth century Walter Bailey lists the three types of pepper in common use as black white and long. He adds that "many herbs of our writers are termed by the name of pepper," and gives such examples as water pepper, hill pepper, mouse pepper, herb pepper, and savoury pepperwort. But authors in England (he says) describe true pepper by using the single word *Piper* without any addition.[10] In

---

*Socage was a form of land tenure held by certain determinate services other than knight-services.

discussing the black, white and long peppers Bailey refers to the confusion of thought regarding whether or not all three sorts grow on the
same plant.[11] The ancient writers believed that they were all three the
fruit of one tree, saying that the long pepper is the first growth or
"rudiment" of the pepper and that the terms "white" and "black"
referred to the degree of ripeness of the pepper grains.[12] A later version
was that black pepper was blackened by fire because, according to the
story, the serpents which lived under the pepper trees had to be driven
off by fire before the pepper could be harvested.[13] Sixteenth century
writers concluded that black and white peppers came from the same
sort of tree, but that the difference in colour was unrelated to ripening;
rather it was similar to that of white or red grapes, both of which grow
on vines and are unchanged in colour by the degree of ripening.[14]
Bailey forgives the Greeks for their error but berates the Arabs for their
negligence in not observing the truth when they lived near to where
pepper grows.[15] Gerard states quite clearly that

> The tree that beareth long Pepper, hath no similitude at all with the
> plant that bringeth blacke and white Pepper . . . for they grow in
> countries far distant one from another.[16]

A variety of names is used to describe long pepper. One description
used in England is "pepper from Ethiopia." This term seems to cover a
multitude of varieties when used by sixteenth century writers. Included
is *Amomum melegueta* (see cardamon, below).

Bailey writing in 1588, says that he has seen "whole clusters of pepper preserved in brine and in salt" at Poole in Dorset and in London. He
adds: "Long pepper is to be seene in every shop."[17] Unfortunately, the
price paid for pepper in the shops is not available. *The Northumberland
Household Book* gives a price of 16 pence per pound for the year 1512,
while *The Rate Book* for 1604 gives a valuation of 2/6 per pound for
long pepper. The price is likely to have fluctuated considerably in the
period.

"The operation of al sortes of Pepper differ little," says Cogan,
though white pepper ("as Galen writeth") is best for the stomach.[19] All
kinds of pepper heat the body, contrary to the prevalent view that pepper is cold in operation. Bullein also makes a point of contradicting the
view that pepper is hot in the mouth and cold in the stomach.[19] This
striking difference of opinion as to whether pepper is hot or cold is
referred to by Gerard, who explains that Arab and Persian physicians

say that pepper is hot in the third degree but that Indian physicians, "which for the most part are Empericke,"[20] say that pepper is cold.[21] It is perhaps of interest that the general idea of pepper (by the "vulgar") should follow the Indian physicians rather than the Arabs, particularly when the apparent effect of pepper is far from cooling and the traditional *Regimen Sanitatis* described pepper as hot and dry in the third degree.[22]

The degree of heat ascribed to pepper varies from the fourth to the third degree. This change is illustrated in Batman's edition of the *De Proprietatibus Rerum*[23] of Bartholomeus Anglicus, where the original says that pepper is hot and dry in the fourth degree and Batman's addition (clearly indicated) says hot and dry in the third degree. In terms of the general value of pepper such a change in degree would not seem to be of very great significance as regards its value. However, sixteenth century writers did take the trouble to correct the value from the fourth to "the end of the third degree." Buttes compromises and says that pepper is "hot and dry in the third [degree] and almost in the beginning of the fourth."[24]

The general value of pepper is most often described in rather vague terms, such as: it has the virtue to temper and dissolved, to consume waste and to draw.[25] It also does certain other things: (i) it comforts the stomach and helps digestion; (ii) it helps the colic or any discomfort caused by wind, and expels urine; (iii) it helps a cough, dissolving phlegm and helping to overcome diseases of the breast caused by cold; (iv) it "withstands the causes of a cold fever being given before the fit" (the timing of taking foods during the progress of a fever was considered critical; (v) it eases the "shakings" caused by fevers.[26]

Besides these main benefits pepper also cleared the head of "phlegms and rheums," by causing the person to sneeze after powdered pepper had been put up the nose. It also resists poisons and is a good mendicament for the eyes, as it cleanses the dimness of sight. A number of powerfully aromatic spices were considered to be helpful in improving the sight.

Pepper is hurtful to hot constitutions especially if taken in hot weather. and if used without moderation it "burneth the blood."[27] Blood was of course, recognized as being hot and moist in a temperate degree; any heating of the blood would badly affect the body's balance of humours.

Pepper was taken both in the spicing of everyday foods, as in "to boile chickens," "to bake Calves feet," and "To make peascods,"[28] and also in a "special confection" (Cogan's term) made of all these types of peppers and called *"Diatron piperion."*[29] This was considered particularly good for a cold windy stomach and could be taken at any time of the day, preferably after food. The ingredients were usually such things as white, black, and long pepper, thyme, ginger, aniseed, and parsley seed, all pounded and boiled in a solution of sugar and hyssop water. The recipe, as given in *The Widdowes Treasure,* has an additional few verses extolling the virtues of *Diatrion piperion* and includes the information that it will restore memory.[30] Bailey reminds his readers that it can be obtained from apothecary shops.[31] The cost of pepper would have prohibited its use by the poor, but those who could afford it recognized that its dietary velue went far beyond the flavour it added to a great variety of dishes.

Cinnamon. True cinnamon is the dried inner bark of *C. Zeylanicum,* a small evergreen tree native to Ceylon. Gerard calls it the "Cannell or Cinnamon tree," and explains that *Cassia* and *Cassia lignea* are also "unproperly" called cinnamon by some.[32] This confusion between cinnamon and cassia is of ancient origin.[33] Among sixteenth century writers on foods, some recognize the difference, and others do not. Cogan appears to confuse the two materials when he says, describing cinnamon,

> That which we have is the barke or rinde of a certaine tree growing in the Indies, and is the right Cassia, as *Math.* thinketh.[34]

Buttes recognizes that the "cinnamon" usually available in England is "not the right and true spice," but explains that true cinnamon is rare and scarce and therefore little is brought to England.[35] This scarcity was in fact partly due to the monopoly held on cinnamon by the Portuguese whereby the English could obtain it only from Lisbon instead of directly from the East. Gerard, in describing *Cassia fistula* or pudding pipe, states categorically that the "old cassia fistula" is now called canella by the apothecaries, "which they use instead of the right Cinnamone, but deceitfully." Gerard describes the pulp of this cassia as being moist in the end of the first degree and a little more than temperately hot.[36] However, other writers, when describing cinnamon (whatever its true identity),[37] class it as hot and dry in the third degree. All acknowledge its considerable use in medicine and in food.

Cinnamon is accepted as "very comfortable to the stomacke and principall parts of the bodie."[38] The parts actually referred to by various authors include: the brain, breast, liver, spleen, entrails, kidneys, and sinews. Cinnamon is also important in easing inflamed intestines, wind, dropsy, and coughs. It causes the menses, provokes urine, resists poisons, preserves sight, makes sweet breath, gives a good colour to the face, and preserves from putrefaction. In general, it restores and preserves "the debilities of nature."[39] The list of benefits attributed to cinnamon seem remarkably wide even by sixteenth century standards.

The method most frequently recommended for taking cinnamon was as "cinnamon water." A number of recipes are available. Gerard mentions the distilled waters of the flowers of the cinnamon tree; he also refers to oil from cinnamon berries, but the most common cinnamon water was made by an infusion of the dried bark.[40] Cogan suggests taking a pound of cinnamon (well beaten), a gallon of sack, a pound of "sugar-candie" (sugar clarified and crystallized by slow evaporation). Mix them together and put "to steepe all together and so distill [infuse] them." Students are advised to keep some of this valuable remedy to hand in their closets and to take "now and then a spoonefull."[41]

Cinnamon seems to have been a popular flavour in cookery. *The good Huswives handmaid* includes cinnamon in the following recipes: (i) boiled leg of mutton with a pudding, (ii) mutton for the sick, (iii) quails, (iv) sweet pies made of veal, (v) oysters, (vi) cream, (vii) ipocras, (vii) posset curd, and (ix) pancakes.[42] It was also widely used when cooking fruits.

The Countess of Leicester's private accounts in the year 1265 show prices for cinnamon ranging from 10d. to 1/– per pound, a price range that remained constant throughout the century.[43] The references used here for prices of spices during the sixteenth century do not include cinnamon. It is probable that the cost of cinnamon was of the same order as other imported spices, and it appears to have been well liked and considered a valuable item from the dietary point of view.

Cloves. Henry Buttes, in his lighthearted notes called "storie for Table-talke," referring to cloves (or clowes as he spells them), suggests that the word is derived from "glowes" because the "vehement and ardent heat of clowes" causes a glowing in the mouth.[44] Be that as it may, the accepted virtues of cloves throughout the Middle Ages had made them a valuable commodity. Cogan says "no spice is of more force,"[45] but unfortunately does not elaborate further.

Authors agree that cloves are hot and dry in the third degree and have the following beneficial effects:

Help those afflicted by wind and stoppages of the liver.

Comfort the stomach and principal parts of the body, including liver, spleen, and sinews.

Strengthen the brain and entrails.

Stop diarrhoea.

Help those with dropsy.

Provoke urine.

Act as an aphrodisiac.

Resist poison.

Aid the sight.

Amend stinking breath.

Preserve from "putrification."

In general, cloves help to restore and preserve. They should, however, be avoided by choleric people.

The cloves used in sixteenth century England were the same types as are used today — namely, the unopened flower buds of the clove tree, which "when they be dried in the sunne, they become of that dustie blacke colour which we daily see."[46] In view of their virtues and the degree of their qualities, cloves were used in many ways, both as a medicine and as a food.

Used *whole*, cloves were put into many dishes for flavouring, though it was recognized that too much clove causes an unpleasant bitter taste.[47] Examples of dishes in which cloves were used are: (i) boiled duck, (ii) stewed birds, (iii) a "florentine," (iv) a good custard, (v) eel pie for Lent, (vi) stewed hare, (vii) roast venison.[48]

In *powdered form* cloves were also used widely for their "sweet savours" in hot milk and for distilled waters, i.e. in aromatic drinks.

Oil of cloves was extracted from cloves (according to Gerard) in the form of a "thicke butter of a yellow colour." This material, he says, was used by Indians to cure wounds in the same way the English used balsam.[49] The oil of cloves generally used in England seems to have been in a more liquid form, because reference is made to oil or water of cloves being dropped in the eyes (it is to be hoped much diluted) to increase the sharpness of sight.[50]

According to Gerard, cloves are one of the commodities not known to the Greeks and therefore might not be as familiar to Europeans as many other spices.[51] Clair suggested that they must have been rare in England before the discovery of the Cape of Good Hope. Cloves were always costly in England; those reaching England before this time were fantastically expensive, sometimes "nearly four hundred times their first cost."[52] It is known that the Countess of Leicester bought cloves in comparatively small amounts (a pound or half a pound) in 1265 at the very high price of 13/– per pound. However, later in that century the price fell to around 2/– per pound.[53] Prices for cloves in England in the sixteenth century are not easy to find. *The Northumberland Household Book* gives a price of 8/– per pound for "mace and cloves." Roberts does not list cloves in his *Rate Book* figures (1604). Writing in 1623, Gerard Malynes gives 9d. per pound as the cost of cloves in the East Indies and says they were valued in England (excluding various import charges to be paid at 5/ per pound.[54] These figures, of course, refer to the period when the Dutch held the monopoly from the East Indies.

In view of the high cost of cloves and the range of dishes in which they might have been included it is fortunate and of interest that recipes are available which give some indication of the quantity in which they would have been used. The following recipe "To make a good Gellie" illustrates the proportions used of a number of spices.[55]

Jelly water is made from four calves' feet, scalded (to remove hair), and then boiled until tender. To this is added some claret wine and a little malmsey. The following ingredients are then added:

> 1 pottel (2 quarts) of gelly water
> 1 quart wine
> 1 pint malmsey
> salt for "seasoning"
> 1 lb. sugar
> 1 oz. ginger
> 1½ oz. cinnamon
> 12 cloves
> 12 pepper corns
> a little saffron.

All these ingredients are to be boiled together. Then add a saucer full of vinegar with "turnsall"[56] in it, and the whites of eggs (no quantity given). The whole mixture is boiled again and strained. These proportions of ingredients suggest quite a highly flavoured dish compared to modern English standards, which (except in curried dishes) usually use spices in such large proportions only for spiced drinks.[57]

Ginger and Galingale. Ginger is one of the earliest Oriental spices known to Europeans.[58] It was mentioned in leech books in England in

Anglo-Saxon times.[59] It was frequently recommended in recipes of the thirteenth and fourteenth centuries. The "Goodman of Paris" distinguishes between the quality of ginger from various sources.[60] Gerard describes his difficulties in getting an accurate drawing of the ginger plant and is indebted to Mathias L'Obel for his information.[61] The difference in gingers noted by writers in the sixteenth century was between dry ginger and green ginger, the latter being candied with sugar or honey. The frequent references made to the fact that ginger should not be rotten indicates some difficulty in keeping it.

Though most authors differentiate clearly between the qualities of dry and green ginger (dry ginger is hot in the third and dry in the second degree; green ginger is similarly hot but moist in the first or second degree), they are not so specific in allocating benefits to the two kinds. In general, ginger has these virtues:

It makes food go down into the stomach easily.

It heats the stomach (more slowly than pepper).

It aids digestion.

It removes phlegm.

It "provoketh sluggish husbands" (according to Buttes).[62]

It quickens the memory; it is especially recommended for students, to be taken as green ginger, before food, first thing in the morning.[63]

It aids sight.

The references to aiding the sight are fairly precise. Ginger helps against the "darkness of the sight."[64] Dioscorides had recommended it for those things "which darken the Pupillae."[65] Cogan gives the quantities of sugar and spices required to make an eyewash which in a short time will (he says) have "worne away a fleume growne over the eye."[66] On the other hand De Laurens,[67] writing about sight, says that strong spices such as ginger, pepper, and mustard hurt the eyes. It is not clear if this refers to an external application, or an oral one.

The prices of ginger available do not always indicate the type of ginger referred to. It does not seem to be one of the most expensive spices, though it certainly was not cheap. *The Northumberland Household Book* gives a price of 4/– per pound, and the *Rate Book* of 1604 lists green ginger at 1/– per pound.

Ginger was much used for making *ipocras*, but was also added to a wide variety of dishes, including meat, fish, and fruit. Some examples are: (i) stewed mutton, (ii) pheasant, (iii) baked pork, (iv) apple tart, (v) hare, (vi) boiled bream, (vii) baked fresh salmon (in pastry).[68] Ginger was also an ingredient (with sugar and cinnamon) in "Blanch powder," which was sprinkled on cooked dishes such as baked apples.

An alternative sometimes used in England is *galingale* which, according to the *Oxford English Dictionary*, can refer either to an oriental root (the name being derived from the Chinese meaning "mild ginger from KO"), or to a type of English sedge, the root of which has properties similar to the oriental variety.

The galingale generally referred to by sixteenth century English authors is a variety of sedge (e.g. *Cyperus longus*). The term "galingale" was also sometimes applied to a variety of sea-grass. Bullein refers only to 'galingell" without identifying it.[69] Cogan says "galingale or rather Cypresse roots," and adds "though it be rare yet is found in some Gardens."[70] Gerard describes four varieties — namely, English galingale, Spanish galingale (or sweet cyperus). round cyperous and cat-taile grass *(Cyperus Typhinus).*[71]

It is generally agreed that galingale is hot and dry in the second or the third degree. Taken by mouth it helps to:

break down and expel the stone.

aid in digestion.

warm the body.

provoke urine.

ease dropsy.

cause the menses.

act as a remedy against snake venom.

refresh the spirits and mind.

improve the colour and make sweet breath.

Applied externally, it is helpful for dropsy in a limb, or when applied to persistent ulcers in the mouth or anal region. The mixture to be applied includes powdered galingale, liquorice roots, and bayberries, mixed with the urine of a boy under fourteen years of age.[72] Cogan (referring to Fernal) also says galingale is beneficial when added to baths.

No records have been found of a household price for galingale; it appears that its uses were predominantly medicinal.[73] A survey of contemporary cookery books suggests that galingale was rarely used in cooking.

Mace and Nutmeg. Mace is the outer covering or husk of the fruit of the nutmeg tree, the kernel being called the nutmeg. Gerard describes this difference accurately, but lists only the virtues of nutmeg.[74] Boorde also omits mace, but some authors attempt to differentiate between the two spices.

Mace. Mace is hot in the second degree and dry in the third.[75] Its main benefit to man seems to be related to the stomach, which it comforts and restores; for this it should be taken "boyled whole in brothes or coleies [a sort of broth] or milke."[76] Mace is also good against bloody fluxes, colic, and the spitting of blood.

Prices for mace are not often listed. In *The Northumberland Household Book* mace is included with cloves at 8/– per pound. In the figures given by Malynes in 1623 mace is valued in England, without import charges, at 6/– per pound.[77] In the same list nutmegs are valued at 3/– per pound

In cookery, mace was included in a wide variety of recipes, such as: (i) stewed cock, (ii) stewed beef, (iii) veal, (iv) hare, (v) venison, (vi) bream, (vii) stewed herring.[78] Mace seems to have been used to a much greater extent with meat and fish dishes than in the cooking of fruits or vegetables.

Nutmeg. Nutmegs are hot and dry, both in the second degree.[79] If chewed they will cause sweet breath and "amend those that do stinke." Nutmeg is good against freckles; it quickens the sight, eases diarrhoea, breaks wind, provokes urine, strengthens the belly and weak livers, and "it taketh away the swelling in the spleene."[80] This specific reference to an effect of nutmeg on the spleen is unusual, being more precise than the other vague terms more commonly used, such as "comforts" or "strengthens."

Cogan believes nutmegs are particularly beneficial to students; in fact, he says "And in my judgement it [nutmeg] is the best spice for students of all other."[81] He bases this view on the fact that it comforts the brain and sight as well as the stomach and spleen. For "weake heades" he advocates nutmegs taken in a caudel[82] of almonds or hempseed, as this will send the person to sleep. (He makes no comment here on the part hempseed plays in this operation.)[83] His final advice is that students should keep a supply of candied nutmegs, available from "apothycaries" by them always.

The household books examined for this study do not provide prices of nutmeg. The *Rate Book* of 1604 gives a valuation of 4/– per pound for candied nutmegs, which were the most commonly used. Cookery recipes show only a limited use of nutmegs, though this use does range from a stuffing for pork to *ipocras.*[84]

Saffron. By the sixteenth century the growing of saffron was well established in England. Harrison describes it at some length.[85] He says it was first planted around Saffron Walden in the time of Edward III (1312-1377),[86] and describes the crop from both its botanical and various agricultural aspects, including yields per acre and monetary returns. Gerard, in his index to his *Herball,* lists several kinds of saffron. These include the common saffron, vernal saffron, bastard saffron, and wild bastard saffron.[87] This study concentrates on the common variety.

Saffron is described as hot in the second degree and dry in the third (Gerard), or dry in the first degree (Cogan and Buttes). It is a little astringent or binding, but the hot quality overrules, and this gives saffron "a certain force to concoct."[88] Considerable stress is placed on the harm that an excess intake of saffron can cause The emphasis here is greater than for other spices which could also be harmful taken immoderately. Too much saffron can cause headaches and sleeplessness. and could be deadly.[89] However, the list of saffron's virtues is very long and (briefly) is as follows:

It strengthens the heart.

It concocts raw humours of the chest.

It removes obstructions in the lungs.

It is good for consumption.

It is good against surfeit.

It is good against the yellow jaundice or a "stoppage" of the liver.[90]

It is good for internal diseases [in general] and after childbirth.

It provokes urine.

It provokes Venus.

Used in a poultice, it is good for aches and swellings, including those of St. Anthony's fire.[91]

It can be added to eardrops.

Added to milk, it is valuable as an eyewash.

Taken with walnuts, figs, sage, mithridatium, and pimpernel water, it acts as a prophylactic against the pestilence.

(Harrison points out that, in addition to its medicinal virtues, saffron kills moths.)

Cogan puts saffron in his section on herbs and gives as his reason that saffron "is so usuall in meates."[92]

A random selection of recipes using saffron are: (i) baked oranges, (ii) calves' head, (iii) Lenten pottage with eels, (iv) almond butter (one of many sorts), (v) apple fritters.[93] Saffron was also used in breads and buns, and for colouring matter.

As far as can be judged from the somewhat limited records available, saffron appears to be the cheapest of the spices in the sixteenth century. This is likely to have encouraged its widespread use.

In 1556 there appears to have been a glut of saffron, followed by a shortage. Harrison emphasizes that (around 1577) more saffron ought to be grown.[94] Through the century the price of saffron generally seems to have been low. *The Northumberland Household Book* quotes 4d. per pound, and the Petre family accounts refer to "2d. for saffron for the kitchen," no quantity being specified.[95] Drummond and Wilbraham quote a high price for saffron — 20/— per pound.[96] This is derived from Harrison's references to yields per acre. The original text is not quite as specific about the exact quantity of saffron equivalent to £20 as the marginal notes in Furnivall's edited version[97] indicate. This price certainly contradicts the other prices quoted above. Imported saffron was one of the most expensive spices[98] but in the sixteenth century its widespread use indicates a marked lowering in price.

It is of interest that by the sixteenth century the garbelling (inspection, cleansing and purifying) of spices was recognized as requiring the control of the Grocers Company of London; Saffron is not listed in the instructions provided by "divers grocers" (written about 1592).[99] Harrison believes that the sale of saffron was open to much abuse; he says "there is no more deceit used in anie trade than in saffron," and describes some of the tricks used to deceive customers.[100]

Cardamom. Today cardamom seeds come from the cultivated perennial plant *Elettaria cadamomum*. The ripe fruits contain small, dark brown, highly aromatic seeds used in the preparation of curry powder, gingerbread, sausages, pickles, and as a flavour for cakes. They are also used in the preparation of some aromatic drugs.

In earlier times the Latin name *cardamomum* was linked (according to Gerard)[101] in Bengali with a number of names, including "Guzarata," "Decan Hil," and "of some Mileguetta and Milegetta." In English they are referred to as "Graines" and "Graines of Paradise." Whatever the confusion between varieties of peppers and wild cardamom in the sixteenth century there was a clear understanding of the benefits of grains of paradise or cardamom among writers on diet. They were hot and dry in the third degree and similar in operation to pepper. If chewed, they draw out the watery humours from the head and stomach. They are good for women. Taken in sack, they "helpeth the agewe, and riddeth the shaking fits."[102] All who have cold stomachs should take them, and Cogan says "Olde folks use them often in their drinke either for some speciall propertie, or else because they are better cheape than other spices."[103] However, *The Northumberland Household Book* quotes them at 12d. per pound, which is not the cheapest spice.

Liquorice. Neither Cogan, Bullein, or Buttes makes any specific reference to liquorice. Boorde says briefly, "Lyqueryce is good to clense and to open the lunges and brest and doth loose fleume."[104] Gerard describes two types — the common variety, and "Hedgehogge Licorice."[105] He says he grows common liquorice in his garden and that a good crop is obtained by the poor people in the north of England, who manure the plants diligently. The fresh root is sweet, of "temperate" heat, and more moist than dry. Like Boorde, Gerard advocates it for clearing the lungs and for sore throats.[106] This is done by sucking a lump of the hardened juice. When drunk with (raisin) wine liquorice, it helps "infirmities" of the liver and chest, as well as scabs or sores of the bladder and ulcers of the mouth. It is helpful in diseases of the kidneys and "mitigates" the sharpness and saltness of raw humours. Applied externally the juice is good for new wounds, and the dry, finely powdered root benefits the eyes. Langham, in his *The Garden of Health,*[107] which deals with the medicinal properties of "simples and plants"), gives 23 suggestions for the benefits and use of liquorice. (This is a comparatively small number for Langham, who gives 63 sections under pepper and 114 under onions.)

Though liquorice is used in the making of ginger bread its main use is medicinal, particularly related to the respiratory system. *The Northumberland Household Book* gives a price of 6d. per pound for "Licoras powder," but no prices for what we would now call "liquorice sticks" have been found.

Sauces

When the term "sauce" is used in the sixteenth century manner — i.e., to include salt, vinegar, mustard, common and green sauces, oils, sugar, and honey — then naturally there are very few dishes likely to be eaten without some sauce.[108] However, in the narrower sense of a particular flavour, or mixture of flavours, to be served with certain dishes, a number of specific rules were advocated. *The Booke of Carving and Sewing,*[109] in describing the serving and carving of meats, indicates which sauces should or should not be served with particular dishes. For example, under "Sauce that capon" we read "chickins shal be sauced with greene sauce or vergris." Under "Aley that fesant" the instructions end ". . . and no sauce but only salt." Though the advice given is not always quite clear to a modern reader, some indication of the sauces to be used is given. There follows a selection from the many examples available:[110]

Sauce	Meat	Fish
White salt	snipes, pheasant	
Salt & cinnamon	sparrows, thrushes	
mustard	brawn, beef, bacon, mutton	salt herring, other fish, eels.
mustard & sugar	lamb, pig, fawn	
mustard, garlic & pepper	ribs of beef	
green sauce	capons	halibut, fresh turbot.
vergis (verjuice)	boiled chickens, capons	
sauce gamelin	woodcock, lark, quail, venison	

All these items are discussed below in this section, except "sauce gamelin." This may also be referred to as "gamelyn" or "camelin," and according to the *OED* it is a "dainty Italian sauce." It usually contained raisin, nuts, bread crusts, cloves, ginger, and cinnamon, all powdered together and mixed with vinegar.[111]

In general the meat or fish dishes were served to a mess, each member helping himself from the main dish. The sauces were served separately, each for the appropriate meat.

The instructions in *The Booke of Carving*. . . were intended for noble households, but many of the sauces would be available to poorer establishments in a comparable if not an exactly identical form. The number and variety of the sauces used to match the number of dishes and individual tastes must have been very large indeed so that, as Cogan says, "it were an infinite matter to fully discourse therein."[112]

Salt. According to the *Encyclopaedia Britannica* (14th edition), "the habitual use of salt is intimately connected with the advance from nomadic to agricultural life." The importance of salt in the life of men through the centuries is reflected in the ideas and terms related to salt in our language today. These range from the idea of the "covenant of salt" in the Bible (Num. xviii, 19) to the *salarium* or a monetary allowance given to a Roman soldier in lieu of his salt ration.

In sixteenth century England "the sawce most common of all other is

Salt."[113] Salt is so necessary to man (says Cogan) that he cannot live without it, and it is for this reason that salt is the first thing to be set on the table and should be the last to be removed.[114]

The two kinds of salt in general use were Bay salt and White salt. Other salts were used by physicians, but as they were not used for food they are not included by writers on diet. Bay salt was produced from sea water, while white salt came from the evaporation of the brine from natural brine springs and wells, particularly those found in Cheshire "at the townes called the wiches," and in Lincolnshire, and near Newcastle.[115] The boiling of this brine gave a good white salt suitable for salting all kinds of flesh. Two representative prices of white salt are: from *The Northumberland Household Book*, 4/– per quarter, and from the Petre household 2½d per ½peck (by volume, this is one gallon).[116]

Despite the very widespread use of salt, it was well recognized that too much was harmful. Salt is hot and dry, and this dryness makes it useful in resisting poison and gives it the power to consume all corrupt humours and dry up superfluous humours such as blood and water; but care must be taken by lean and choleric people regarding the amount of salt they take. Too much salt makes the body "appear aged and to be angry."[117] Excess salt can also cause a variety of skin irritations because it engenders sharp and biting humours. Cogan explains that he cured an "Itche" from which he had suffered for a number of years at Oxford by abstaining from salt for a year.[118]

It is noteworthy that despite, or perhaps *because* of the widespread use of salt, advisers on diet emphasize the harm it can do rather than stressing its virtues. The correct approach to the eating of salt is summed up by Bullein when he says "The verie use of it is onely to season meates not to be meate."[119]

Vinegar. Today vinegar is described as a product of the alcoholic and subsequent acetic fermentation of a wide variety of saccharine liquids. Basically it is dilute acetic acid flavoured and coloured by materials extracted from its source material. In the sixteenth century "right Vinegar is made of wine onely."[120] There were two kinds of wine vinegar available, namely red and white, but provided the vinegar had been properly made, the colour was not significant. At the same time, "vinegars" were also made from a mixture of ale and wine, or from ale alone (coloured with turnesol and called by Cogan "Aliger"), or with beer alone. Bickerdyke refers to officials appointed to inspect breweries to see if "vyneagre" or "al-eagre" or "bear-eagre" were being made.[121]

The cost of vinegar depended in part on its origin, and it fluctuated according to market conditions. A recorded price in 1590 was red wine vinegar 24 gallons for £2, while the best white vinegar was slightly dearer at 2/— per gallon.[122]

In general all writers agree regarding the effects of vinegar on the body, but there are some conflicting references to quality. *Regimen Sanitatis* describes vinegar as dry and cold; Cogan says it cools and binds, but Buttes lists it as cold in the first and moist in the second.[123] The confusion would seem to arise from the accepted effects of vinegar (i.e., drying) and its obviously fluid appearance, which was recognized as able to quench thirst. The difficulty of reconciling the observable characteristics of a material with its characteristic effects has already been referred to.[124]

In describing the effects of vinegar, our authors seem to put stress on the less beneficial aspects. The following basic points come from *Regimen Sanitatis*. Vinegar: dries, cools, makes lean (taken fasting, it hurts the sinews), engenders melancholy (it should not be taken by melancholic people), diminishes the "seed of generation."[125] A later version of the *Regimen Sanitatis* adds that vinegar, taken continually, hurts the sight, the breast (causing a cough), the stomach, the liver, and may vex the joints with "arthritical griefes trembling and shaking."[126] On the more positive side, vinegar is said to be good for the stomach, preserve the appetite, act as a protection against the pestilence, and (taken with rose water) make a good mouthwash.[127]

Whatever its benefits or defects vinegar was widely used by those who could afford it, both in cookery and in medicine. It was used medicinally to wash wounds and in making plasters, and as an inhalant.[128] It also had what might be termed a cosmetic application; some maidens are reported as drinking vinegar "to abate their colour and to make them faire," or, as the marginal note puts it (somewhat cryptically), "a practice to make one lean and low coloured."[129]

The place of vinegar in the public esteem can probably be best illustrated by the fascinating reference to "Dry vinegar to carrie in your pocket!" (1615). [130] This, despite the comment of Buttes that "vinegar nourisheth nothing at all."[131] An alternative to vinegar was the acid fruit juice called *verjuice* (there are many ways of spelling this word). This is found in many recipes and was considered to have the same, but weaker, characteristics as vinegar. In France it was made from grapes, but in England pressed and strained crab apples were usually used. As it could be made from any sour fruit it could have been made at home by

the country poor. *The Northumberland Household Book* gives a price
of 3d. per gallon.[132]

Mustard. Mustard is the third most common sauce used in England.
Gerard describes a number of varieties, dividing them into the "treacle"
or wild mustards and the "tame" ones.[133] Of the tame, servie or field
mustard seems to have been the variety referred to generally as "common mustard." Cogan says the best mustard is grown round Tewkes-
bury in Gloucester and in Yorkshire.[134] There is a noticeable absence of
references to the cost of mustard in the records consulted, presumably
because it was collected locally.

Mustard is hot and dry. Most authors merely explain that mustard is
hotter than salt, but *Regimen Sanitatis* describes it as hot and dry in the
fourth degree.[135] The virtues of mustard are many. It pierces and clears
the brain (by causing sneezing), purging the head, teeth, and throat; it is
good against all diseases of the stomach, lungs, wind, phlegm, or
"rawnes of the guts"; it acts as a diuretic, helps in the palsy, and in
fevers. With honey, mustard helps a cough and the falling sickness. It is
bad for the eyes.[136]

Mustard was considered efficacious when applied externally in a
plaster. The main use in cookery was as a mustard sauce, where it was
widely used with both flesh and fish, particularly with brawn at the
beginning of a meal. Austin's collection of recipes does not include one
specifically called mustard sauce, though mustard is frequently incorporated in other recipes, e.g., mixed with the liver of capons or fish. Of
the two recipes provided by Sir Kenelm Digby,[137] "Lady Holmeby's
quick fine mustard" is made by taking true mustard seed dried in the
bread oven after baking, beaten to a fine powder, and mixed together
with sherry-sack. Then add five or six spoonfuls[138] or more of sugar to
a pint of mustard, and mix well. This will keep a good long time. (Some
very sharp wine vinegar can be added.)

Common and green sauces. By tradition a common sauce should be
made with six items – namely sage, salt, wine, pepper, garlic, and parsley.[139] Cogan believes that each of these things is valuable taken in
various sauces, but he feels that the mixture of the six is a "mingle
mangle" and is not good.[140] The sauce that he advocates for a number
of dishes is made from onions sliced very thinly, good water, and
"grosse pepper." The onions are improved if boiled in water and then
dripping is put on them.

Another name for a green sauce is "sauce vert." Buttes includes green sauce as a separate item in his list of foods. He says it is made of sweet herbs such as betony, mint, basil, with rose vinegar, a clove or two, and a little garlic.[141] This sauce, which could be taken with a variety of dishes, improved the savour and increased the appetite. Green sauce also helps concoction and breaks phlegm in the stomach. It should not be taken during fever or in hot stomachs.

Oils. "Oyles" do not seem to have a precise meaning in the fifteenth and sixteenth centuries. Austin quotes three "oyle soppes,"[142] of which two have onions fried in oil, and the other has milk and no oil at all. Boorde classes "oyle, grese, or fat" as "buttyresshe."[143] Frying was one of the accepted methods of cooking (as in the making of fritters), and the term often appears in cookery instructions. Materials used for frying seem to have been butter, oil, suet, lard, and "drippings" from the joints roasted on spits. Butter has been referred to elsewhere and only "oil" and "fat of beasts" will be discussed here. Though references to oil are usually found under the heading of olives, Bullein does have a section on "the vertue of oile." He says that green olive oil is the mother of all oils and draws into itself the virtues of the materials it is mixed with.[144] Salad oil (which generally meant olive oil) is good to digest the cold herbs in salads, when tempered with sharp vinegar and sugar. There are "many goodly vertues in compounded oils both to callifie and make hote."[145] New oil moistens and warms the stomach but old oil corrupts the stomach and makes the voice hoarse. The oils most frequently mentioned are "flower oils" such as the oil of roses or violets. Gerard mentions a number of edible oil plants such as arachis, sesame and sunflower, but the development of the use of a range of edible oils came later. Commercial records refer to "Spanish oil" and "Seville oil," with a mention of "argan oil" (a plant seed oil) in small quantities, "fish oil," and "train-oil" *(lachrymae arborum).* [146]

The emphasis in describing the fat from animals is that it should not be eaten alone with the lean. Fat alone "cloyeth the stomacke, and causeth lothsomnes."[147] Countrymen are known to eat the fat from bacon, beef and pork, without any lean, but it was recognized that rural stomachs had remarkable digestive powers. From the cookery point of view several methods of preserving lard are available.[148]

Sugar, Honey, and Sweet Things

In recent years new work has been done on the special significance of sugar in the diet.[149] The importance of sweet things in man's diet is of long standing, both because of physiological effects and the satisfaction provided in terms of taste.[150] According to the ancients, tastes were linked with elemental qualities, sweetness being linked with heat. Honey was considered to be far the sweetest of all things. Galen points out that the heat in honey is the right amount to produce its sweetness.[151] Any additional heat will be in excess and cannot produce more sweetness, but will make the honey bitter. According to English writers in the sixteenth century, sugar was hot and moist in the first degree, or, "as some thinke, possessing an equall temperature of all qualities,"[152] while honey was hot and dry in the second degree. Apparently, judging from Bullein's reference to such an error, there were some who thought that honey was hot and moist. Bullein goes on to point out that if honey is clarified and kept in a closed vessel "there is nothing that is liquid upon earth that remaineth longer."[153] Both honey and sugar were widely used and were valuable both in the diet and medicinally. On the whole, their benefits and disadvantages were similar, the effect of honey being stronger in each case.

Honey: hot and dry in the second degree, causes thirst, turns to choler,[154] inflames blood, operates against phlegm, is to be avoided by the young and by those with hot natures, is good in winter for the old, cold, and rheumatic.

Sugar: hot and moist in the first degree, causes thirst, turns to choler, operates against phlegm (sugar candy does this best), can be given to all ages and all complexions (bearing in mind its choleric effect).

Thomas Hill gives four pages on the virtues of honey for many parts of the body. Some aspects of the widespread use of honey and sugar in sixteenth century England are referred to below. As regards availability, the exact quantity of honey (wild and cultivated) produced or imported is impossible to determine. The importance of the cultivation and care of bees was recognized from Anglo-Saxon times and is illustrated by the advice provided in the sixteenth century on apiculture.[155] A figure for the cost of honey in 1594/95, is 6d. per pint.[156] *The Northumberland Household Book* quotes 4½d. per pound for sugar (type unspecified).[157] Prices during the century fluctuated around 1/– per pound. Sugar had been imported into England "at least two and a half centuries before 1500."[158] It was first refined in England about 1544. In the sixteenth century a number of sources were available – e.g. through Antwerp, from Morocco, and from Brazil. Six different types of sugar are recorded in consignments from Morocco. The terms "molasses or sugar syrope" are used in their present meaning, but the

use of the word treacle did not then refer to a byproduct of sugar refin-
ing, but to "theriac," an antidote against poison (see below).

Willan calculates the consumption of sugar in England in the sixteenth century as about 1 lb. per head per annum (as compared to the
calculated figure of 105.6 lb. per head per annum in 1972). Travellers
commented on the black teeth of the English as being due to their high
sugar intake.[159] The intake of sweet substances must certainly have been
high, to judge from the recipes in cookery books for dishes and drinks.
Sugar was added to wines and it or honey was an important ingredient
of such drinks as oxymel (both in *oxymel simplex** and *oxymel com-
positum*, to which roots, seeds and herbs were added). Digby, in the
next century, gives 52 recipes for meath or metheglin,[160] all of which
contain honey or sugar or both; besides this group of drinks there were
numerous varieties of honey waters.

Similarly, in previous centuries sweetening agents had been used in
a wide variety of dishes. Of the 196 recipes listed in *The Forme of
Cury,* about one third had added sweetening.[161] So too in the sixteenth
century sugar was added to such dishes as (i) boiled leg of mutton with
lemons, (ii) veal tart, (iii) stewed herrings, (iv) spinage fritters, as well as
to fruit and conserves.[162] Candied fruits and plants (e.g. roses and violets) were considered valuable items. The conserving and preserving
effects of sugar and honey were an important characteristic of both
foods. Honey had been used for preserving food materials from ancient
times. Some elaborate sugar confections were prepared for banquets in
the sixteenth century, but a study of cookery books shows a marked
increase in recipes for conserves and confections in the seventeenth and
eighteenth centuries.

Theriac and Methridatium.[163] These substances were both of ancient
origin, each being a mixture of many ingredients and considered to be
antidotes against poison or the venom. They are frequently referred to
by sixteenth century writers in relation to poisons and the pestilence,
both of these subjects providing a continual source of anxiety. The
word "treacle" or "triacle" is often used to refer to theriac. The differentiation between the older meaning and the sugar product is not
always made clear in modern commentaries on Elizabethan trading
records. According to the *OED*, the first use of the term treacle to
describe an uncrystallized sugar product was in 1694. At that time the

Oxymel simplex contained water, honey and strong white vinegar.

word still had the other meanings of a "triacle" or "sovereign remedy," and could also refer to the names of plants (see wild mustard, above). In the sixteenth century "Venetian treacle" or "treacle from Amsterdam" referred to a therapeutic material carefully prepared, sometimes with elaborate ritual.

Basically, the flavours discussed in this section provide the qualities of heat and dryness in differing degrees, two qualities recognized as being particularly valuable to the English with their rheums and their cold, damp climate. Therefore, spices and condiments were considered valuable for their dietetic and medicinal virtues as well as for their characteristic flavours.

Some social historians have explained the widespread use of spices and seasoning in the sixteenth century as being mainly due to the need for masking the flavour of tainted or preserved meats, in times when the transport and keeping of foods was difficult. Drummond and Wilbraham observe that the "popularity of strong seasoning for meat was undoubtedly due to the frequency with which it was necessary to mask taint."[164] Few have commented on the recognized value of spices in the dietary regimen. Mead is an exception, for he points out the use of spices in order to stimulate the action of the stomach, in a time when people realized the burden that the enormous amounts of meat eaten would put upon the digestion.[165]

Before we can confirm or dismiss the idea that seasonings and expensive spices were primarily masks for bad food, we need further information on the Elizabethan agricultural situation, the conditions and mode of transport of foodstuffs, and market facilities. The "masking" theory is, however, questionable on the basis of present knowledge, for the greater proportion of the population lived in the country near to their food supplies. Those who could afford spices were also liekly to have local fresh foods from domestic animals, game and fish, easily available, and, as has already been indicated, the quality of such food had been praised by foreigners and Englishmen alike. It is also of interest that *Le Cuisinier François*[166] of La Varenne, which set aside the heavy use of spices, appeared in the middle of the next century when facilities for transporting and keeping foods had not notably improved. This suggests a change in taste rather than in storage facilities.

Whatever the conclusions of further study, the appearance of detailed advice on spices in books on the preservation of health, seems to indicate that this aspect should not be overlooked.

POSTSCRIPT

In spite of the great strides forward in recent years in the production of food, malnutrition remains one of the most important public health problems of the world. Vast numbers of people, especially in the developing countries, suffer from protein-calorie malnutrition or from specific deficiency disorders. The magnitude of the task of providing them with food both sufficient in proteins and calories and containing the required nutrients cannot be over estimated, nor can the need for more thorough research on the malnutrition diseases themselves be minimized.

Director General, World Health Organization (1970)

MAN'S ABILITY to explain the same situation in a variety of different ways is clearly illustrated by a comparison of Elizabethan and modern approaches to diet. The Elizabethan dietary of health was developed through the strict attention to logic and careful observation which were characteristic of the period. This, combined with a close conformity to the ancient teachings of Hippocrates and Aristotle, and firmly based on concepts postulated by Galen more than one thousand years before, provided theories of diet which were formal and complex though lacking in precision because of their philosophical roots. Modern nutritional science is based on a reductionist philosophy, with the acceptance of biochemical laws. This, when combined with sophisticated laboratory techniques, enables nutrition to encompass such diverse fields as the micro-research of cell nutrition and the worldwide study of population needs. The basis of modern theory is recent, being provided by changes in thought and skills first developed at the beginning of the last century. The following extremely selective (consciously biased toward conditions in the U.K.) and severely truncated outline gives some indication of the path of nutritional thought from the sixteenth century to modern times.

The disappearance of Galenism, * after exerting so profound an influence for so long was not a sudden change but a gradual process,

---

N.B. Footnotes to the Postscript appear on pages 351-355.

with many causes and conditions which initiated and facilitated its replacement by a "chemical" approach to foods and medicines. Important influences were the rise of the iatro-chemists and iatro-physicists.[1] Temkin has pointed out that "so great was the impact of physics on the other sciences, from chemistry to biology, that the beginning of modern physics in the seventeenth century appears as the beginning of modern science in general."[2] Besides this overall influence on the foundations of science, William Cullen,* writing in the eighteenth century, believed that it was the general knowledge about, and acceptance of the circulation of the blood, together with the discovery of the *receptaculum chyli* and the thoracic duct, through the work of Aselli and Pequet, which "finally exploded" Galenic ideas in about the middle of the seventeenth century.[3] As a science, Galenism could hardly have survived past the middle of the seventeenth century, but it did survive, despite the new philosophy, as a guide to medical practice.

Lester H. King, in his discussion of Friederich Hoffman's *Fundamenta Medicinae*, has summarized the chief schools of metaphysical explanation at the end of the seventeenth century. These include Galenic (derived from Aristotle), Neoplatonic, Spagyric, Helmontian, and the two Atomist philosophies of Descartes and Gassendi. Though influenced by all these approaches, "yet in his specific discussions of physiological and pathological features, Hoffman adhered to a Galenic schema as modified by mechanical principles."[5] Louis Lémery's *Traité des Aliments* (1702) shows a mixture of Galenic, Cartesian, and chemical ideas in its introductory theory.[6] It was within this framework that Hoffman set the ideas which were later developed by Cullen who, while acknowledging his debt to Hoffman for being the first to provide in "a tolerably simple and clear system" a theory which included the powerful influences of the nervous system and their application to disease, also rejected the fact that Hoffman's fundamental doctrines were mixed up with humoral pathology, which was unacceptable to Cullen, who described it "as incorrect and hypothetical as any other."[7]

In the main stream of the development of nutritional science Cullen's importance lay in his influential doctrine of neuropathology and in his *Materia Medica.*[8] His theories were based on the belief that the essential vital phenomenon was nervous excitation, and because the nervous power appears only in the living and disappears at death it "may be otherwise properly enough termed the *vital principle.*"[9] He postulated

---

*William Cullen (1712-90), foremost teacher of pharmacy and medicine in eighteenth century Britain.

that after digestion the nutritive parts of foods, whatever their origin, were formed in the blood into a single alimentary principle or *"animal mixt."* [10] This supplied the material for the maintenance of all body solids and fluids, but Cullen says "In what manner the nutritious fluid, thus carried to the several parts is there applied, so as to increase the length of the nervous fibre itself or in what manner it becomes solid we cannot explain; nor can these particulars be explained upon any other supposition that has been formed with respect to nutrition." [11] Cullen's time and talents put him in the unusual position of being able to look backward at the remnants of Galenism and forward towards the new ideas of chemical analysis, though he rejected these in the form in which he knew them, [12] saying in his *Materia Medica*: "I judge it [the chemical analysis of substances] to be of no use in explaining or ascertaining the virtues of medicines." [13]

Though diet was still acknowledged to be an important factor in the maintenance of health, the division between diet and medicine had widened since the Elizabethan period, producing some conflict over diet's place in the treatment of disease. [14] A compromise generally accepted in the eighteenth century was that diet could be useful in the treatment of chronic diseases. John Quincy, author of *Pharmacopoeia Officinalis* (1718), said:

> In all chronic Cases medicines are to be contrived as near to a Diet as can be; and therefore the common Drinks and Foods are to be medicated as far as they will admit and the Case requires... But in acute cases, which are generally dangerous, there is required no such regard. [15]

This view was supported by George Cheyne, author of *An Essay of Health and Long Life*, 1724. It is significant that until recent times leading writers on diet were frequently authorities on *materia medica* (outstanding examples are Cullen, J. Paris [1785-1856], and J. Pereira [1804-1853]), and the two subjects were commonly considered together. However, the rise of chemical ideas, together with the trend towards systematization, was tending to cause the separation of aliments (considered here to include food and drinks) from medicines. [16] Like contemporary writers on *materia medica,* Cullen was a systematizer, but he differed from other authorities in making a complete separation of aliments and medicines. [17] He acknowledges that there would be some overlap, but supports his separation on the basis of practical effectiveness, saying, "... yet I maintain, contrary to the practice of writers on materia medica; that such instances should be considered under the different views that may be taken of them as aliments or medicines and these should be considered separately to avoid distracting the student by different views presented at the same time."[18]

The year of Cullen's death (1789) saw the publication of the *Traité élémentaire de Chimie, présenté dans un ordre nouveau et d'après les découvertes modernes* by Antoine Lavoisier, which provided a basis for our present biochemical theory of nutrition. In this work Lavoisier "refuted the phlogiston theory and reconstructed chemistry by the discovery of the compositions of air and water and by the recognition of the chemical elements as the ultimate residues of chemical analysis."[19] In his *Table of Simple Substances* (belonging to all the kingdoms of nature, which may be considered as the elements of bodies) were included:

New Names	Correspondent Old Names
Light	Light
Caloric	Heat
	Principle or element of heat
	Fire. Igneous fluid
	Matter of fire and of heat

Other "new names" included in this group were: Oxygen, Azote [nitrogen], and Hydrogen. Lavoisier's research with Laplace* had enabled them to conclude that respiration was a kind of combustion. The heat evolved in respiration was suggested as a sort of animal heat.[21]

Great advances were made in both the theory and techniques of physiological chemistry in the first quarter of the nineteenth century. J. A. Paris, in *Elements of Medical Chemistry* (1825), says: "But there are changes perpetually going on in the animal body that are beyond the control of the living principle and therefore the Physiologist who is not a chemist will be utterly at a loss to comprehend them."[22] An important step towards modern theories of nutrition was the work of William Prout "On the ultimate composition of simple alimentary substances" (1827)[23] in which he rejected the traditional idea of one alimentary principle. He reduced "all the principal alimentary matters employed by man" into three classes, viz. *saccharine, oily* and *albuminous.* This group of foods in relation to their chemical composition was used as a starting point by a number of later workers.

---

*Pierre-Simon de Laplace (1749-1827).

In 1842 Justus von Liebig published his *Animal Chemistry*.[24] In this
extremely influential book he grouped foods according to their chemical content and function. Albuminous or nitrogenous foods were described as "plastic" and were considered to provide material for growth
and movement. Liebig called the non-nitrogenous foods (i.e. carbohydrates and fats) "respiratory," and postulated that body temperature
was maintained by their breakdown, thus separating movement and
heat. A number of his contemporaries disagreed with this theory, which
was finally disproved by Fick and Wislicenus,[25] who climbed the Faul-
horn mountain in 1866, despite an abstinence from nitrogenous foods
for thirty-one hours, thus showing that the breakdown of albuminous
foods was not essential for movement. The work of Mayer, Helmholtz
and Joule[26] led to the acceptance of the notion that heat and movement in the body were manifestations of thermal and mechanical
energy, which were inter-convertible.

Writing in 1843, Jonathan Pereira[27] classified the chemical elements
of the food of man, equating them to the essential constituents of the
human body. He listed thirteen (in modern notation they are: C, H, O,
N, P, S, Fe, Cl, Na, Ca, K, Mg, F). Of the fifty-five elements known at
that time, nineteen had been found in "organized or living bodies,"[28]
leaving six which were not essential. He points out that "A living body
has no power of forming elements or converting one elementary substance to another." This had formerly been a matter of controversy.
The immutability of elements was an essential premise in the use of
"balance" studies of the intake and excretion of elements (and the later
studies of nutrients) to determine man's nutritional needs.

The first workable quantitative basis for calculating the food requirements of man was established in the mid-nineteenth century. These
were the "figures" of Jacob Moleschott[30] which referred to the
amounts of nitrogenous (albuminous) material and nitrogen-free materials (fat and "fat-formers")[31] required per day for a working man
weighing 63.65 Kg. The basis of his calculation and the methods used
have been discussed elsewhere,[32] but it is significant that besides building on the current physiological theories and techniques, Molescott
used the new concept of Quetelet's *homme moyen*[33] or average man.
He also used a number of dietary intake records available at the time.
The use of food-intake analysis as a research tool had only become
feasible when physiochemical theory and techniques enabled the analysis of foodstuff to be matched directly with the material needed by the
body. This meant eventually an acceptance of the uniformity of action

in chemical laws, which in turn predicated the rejection of a philosophy which included "vital power." The nineteenth century saw the decline of vitalism and an increase in a materialistic or reductionist philosophy. A much quoted phrase which expresses the latter is "Ohne Phospher kein Gedanke" ("No thought without phosphorous") from Moleschott's *Lehre der Nahrungsmittel.* [34] Basically, Moleschott's pattern of investigation followed that used today to determine Recommended Intakes of Nutrients. [35] These depend fundamentally on the results of dietary surveys and metabolic balance studies, which are related to the population as a whole through statistical techniques.

The accuracy of the diet records used by Moleschott[36] cannot be judged because methods used for the surveys are seldom available. However, the increasing number of recorded dietary intakes reflected a marked interest in the study of diets in various countries. The reason for this cannot be pinpointed, but it is likely that, besides the effects of the developments in scientific thought and techniques, the interest was influenced by an increasing public awarenesss of the ordinary man and his problems. [37] Also, practical reasons forced authorities to consider the diets of various groups of the population. Examples in Britain are: The Naval Mutiny of 1797, which caused far-reaching reforms, including a sequence of changes in naval rations. [38] The dietary conditions in the Army were brought to the notice of the country through the Crimean War (1854-56). Investigations into the standards of living of labourers and agricultural workers had to be made in order that "the ordinary levels of subsistence of the labouring classes of the district" should not be less than the diet provided in the Poor Law Institutions. [39]

In his chapter "On Dietaries"[40] Pereira insisted that "An accurate acquaintance with the quantity and quality of food necessary to the maintenance of human health and life under different circumstances is a matter of interest to everyone." This interest was especially important for those who had responsibility for the care of others. He listed: statesmen, magistrates, naval and military officers, physicians, surgeons, governors of hospitals or other public institutions, and guardians of the poor. His "dietaries for the healthy" included ration scales for:

Children: in the care of foundling hospitals, orphanages, and asylums.

Adults: Dietary for the naval service also included "Dietary for Emigrants" as fixed by their Majesties' Colonial Land Emigration Commissioners; Army Rations; Dietary for able-bodied Paupers; Dietaries for Prisoners.

Pereira question the attitude which stated that prisoners should not have a better diet than that which can, in general, be obtained by an honest labourer for his family. "The question is," he said, "not what the honest labourer can obtain, but what is necessary for the prisoner."[41] The quality of the diets was calculated in terms of the average quantities of dry matter, moisture, Carbon, and Nitrogen.[42]

In the treatment of many diseases, attention to the diet was considered to be important. Pereira particularly stressed non-febrile disorders of the digestive and urinary system. Diet was not so significant in acute illnesses where a "low diet" would be prescribed anyhow because of the patient's poor appetite. The appetite was used as an appropriate guide to the amount of food required.

"Dietaries for the sick," selected from twelve major hospitals, were designated: Full common or meat diet (this was the usual diet), Animal diet (exclusively or principally composed of animal foods), Vegetable diet, Spare or Abstemious diet, Fever diet, Low diet, Milk diet, Dry diet. Also, Dietaries for the Insane and Dietaries for the Puerperal Woman were provided.

F. W. Pavey, in his *Treatise on Food and Dietetics*,[43] *physiologically and therapeutically considered* (1875), writing about the amount of food required, discusses the overall weight of food to be eaten. In his own case (height 5 feet 9 inches, weight just over 140 pounds), he found about 30 ounces (gross) of food daily to be sufficient. For the amount of constituent alimentary principles he referred to the "model diet of Moleschott,"[44] dividing the diet in the following proportions:

Nitrogenous matter should be about 1/r of the water free food — i.e., about 405 ounces daily.

Fat, about 2½ ounces daily.

Carbohydrates, between 15 and 22 ounces daily. The quantity should be enough to "fill up what is defective for force production — heat and mechanical work — in other principles."[45]

Mineral matter, ¾ to one ounce daily.

Extra water is needed beyond that in the food.

In the last quarter of the nineteenth century, research in nutrition concentrated mainly on calorimetry and energy metabolism, as in the work of M. Pettenkofer (1818-1901), Carl Voit (1831-1908), M. Rubner[46] (1854-1932), and W. O. Atwater[47] (1844-1907). Also, the study of proteins and amino acids was undertaken by such investigators as T. B. Osborne (1859-1929) and R. H. Chittenden[48] (1856-1943).

Concurrently, important advances were made in other aspects of human physiology. The work of Claude Bernard (1813-78) had far-

-reaching effects on concepts in nutrition. His *Introduction à l'étude de la médecine expérimentale* (1865),[49] was a guide to research methods, while his concept of the *milieu interieur* pointed the way to the discovery of the endocrine glands and to the later concept of *homeostasis* (Cannon, 1932).[50]

At the turn of the century, assessment of the *quality* of the diet was made in terms of protein, carbohydrate, fats, and an ill-defined supply of inorganic salts. Striking progress had been made in the field of energy requirements, providing a foundation for the *quantitative* side of human nutrition which has remained substantially unaltered. However, the importance of nutrition to health and the role played by faulty diets in producing disease was not fully realized by scientists and doctors. In his lectures on "Disorders resulting from defective nutriment," given in 1842, George Budd had referred to diabetes, scurvy, a condition (unnamed) of which "the most distinctive character is a peculiar ulceration of the cornea," and finally a disease "chiefly marked by the softness, or imperfect development of the bones." Budd added a possible fifth disease in which diarrhoea was the most striking symptom.[51] It was appreciated that each of these diseases was different and arose as the result of different defects or errors in the diet. Though at that time it was not possible to state the exact "element" which would prevent the various diseases, it was recognized that the treatment needed to be dietetic.

In 1881, N. Lunin, following an animal feeding experiment using an artificial mixture of the individual constituents of milk, said that "a natural food such as milk must therefore contain besides these known principal ingredients small quantities of unknown substances essential to life."[52] Commenting on this situation, Lunin's teacher, G. Bunge (according to the *Textbook of Physiological and Pathological Chemistry*) added: "It would be worth while to continue the experiments.[53] The matter was not pursued at that time and it was Gowland Hopkins who, in his paper entitled "Feeding Experiments illustrating the Importance of Accessory Factors in Normal Dietaries,"[54] reported carefully controlled experiments and convinced other workers of the importance of accessory food factors, later called vitamins. Ihde and Becker, in "Conflict and Concepts in Early Vitamin Studies," explain that the recognition and understanding of deficiency diseases was delayed as a result of having to compete with more attractive medical concepts.[55] This can be easily understood when it is realized that the amount of a vitamin required to prevent a deficiency disease may be very small.[56]

The speed with which vitamin research proceeded is illustrated by reports of the U.K. Medical Research Council on Accessory Food Factors (Vitamins). The first report appeared in 1919 when "the importance of vitamins was by no means recognized."[57] A new edition, nearly double in size, was issued in 1924, and a third in 1932. The latter referred to the new periodical, *Nutrition Abstracts and Reviews,* as being required as "a regular means of bringing together and making more readily available the results of research work as they accumulate in the now widely distributed and often disconnected fields of work, medical, agricultural, dietetic, and commercial, in which the subject of nutrition is being so rapidly developed."[58] As the distinguished nutritionist, C. A. Elvehjem has pointed out, by 1920 the science of nutrition had not yet been fully recognized,[59] but in the next twenty years many vitamins were identified and synthesized and there was such a proliferation of therapeutic diets (some were designated by the name of the individual who planned them) that a plea was made for "fewer and better diets."[60]

Important steps were taken in applying nutritional knowledge to the problems of maintaining health in the poorer sections of the population, both on national levels and through the League of Nations on an international plane.[61] The Second World War gave extra impetus to the study of nutrition both in research[62] and in its application. In some countries a knowledge of nutrition was effectively used to ensure that restricted food supplies were used in the best way to maintain the health of the population. Two important tools were developed:

(i) The table of *Recommended Dietary Allowances,* published by the United States National Research Council in 1943.[63] Many countries have followed this pattern when preparing Recommended Allowances for their own population groups and particular circumstances.[64] The U.S. Tables have been revised regularly. The extension of knowledge about nutrition has been aided by increasingly sophisticated techniques. Schoenheimer's use of deuterium (heavy hydrogen) enabled him to postulate the concept that body constituents are in a dynamic state of equilibrium.[65] The use of radioactive isotopes and improved laboratory equipment for microanalysis have helped to clarify metabolic pathways and speed up analytical procedures. A comparison of the first and the seventh (1968) published U.S. tables of Recommended Dietary Allowances gives some indication of the advances in nutritional science since World War II:

1943

Nutrients tabulated: total 10: K calories, Protein, Calcium, Iron, Vitamin A, Thiamine, Riboflavin, Niacin, Ascorbic Acid, Vitamin D.

Population Groups: total 17:

   Men and Women – by activity: very active, moderately active, sedentary. Also Pregnant and Lactating women.

   Children – by age: under 1 year, 1-3 years, 4-6 years, 7-9 years, 10-12 years.

   Boys – 13-15 years, 16-20 years.

   Girls – 13-15 years, 16-20 years.

1968

Nutrients tabulated: total 17: K calories, Protein, Vitamin A, Vitamin D, Vitamin E, Ascorbic Acid, Folacin, Niacin, Riboflavin, Thiamine, Vitamin B_6 Vitamin B_{12}, Calcium, Phosphorus, Iodine, Iron, Magnesium. Additional comment is given on trace elements such as chromium, cobalt, manganese, zinc, and selenium. Sodium, potassium, and chloride are also discussed.

Population Groups: total 26:

   A Reference Man – 70 Kg. aged 22 years, plus 6 more groups.

   A Reference Woman – 58 Kg. aged 22 years, plus 9 more groups.

   Infants – 3 groups.

   Children – 6 groups.

   The inclusion of sodium, potassium and chloride indicates the advances made in the study of electrolyte balances in the body. These series of mythical "statistical" individuals, taken as representative of the various groups, are used as guidelines for the estimation of the needs for nutrients of both the population in general and (with the appropriate adjustments) of single individuals.

   (ii) The second "tool" is the development of large scale long term food intake surveys. These provide information related to the preparation of Recommended Daily Allowances and enable regular checks to be made of the level of dietary intake for a whole population. The most comprehensive example is the British *National Food Survey,* which was initiated in 1940 and has provided a continuous sampling inquiry into the domestic food consumption and expenditure of private households in Great Britain. The latest *Household Food Consumption and Expenditure: 1970 and 1971*[66] gives estimates of household food consumption related to income groups, family composition, and geographical area. The information obtained provides a basis for a National Food Policy. Besides care for the "vulnerable groups," special surveys are set up when the authorities have reason to think that the nutritional level of a particular group may be threatened by social or economic circumstances. Present examples in the United Kingdom are studies of the elderly and schoolchildren.[67] Practical measures to improve nutrition have been introduced; these include the addition, by law, of nutrients to particular foods,[68] the provision of nutritionally valuable foods at reduced prices for vulnerable groups, and facilities for nutrition education.

An essential part of *applied nutrition* is a knowledge of the nutritional value of different foods. This can be obtained from published Food Tables[69] which now include an increasing number of items from many parts of the world. The use of standard food tables of chemical composition implies the acceptance of the idea of an intrinsic value in the food itself unrelated to the condition and circumstances of any individual who may eat it.

Today Nutrition has become a profession, with nutritionists and dietitians working in a variety of areas of the subject. but with the main objective of ensuring that people, in their homes or in institutions, receive the diet they need for good health. The physician's part is predominantly curative The present day trend is for therapeutic diets to be a close adaptation of the normal diet, with adjustments of one or more nutrients, but otherwise containing the correct amounts and proportions of them. A nutrition textbook widely used in the United Kingdom[70] now lists eighteen diet sheets. In general terms, they deal with:

Convalescence and under weight.

Obesity and weight reduction.

Diabetes mellitus.

Diseases and failure of the liver.

Diseases and failure of the kidney.

Cardiac conditions.

Intestinal conditions. including constipation.

The control of cholesterol levels in the blood (this is considered to contribute to cardiac failure).

Coeliac disease (this is due to an idiosyncracy or sensitivity to gluten).

A number of genetic deficiencies, which can lead to irreparable harm if not diagnosed and treated dietetically, have also been recognized. One of these – *Phenylketonuria* – is due to an inborn metabolic error through which the amino acid *phenylalanine,* present in all dietary proteins which would normally be broken down by enzymes, remains in the blood. The accumulation of this substance damages the brain, causing mental deficiency to a marked degree.[71] This list of common dietetic treatments is applicable to conditions in technically developed countries. It is notable that "deficiency diseases," as such, are not included in the list of therapeutic diets. Recently a comprehensive definition of deficiency diseases has been made by W. R. Aykroyd in *Conquest of Deficiency Diseases* (1970). In the narrowest terms they can be described as "pathological states with characteristic clinical signs, which are due to deficiency in the diet of a nutrient and can be prevented or cured by providing the missing nutrient."[72] Lack of essential nutrients is more usually found in the developing countries, where diseases due to the lack of one or more nutrients, and an inadequate amount of total calories, may be a serious obstacle in the development of the nation as a whole.

It is recognized that the effects of nutritional inadequacy are more than physical, and prolonged conditions of semi-starvation profoundly affect behavourial patterns. For moral and political reasons it is considered desirable and necessary for the technically developed countries to aid the poorer peoples of the world to reach a standard of nutrition which will enable them to use to the full their potential initiative and effort. International agencies are attempting to ameliorate bad conditions through Applied Nutrition Programmes. United Nations Agencies* work closely with the National governments in planning these programmes, and they call upon the expert advice of workers in the fields of medicine, agriculture, education, economics, marketing, anthropology, sociology, and food technology, as well as nutrition.

H.M. Sinclair, in the latest edition of Robert Hutchison's *Food and the Principles of Dietetics,* points out that the first edition (1900) was intended for students and practitioners of medicine in view of "the almost total neglect of the subject of dietetics in ordinary medical education" – a situation (says Sinclair) that has remained unchanged to the present day.[73]

The vast increases in the store of information in medicine, nutrition, and allied subjects has led to an ever greater degree of specialization, with a marked lessening of the study of the *whole man* advocated in the Elizabethan period. In the 400 years separating the Elizabethan and the twentieth century concepts of the relationship of man and his food, the

---

*Particularly World Health Organisation (WHO) Food and Agriculture Organisation (FAO) U.N. Childrens Fund (UNICEF).

changes have been so great that they seem to have little in common beyond the unchanging factors of man and foods. The present speed of the changes in fundamental ideas of life and environment make it probable that many of the theories held in the first half of this century will at its end be looked back at with curiosity and disbelief.

Modern researchers in nutrition are well aware that our present biochemical "model" for explaining nutritional functions is inadequate. Nevertheless, most workers subscribe to the belief expressed by the late President John F. Kennedy in 1963 at the twentieth anniversary of the Hot Springs Conference:

> So long as freedom from hunger is only half achieved, so long as two thirds of the nations have food deficits, no citizen, no nation, can afford to be satisfied. We have the ability, as members of the human race. We have the means, we have the capacity to eliminate hunger from the face of the earth in our lifetime. We need only the will.[74]

FOOTNOTES

CHAPTER I

1. C. D. O'Malley, *English Medical Humanists*, 1965, p. 40.
2. W. Pagel, *The Religious and Philosophical Aspects of Van Helmont's Science and Medicine*, 1944. W.P.D. Wightman, *Science and the Renaissance*, 1962. A.G. Debus, *The English Paracelsians*, 1965.
3. Arnald of Villanova (1235-1312), famous for (among other works) his commentary on the *Regimen Sanitatis Salerni*, frequently stressed the medical aspects of alchemy. See E.T. Withington, *Medical History*, 1964, p. 99.
4. P.H. Kocher, *Science and Religion in Elizabethan England*, 1953, Chapter 10 "Astrological Fate."
5. Kocher, p. 206.
6. A. Arber, *Herbals Their Origin and Evolution*, 1938.
7. Langton, Sig. A7^r.
8. W.G. Spencer, *Celsus de Medicina*, 1935, Vol. I, p. ix.
9. Galen (Daremberg), Vol. II, pp. 376-397.
10. *Empiricists* had philosophical roots in the doctrine of scepticism. They held that all knowledge was uncertain, that all causes could not be investigated, that the only valid reasoning in medicine was by experience, experiment, and analogy. *Methodists* rejected the study of anatomy and physiology as having no bearing on the practice of medicine. They advanced the concept of "atomic" structure. Diagnostic criteria were limited to the recognition of either an abnormally dry, tense and constricted state *(status strictus)* or conversely an excessively moist, relaxed, or fluid state *(status laxus)*. This very much simplified treatment. *Dogmatists*, also called Rationalists, emphasized theoretical principles and believed it was essential to study the structure and function of the body to know the cause of disease.
11. Langton, Sig. A8^r.
12. Langton, Sig. A8^v.
13. Langton, Sig. B1^r.
14. Clearly a reference to Hippocrates' *Airs, Waters and Places*, Vol. I, pp. 71-137.
15. Langton, Sig. B2^r. Here reference is made scathingly to those physicians (recognizable in every century) who are prepared to write prescriptions for patients without adequate sight or sound of them. Diagnosis from urine was an important aspect of medical practice. Robert Recorde, a famous writer on the urines, also stresses the importance of the doctor seeing the patient. R. Recorde, *The Urinall of Physick*, London, 1567 (1st edition 1548), Sig. B3^v. The *DNB* refers to a *Treatise of the Urines* (London, 1552) by Christopher Langton. No other reference to this book has been found in other standard reference books.
16. O. Temkin, "Nutrition from Classical Antiquity to the Baroque," *Human Nutrition Historic and Scientific*, ed. I. Galdston, New York, 1960.

17. J. Thirsk (ed.), *The Agrarian History of England and Wales (1500-1640)*, Vol. IV, 1967, p. 162. W. K. Jordan (*Philanthropy in England*, 1959) also comments on this (pp. 61-63).

18. Jordan, pp. 56-76.

19. O. Temkin's *Galenism*, 1973, was not available at the time of the writing this study. Galen's views as outlined here, are derived chiefly from the following works: Clifford Allbutt, *Greek Medicine in Rome*, 1921; H.P. Adelmann, *The Embryological Treatises of Hieronymus Fabricius of Aquapendente*, 1942; H.P. Adelmann, *Marcello Malpighi and the Evolution of Embryology*, 1966; M.T. May, *Galen on the Usefulness of the Parts of the Body*, 1968.

20. Temkin, "On Galen's Pneumatology," *Gesnerus*, 1950, *8*, pp. 180-189.

21. May, p. 48.

22. May, p. 52, footnote 223 gives reference to *De tremore*, chap. 6 (Kühn, VII, 614, 616).

23. Galen (MTM), p. 207.

24. *Anadosis* (or giving up) is the term used to describe the action in the intestines in the English translation: Galen (May), p. 239. It is equated with absorption and distribution in the Index.

25. Galen, p. 237.

26. May, p. 301, footnote 43.

27. Semen originated from the blood and in the last analysis from the aliment. Adelmann, *Malpighi*, p. 745.

28. Galen (Kühn), Vol. IV, pp. 652-702.

29. Edwin Clarke, "Aristotelian Concepts of the Form and Function of the Brain," *Bull. Hist. Med.* 1963, *37*, pp. 1-14.

30. Adelmann, *Fabricius*, p. 44.

31. Galen, p. 31.

32. Galen, p. 31.

33. Galen (Kühn), Vol. VI, pp. 453-784.

34. Galen (Kühn), Vol. XI, pp. 379-892 and Vol. XII, pp. 1-377.

CHAPTER II

1. See T.O. Cockayne (ed.), *Leechdoms, Wortcunning and Starcraft of Early England*, 1844-1846; W.R. Dawson, *A Leechbook or Collection of Medical Recipes of the Fifteenth Century*, 1934; C. H. Talbot, *Medicine in Medieval England*, 1967, refers to late fourteenth and early fifteenth century treatises in English (p. 189).

2. Talbot, *Medicine in Medieval England*, 1967.

3. Thomas Wright, *Popular Treatises on Science Written during the Middle Ages*, 1841, in the preface.

4. For a discussion of texts see: Sandford V. Larkey, *The Versalian Compendium of Geminus and Nicholas Udall's Translation: Their Relation to Versalius, Caius, Vicary and De Mondeville*, 1933; also C.D. O'Malley, *Thomas Geminus Compendiosa totius anatomie delineatio*, Introduction, 1959; Thomas Geminus (trans. Nicholas Udall), *Compendiosa Totius anatomie delineato*, London, 1553, (Compendious Anatomy); Thomas Vicary, *A profitable treatise of the Anatomie of Man's Bodie*, London, 1577.

5. Wellcome MS. No. 564 (formerly No. 632), S.A.J. Moorat, *Catalogue of Western Manuscripts on Medicine and Science in the Wellcome Historical Medical Library,* 1962.

6. D. Singer and A. Anderson, *Catalogue of Vernacular Alchemical Manuscripts in Great Britain and Ireland Dating from before the Sixteenth Century,* 1928-31; also *Catalogue of Latin and Vernacular Plague Texts . . .,* 1950.

7. H.S. Bennett, *English Books and Readers 1558-1603,* 1965, p. 179.

8. See G. H. Putnam, *Books and their Makers during the Middle Ages,* 1962 (reprint of first edition of 1896-7), Vol. II (1500-1709), pp. 464-470.

9. Bennett, p. 168. Richard Day also alleged, in 1585, that "thousands" of this book had been printed and sold by various men, none of whom were entitled to do so.

10. See J. Gairdner (ed.), *The Paston Letters, 1422-1509,* 1904, 6 Vols.; C.L. Kingsford (ed.), *The Stonor Papers,* 1919, 2 Vols. only.

11. It is of note that the Lollards (originally followers of Wycliffe, who questioned the actions of the Church), who were often drawn from the artisan class, were accused of distributing and reading their texts.

12. H.S. Bennett, *English Books and Readers 1475-1557,* 1952, p. 27. John Strype, in his *Memorials of Thomas Cranmer,* 1812, Vol. I, pp. 141-142, explains that "the Archbishop [Cranmer] resolved on this occasion to do some good service again for religion. . . . His endeavour now was to moderate the severe act about religion, and to get some liberty for the people's reading of the Scripture." He was violently opposed by the Bishop of Winchester, but the bill passed in a weaker form than Cranmer had intended.

13. L.B. Wright, *Middle-class Culture in Elizabethan England,* 1935.

14. J.W. Adamson, *The Illiterate Anglo Saxon,* 1946, p. 61.

15. Cogan, *The Haven of Health,* 1589 edition.

16. T. Elyot, *Castel of Helth,* London [1539]; G. Gratarolus (trans. T. Newton), *A Direction for the Health of Magistrates and Studentes,* London, 1574.

17. Christopher Langton, *An introduction into phisycke,* London [1550].

18. Henry Buttes, *Dyets Dry Dinner,* London, 1599.

19. *A Proper Newe Booke of Cokerye.* The earliest undated edition [1545] was published in London. A reprint of the original edition with notes by C.F. Frere is available (Cambridge, 1913). The 1575 edition is used for reference in this study.

20. T. Tasso (trans T.K.), *The householders philosophie,* London, 1588.

21. J. Partridge, *The treasurie of commodius conceites and hidden secrets,* London, 1573.

22. P.H. Duffy, *The Theory and Practice of Medicine in Elizabethan England as Illustrated by Certain Dramatic Texts,* unpublished Ph.D. Dissertation, Harvard University, 1942.

23. John Caius, *A boke or counseill against the disease called the sweate. . .,* London, 1552. The Latin work is *De Ephemera Britannica,* written about 1552 (printed in *Joannis Caii Opera,* Louvain, 1556).

24. Caius, *Counseill against the sweate,* Introduction.

25. R. Burton, *Anatomy of Melancholy,* 1621 (Everymans Library, London, 1932, Vol. I), Introduction.

26. Philip Barrough, *The Method of Phisicke,* London, 1583, Sig. A6^r. The same type of reference can be found in a number of books.

27. William Turner, *A new Herball,* London, 1556, Sig. A3^v.

28. Langton, Sig. D3^r.

29. Anon. (trans. T. Newton), *The Olde man's Dietarie,* London, 1586, from an unknown source.

30. *DNB.*

31. William Ram, *Ram's little Dodoen,* London, 1606.

32. H.M. Barlow, "Old English Herbals, 1525-1640," *Proc. Roy. Soc. Med.,* 1913-1914, *6,* pp. 108-149.

33. Paul H. Kocher, "John Hester, Paracelsian," *John Quincy Adams Memorial Studies,* Washington, 1948, p. 630.

34. Galenic works in the vernacular are listed in H.R. Palmer, *List of English Editions and Translations of Greek and Latin Classics Printed before 1641,* 1911.

35. T. Blundeville, *The Arte of Logike plainely taught according to the doctrine of Aristotle,* London, 1599.

36. A general comparison of the two versions can probably most easily be made in C.G. Gruner and H. Haeser, *Scriptores de Sudore Anglico Superstites,* Jena, 1847. This provides facsimiles of the English edition (1552) and the Latin text published in 1721.

37. Talbot, p. 186, refers to late fourteenth century and early fifteenth century treatises in English.

38. See Talbot, pp. 38-55. One of the earliest references to Salerno as a medical centre appeared towards the end of the tenth century. The apogee of Salernitan medicine was reached in the twelfth century. Montpellier is discussed pp. 56-63.

39. Elyot, Sig. 02^r, refers to Linacre's translation of Galen "call in Latyn 'De tuenda Sanitate' translated moost truely and eloquently out of greke."

40. English versions of the Bible were printed "privately" between 1525 and 1539. *The Great Bible* appeared in 1539.

41. R.J. Durling, *Journal of the Warburg and Courtauld Institutes,* 1961, *24,* pp. 230-305.

42; For a detailed discussion of this work see William Telfer (ed.), *Cyril of Jerusalem and Nemesius of Emesa,* 1955.

43. G. Wither, *The Nature of Man,* London, 1636.

44. Palmer, *Translations of the Classics,* p. xi. The Introduction is by Victor Scholderer.

45. L. Thorndike, *A History of Magic and Experimental Science,* 1941, Vol. V, p. 48.

46. Talbot, p. 42.

47. An English translation of the *Isagoge* is available in H.P. Cholmeley, *John of Gaddesden and Rosa Medicinae,* 1912, pp. 136-166. This translation is from the *Articella* published in Lyons in 1515. Also, E.T. Whithington, in his *Medical History from the Earliest Times,* 1964 (reprint of the first edition of 1894), gives a translation of the *Isagoge,* p. 386.

48. John Ordronaux, *Code of Health of the School of Salernum,* 1870, p. 39.

49. There is some controversy over this and over the date of origin. The matter is discussed by Sir Alexander Croke in *Regimen Sanitatis Salernitanum,* 1830. F.R. Packard and F.H. Garrison refer to Croke's views in their version of Sir John Harrington's *The School of Salernum,* 1920.

50. Norman Moore, "The Schola Salernitana: its History and the Date of its

Introduction into the British Isles," *The Glasgow Medical Journal*, 1908, *69*, pp. 241-268.

51. Moore, p. 267.

52. Thomas Paynell, *Regimen Sanitatis Salerni*, London, 1528.

53. Thomas Phayer, *The Regiment of Life newly corrected and enlarged*, London, 1544.

54. Referred to by Norman Moore, p. 252. Also referred to by Croke as being at Corpus Christi College, Oxford. Not seen.

55. Philemon Holland, *Regimen Sanitatis Salerni*, London, 1617.

56. J. Harington (trans.), *The Englishmans doctor. Or the Schoole of Salerne*, London, 1607.

57. Elyot, Sig. A3^r.

58. Packard and Garrison, p. 30.

59. H. Cameron Gillies, *Regimen Sanitatis*, 1911. This work is taken from a Gaelic Medical Manuscript (British Museum, Add. 15582) said to be part of the *Vade Mecum* of the famous MacBeaths, and dating from the early sixteenth century or before.

60. B. Lawn, *The Salernitan Questions*, 1963. This is subtitled, "An Introduction to the History of Medieval and Renaissance Problem Literature." Statements from material on pp. xi, xii, 171, 173, 177.

61. W. Bullein, *The Government of Health*, London [1558], is one example.

62. Robert Steele, *Mediaeval Lore from Bartholomew Anglicus*, 1924 (1st ed. 1893).

63. Stephen Batman, *Batman uppon Bartholome, His Booke De Proprietatibus Rerum*, London, 1582.

64. Culpepper refers to Bartholomaeus Anglicus in his list of "authors made use of in this treatise" (*The English Physician*, London, 1652).

65. A. Arber, *Herbals Their Origin and Evolution*, 1938, p. 61.

66. J. Stannard, "Dioscorides and Renaissance Materia Medica," *Analecta Medico-Historica*, 1904, *1* p. 1.

67. Arber, Chapter III. An extant manuscript of Apuleius in Anglo-Saxon was probably transcribed between A.D. 1000 and 1066. It is concerned with the virtue of herbs.

68. For the dates of these works see Barlow, "Old English Herbals 1525-1640," footnote 32 above.

69. For a discussion of *Le Grant Herbier*, see E.S.Rohde, *The Old English Herbals*, 1922.

70. J. Gerard, *The Herball or Generall Historie of Plantes*, London, 1597.

71. Matthias de l'Obel was born in Flanders in 1538. After studying at Montpellier he settled at Antwerp, practised medicine, and became physician to William the Silent. He moved to England in 1569 and lived at Highgate until his death in 1616. He received the title of Botanist to King James I.

72. E.S. Rohde, *The Old English Herbals*, 1972 (reprint of the first edition, 1922), pp. 103-104.

73. See introductory matter by J. Britten, B.D. Jackson, and W.T. Stearn, *William Turner* (facsimiles of his works on herbs), 1965.

74. Nicolas Monardes (trans. John Frampton), *Joyfull newes out of the new-founde worlde. Wherein are declared, the rare and singular vertues of divers herbs,*

trees, plantes, oyles and stones, with their applications, ass well to the use of physicke, as of chirurgery. . ., London, 1577.

75. Palladius, Rutilus Taurus Aemilianus, fourth century A.D. See Barton Lodge, *Palladius on Husbandry, 1873.* From a MS. of about A.D. 1420 in Colchester Castle.

76. Hesiod, Greek poet and farmer, fifth-fourth century B.C.; Cato, Marcus Porcius the Censor 234-149 B.C.; Varro, Marcus Terentius 116-27 B.C.; Virgil 70-19 B.C.; Columella, Lucius Junius Moderatus c. A.D. 36; Pliny the Elder A.D. 23/24-79.

77. Donald McDonald, *Agricultural Writers from Sir Walter of Henley to Arthur Young, 1200-1800,* 1908, pp. 6-10, and E. Lamond's translation and transcription of *Walter of Henleys Husbandry,* 1890, from the original *printed* version of about 1510.

78. John Fitzherbert, *The Boke of Husbandrye. . .,* London [1523]. See G.E. Fussell, *The Old English Farming Books from Fitzherbert to Tull, 1523-1730,* 1947, for discussion of authorship of Fitzherbert's book.

79. A.M. Tyssen-Amherst, "On a Fifteenth Century Treatise on Gardening, By 'Mayster John Gardener,'" *Archaeologia,* 1895, *54,* pp. 157-172.

80. T. Hill, *The Arte of Gardening,* London [1563].

81. See Frederick Smith, *The Early History of Veterinary Literature and its British Development,* 1919, Vol. I.

82. T. Tusser, *A hundreth good pointes of husbandrie,* London, 1557. Reynolde Scot, *A perfite platforme of a hoppe garden,* London, 1574. L. Mascall, *The firste Booke of Cattell,* London, 1581; *The husbandlye ordring of poultrie,* London, 1581; *A booke of the arte and maner, how to plant and graffe all sortes of trees,* London [1572]. Hugh Platt, *Diverse new sorts of soyle,* London, 1594. J. Taverner, *Certaine experiments concerning fishe and fruite,* London, 1600. Conrad Heresbach (trans. B. Googe), *Foure bookes of husbandry,* London, 1577. Prudent Le Choyselat (trans. R.E.), *A Discourse of Housbandrie,* London, 1580. C. Estienne and J. Liebault (trans. R. Surflet), *Maison Rustique, or the Countrie Farme,* London, 1600.

83. Marcus Gavius Apicius, a glutton, living in the time of Tiberius Caesar, is said to have poisoned himself for fear of starving. His name became proverbial and is the derivation of "Apicius Coelius," the author of *De re coquinaria,* a collection of recipes from the third century A.D. See also R. Barber, *Cooking and Recipes from Rome to the Renaissance,* 1973, p. 20.

84. S. Pegge (The Younger), *The Forme of Cury,* 1780.

85. T. Austin, *Two Fifteenth Century Cookery Books,* 1888. See also M.S. Serjeantson, in her article "The Vocabulary of Cookery in the Fifteenth Century" (*Essays and Studies* [1938], XXIII, collected by S.C. Roberts), for a discussion of this manuscript.

86. Anon., *This is the Boke of Cokerye,* London, 1500, printed by Richard Pynson.

87. Duffy, p. 66.

88. This is illustrated by the bibliorgaphy, A.W. Oxford, *English Cookery Books to the Year 1850,* 1915.

89. Anon., *The Good Hous-Wives Treasurie,* London, 1588. This title was used, with variations, for many different editions through the years.

90. Austin, p. viii. A change is apparent in form and content of recipes in the middle and later part of the seventeenth century.

91. P. Pullar, *Consuming Passions,* 1970. See Barber, note 83 above.

92. Harrison, p. 144.

93. Hannah Glasse, *The Art of Cookery, Made Plain and Easy,* 1760 (7th edition), p. iv, says: "So much is the folly of this age, that they would rather be imposed on by a *French* booby, than give encouragement to a good *English* cook!"

94. Many modern translations are taken from Renaissance texts.

95. Thomas Lupton, *One thousand notable things of sundrie sorts,* London, 1579, last edition 1815. Two items referring to diet which are repeated word for word in each edition are in the 1579 edition (p. 15, No. 57; p. 49, No. 100), and the 1815 edition (p. 5, No. 36; p. 16, No. 57) respectively.

96. See F.N.L. Poynter, *A Bibliography of Gervase Markham, 1568?-1637,* 1962.

97. J.F. Simon (trans. G.E. Day), *Animal Chemistry with Reference to the Physiology and Pathology of Man,* 1846, Vol. II, p. 144.

CHAPTER III

1. *Regimen Sanitatis,* Sig. A2^r. All the following quotations come from this section.

2. Andrew Boorde, *The Breviary of Health,* London, 1547. This subject is discussed in "Appendix to all premysses."

3. Alexis of Piemont (trans. William Ward), *The secretes of Alexis of Piemont containing remedies against diseases,* London, 1558. This is discussed in the "Epistle." For an analysis of the relationship of religion to medicine see P.H. Kocher, *Science and Religion in Elizabethan England,* 1953, pp. 225-330.

5. L. Lemnius, *The Touchstone of Complexions,* London, 1576, Sig. L6^r.

6. Cogan, p. 21.

7. Catherine Cooper (catalogued thus in the British Museum, translated into English anonymously), *A notable and prodigious Historie of a Mayden, who for sundry years neither eateth, drinketh nor sleepeth, neyther avoydeth any excrements, and yet liveth,* London, 1589. A similar case in the nineteenth century is described by John Cule, *The Wreath on the Crown,* 1967. Here Sarah Jacobs of Wales fasted from 1867 to 1869.

8. Hippocrates, *Regimen I,* p. 227.

9. Hippocrates, *Regimen II,* pp. 307-343.

10. Boorde, p. 277.

11. T. Bright, *A Treatise wherein is declared the sufficiencie of English Medicines,* London, 1580, Sig. A4^v.

CHAPTER IV

1. Langton, *Prin. parts,* Sig. B5^r.

2. David Ross, *Aristotle,* 1964, p. 105. See also J.R. Partington, *A History of Chemistry,* 1970, Vol. I, p. 53.

3. Ross, p. 106. Partington, pp. 92, 93.

4. Langton, Sig. B3r-B5r for information on the elements. Partington (p. 156) gives the Stoic definition as "that out of which at first all things which exist are produced and into which at last all things are resolved." He shows the connection between this and the description of elements given by Aristotle, Plato, Robert Boyle (1661), and Stahl (1723).

5. See J. Cadden, "Two Definitions of *Elementum* in a 13th Century Philosophical Text," XIIe Congrès International d'Histoire des Sciences (Paris, 1968), *Actes*, 1971, *3A*, pp. 33-36. The true element is termed *elementum* and the crude *elementatum*.

6. Peter Lowe, *A Discourse of the whole Art of Chirurgery*, London, 1612, p. 12.

7. L. Figard, in his study of the influential Jean Fernel *(Un médicin philosophe au XVIe siècle*, 1903, p. 114), says that Fernel, following "commentators on Aristotle " introduced the concept of intermediary elements between Aristotle's ideas of perfect elements and the concrete elements. These pure intermediate elements were not perceptible to the senses. This concept, says Figard, is put forward in Fernel's *De abditis rerum causis* (1548). In C. Sherrington's bibliographical list of Fernel's works (*The Endeavour of Jean Fernel*, 1946, p. 191), it says that *De abditis rerum causis* was first printed in 1548, but is referred to by Fernel as *Dialogi*. This was probably available in manuscript form before the first appearance in 1542 of *De naturali parte medicinae* (Sherrington, p. 104). Jean Fernel's dates are 1485 to 1557.

8. Jones, *Growing and Living*, Sig. A4r.

9. Elyot, Sig. B1v.

10. T. Bright, *A Treatise of the Melancholie*, London, 1586, pp. 57-59.

11. Jones, *Galen's Elements*, Sig. B4r.

12. Batman, Sig. E5v.

13. T. Newton, *Approved Medicines and Cordiall Receipts*, London, 1580, does not give any qualities of simples beyond "hot and moist" in the second degree, and "cold and moist" in the third degree, whereas hot:dry and cold:dry are given in the fourth degree.

14. Batman, Sig. E5v.

15. H. Wyngfield, *A Compendious or short treatise*, London, 1551, Sig. A7r.

16. R. Klibansky, E. Panofsky, and F. Saxl, *Saturn and Melancholy*, 1964.

17. The different humours had particular times allotted to them wherein they were dominant. The following information comes from Elyot (Sig. T3v). All times of the year and hours of the day and night are covered. The dates as given by Elyot refer to the eighth "idus" of the month. *Phlegm* is stronger during the winter – that is, from November 13 to February 13. It has dominance from the third hour of the night to the ninth hour of the same night. The phlegmatic person has greatest good health in summer. *The sanguine humour* is dominant in springtime (February 13 to May 15), and the ninth hour of the night to the third hour of the morning. The time of good health is summer and winter, because of the humidity. *Red choler* is strongest in summer (May 15 to August 13), and the third hour of the day to the ninth hour of the same day. Winter is the time for good health. *Melancholy* (or black choler) is dominant in the remaining parts of the year and day. The time of good health is "harvest" time.

18. Philistion (435-356 B.C.), head of the Sicilian school of medicine founded by Empedocles.

19. Euryphon of Cnidus, born about 470 B.C.

20. Alcmaeon of Croton (c. 500 B.C.), a Pythagorean doctor.

21. Klibansky *et al.*, p. 5.

22. C.H. Herford and Percy Simpson, *Ben Jonson*, 1925, Vol. I, pp. 331-357.

23. M.S. Ogden, *J. Hist. of Med.*, 1969, *24*, pp. 272-291.

24. Langton, Sig. F2^v.

25. Elyot, Sig. C4^r-D1^r.

26. Langton, Sig. F2^v-F3^r.

27. Langton, *Prin. parts*, Sig. C6^v.

28. Elyot, Sig. C4^r.

29. Langton, Sig. C3^v.

30. L. Lemnius (trans. T. Newton), *A Touchstone of the Complexions*, London, 1576, Sig. L6^v.

31. Langton, *Prin. parts*, Sig. D1^v.

32. "Taketh a new name" – here the differentiation between an unnatural humour and the circulating blood is not made clear; such terms as choleric blood are more frequently used to describe the "circulating blood."

33. Ogden, p. 276.

34. Batman, Sig. N2^v.

35. Langton, *Prin. parts*, Sig. C8^r.

36. Langton, Sig. F3^v.

37. Lowe, p. 20.

38. Elyot, Sig. D1^r.

39. Langton, Sig. F4^v.

40. Langton, Sig. F4^v-F5^r.

41. Robert Burton, *The Anatomie of Melancholy*, London, 1621.

42. Langton, *Prin. parts*, Sig. D1^r.

43. See Chapter VIII "Advice to Specific Groups."

44. Langton, *Prin. parts*, Sig. D2^v.

45. The use of the term similar can be confusing because it has a number of different meanings. According to Hippocrates a similar meant a drug which produced symptoms similar to those observed in the disease. In the Doctrine of similars a part of the body was considered to benefit from the application of objects which resembled that part in shape or colour. For example, disorders of the stomach could be treated by the use of animal stomachs, or a preparation of the leaves of the cyclamen (supposedly similar in shape to human ears) could be used to treat aural diseases.

46. In some English fifteenth century texts the terms nerves and sinews are interchangeable; see for example, *The Middle English Translation of Guy de Chauliac's Anatomy. . .*, ed. B. Walner, 1964, p. 57/3 and glossary. The last references to the double meaning given in the *OED* is Burton's *Anatomy of Melancholy* (1621).

47. I am grateful to Mr. E.J. Freeman for this information.

48. J. Vigo (trans. B. Traheron), *The most excellent works of Chirurgerye*, London, 1543, Sig. A1^r-A1^v.

49. J. Bannister, *The Historie of man*, London, 1578, Sig. C1^r.

50. J. Vicary, *The Englishman's Treasure. With the true anatomye of mans body*, London, 1586, Sig. B3^v-C4^r.

51. Elyot, Sig. D2^v.

52. Langton, Sig. C3^v-C4^r.

53. Langton, Sig. C4^v. Here Langton follows Galen rather than Aristotle. See also Sig. C8^v.

54. Langton, Sig. D5^v.

55. Langton, Sig. E5^r, refers to Langton's information on the liver.

56. Batman, Sig. L1^r.

57. Galen, p. 295, explains that under appropriate circumstances the stomach easily attracts nutriment from the liver. Lemnius, Sig. M1^v, says the heart is the fountain of the blood, and the liver the "shop of the blood."

58. Langton, Sig. E6^r.

59. Langton, Sig. F3^v.

60. Batman, Sig. M1^v.

61. Batman, Sig. M1^v.

62. Lemnius, Sig. D2^v.

63. Langton, Sig. F7^r, and following. Probably a true estimation of the clarity of ideas about spirits in the sixteenth century is given by Harvey, writing in 1649: ". . . of these points there are so many and such conflicting opinions that it is not wonderful that the spirits, whose nature is thus left wholly ambiguous, should serve as the common subterfuge of ignorance" (p. 141, *Circulation of the Blood*, ed. E.A. Parkyn, 1952).

64. Langton, Sig. F7^v.

65. Langton, Sig. F7^v.

66. Lowe, p. 26.

67. Langton, Sig. F8^v. See also O. Temkin, "On Galen's Pneumatology," *Gesnerus*, 1950, *8* pp. 180-189.

68. Langton, *Prin. parts*, Sig. E1^v and E2^r.

69. Harvey's concept of the circulation of the blood was not published until 1628.

70. Elyot, Sig. D4^v.

71. Langton, Sig. G1^r.

72. Lowe, p. 24.

73. Elyot, Sig. D4^r.

74. Lowe's information on the vital power is given on pp. 24 and 25.

75. Lowe, p. 25.

76. As well as concoction, the word digestion is used frequently by sixteenth century writers.

77. Langton says (Sig. G4^r) that nutrition is assimilation, but elsewhere in sixteenth century writings the words seem to have meanings supplementary to each other.

78. Langton, Sig. G1^r.

79. Langton, Sig. G1^v.

80. Galen, pp. 19, 27-31.

81. Langton, Sig. G1^v.

82. Langton, Sig. G3^r.

83. Langton, Sig. G2^r. Galen, pp. 27, 29.

84. Langton, Sig. G2^v, G3^r. The following section on nutrition can be found between Sig. G2^v and H1^r.

85. Langton, Sig. G4^v. This closely follows Galen, p. 35.

86. The exact meaning of excrement as used by sixteenth century writers is difficult to determine, but in general it means waste material in any part of the body.

87. Langton, Sig. G5^v-G6^v includes this whole quotation.

88. Langton, Sig. G7^v-G8^r.

89. Elyot, Sig. D4^r.

90. Langton, Sig. H1^r.

91. Langton, Sig. H1^v. The adamant stone referred to a loadstone or magnet. The jet stone had its present meaning.

92. Galen (p. 71) refers to these ideas. "Motte" means a mote or speck of dust and refers to the Atomist tradition.

93. Langton, Sig. H2^v.

94. Elyot, Sig. D4^r.

95. Today we still have no clearcut knowledge of the physical and biochemical factors which affect the control of appetite. Modern theories are summarised by E.H. Hipsley, "Hunger and Appetite and the Maintenance of Balance between Energy Intake and Expenditure," *Food and Nutrition Notes and Reviews* (Canberra), 1961, *18,* pp. 33-40. The matter is also usually dealt with briefly in modern books on physiology or nutrition.

96. Overmouth refers to the cardiac opening of the stomach or the throat.

97. Langton, Sig. H7^r, H7^v.

98. Langton, Sig. H7^v. Galen believed that Plato regarded the liver as the seat of the appetitive part. See F.M. Cornford's translation of Plato's *Timaeus,* 1959 (ed. Oskar Piest), p. 86. Later authors, however, also implicated the stomach.

99. Langton, Sig. H7^v.

100. Galen, p. 295, refers to this idea. See also Galen (MTM), p. 301, May's footnote 43.

101. Langton's information is from Sig. H3^r-H4^r.

102. *OED*. The emphasis on heat is interesting.

103. Elyot, Sig. U4^v.

104. C. Sherrington, *The Endeavour of Jean Fernel,* 1946, p. 69.

105. Lowe, p. 21. Chyle or chilus in the sixteenth century meant the product of incomplete digestion and was something similar to chyme (the product of gastric digestion) today.

106. Celsus, Vol. I, p. 13.

107. The effect of the ideas of Paracelsus and van Helmont on Galenic theories of digestion are discussed by R.P. Multhauf in "J.B. van Helmont's Reformation of the Galenic Doctrine of Digestion," *Bull. Hist. Med.,* 1955, *29,* pp. 154-163.

108. Lowe, p. 21.

109. Elyot, Sig. E2^v, E3^r, E3^v.

110. Elyot, Sig. U4^v.

111. Langton, Sig. H4^v.

112. Langton, Sig. H5^v.

113. Modern theories do not consider one organ weaker or stronger than another in this respect, but it is acknowledged that a nutrient may be of greater importance to one part than another — e.g. the maintenance of the calcium balance in the fluids of the body at the expense of the solid structures which contain calcium.

114. The idea of "superfluities" played an important part in Galenic nutritional theory (Galen, p. 35) and thereafter.

115. Langton, Sig. H6^v.

116. Elyot, Sig. P4^v and Q1^v.

117. A clyster means a washout, drench, enema, or sometimes a suppository *(OED)*.

118. Elyot, Sig. Q4^r, Q4^v, R1^r.

119. Elyot, Sig. Q3^v.

120. The "lyttell crafte of Galene" is *Ars medica (ars parva)*.

121. Elyot, Sig. E1^v.

122. Elyot, Sig. E1^v.

123. Lowe, p. 37.

124. H. Cuffe, *The Differences of the Ages of Man's life,* London, 1607, pp. 83-84. For the Aristotelian view see F. Copleston, *A History of Philosophy,* 1962 (Image Books edition), Vol. I, Part II, p. 51.

125. Marshall Clagett, *Giovanni Marliani and Late Medieval Physics,* 1941. See particularly pp. 79-100 "Body Heat and Antiperistasis." This work is concerned with temperature as a scale of intensity, rather than "temperature" as a balance of qualities in the body.

126. C. Sherrington, *The Endeavour of Jean Fernel,* 1946.

127. G.J. Goodfield, *The Growth of Scientific Physiology,* 1960; E. Mendelsohn, *Heat and Life,* 1964.

128. Walter Pagel, *William Harvey's Biological Ideas,* 1967.

129. Jones, *Growing and Living.* See section Sig. A4^v-D3^r.

130. Gabriel Fallopius (1523-62).

131. Jones, *Growing and Living,* Sig. A4^v.

132. R. Multhauf, "J.B. van Helmont's Reformation of the Galenic Doctrine of Digestion," *Bull. Hist. Med.,* 1955, *29,* p. 158.

133. Jones, *Growing and Living,* Sig. B1^r.

134. Jones, *Growing and Living,* Sig. B2^r.

135. Jones, *Growing and Living,* Sig. B2^r.

136. Jones, *Growing and Living,* Sig. B1^v.

137. Partington, pp. 90 and 91.

138. Claggett, p. 92.

139. Jones, *Growing and Living,* Sig. B1^v.

140. Langton, Sig. C4^r.

141. See Aristotle, *Meteorologica,* Book IV, p. 379^b, 6.

142. Jones, *Growing and Living,* Sig. B2^v.

143. The link between exercise and the production of heat from the body had been recognized and taken into consideration by the ancient teachers.

144. Jones refers to the difference of opinion regarding the action of diastole and systole. See Pagel, pp. 89-124 "Circular Symbolism, Heart and Blood before Harvey."

145. Jones, *Growing and Living,* Sig. B2^v.

146. Jones, *Growing and Living,* Sig. B2^v. Jones quotes Galen; see also Galen (MTM), p. 292.

147. Jones, *Growing and Living,* Sig. B2^r.

148. Jones, *Growing and Living,* Sig. B3^r.

149. Jones, *Growing and Living,* Sig. B3^v.

150. Temkin, *Gesnerus,* 1950, *8*, pp. 180-189.

151. Two examples are: F. Solmsen, "The Vital Heat, the Inborn Pneuma, and the Aether," *J. Hell. Stud.,* 1957, *77*, pp. 119-123; *Handbook of Physiology,* 1964 (eds. W.O. Fenn and Herman Rahn), Section 3, Respiration, Vol. I, pp. 1-12.

152. H. Wyngfield, *A compendious or shorte treatise,* London, 1551, Sig. A8^v.

153. Jones, *Growing and Living,* Sig. D3^r. The first alteration "which is made on moisture in our bodies" is made on good matter by natural heat. The second is partly good and partly evil: good because of the natural heat, and bad because of the unnatural heat present. The third alteration is made of "an evell worker in any evell matter," as when the humour is rotten and is acted on by rotten heat.

154. Jones, *Bathes Ayde,* Sig. C2^v.

155. Jones, *Growing and Living,* Sig. C2^v.

156. Jones, *Growing and Living,* Sig. C3^r.

157. Jones, *Growing and Living,* Sig. C3^v.

158. Jones, *Growing and Living,* Sig. C3^v.

159. J.B. Montanus (1498-1552).

160. Jones, *Growing and Living,* Sig. C4^r.

161. Pagel, *Harvey,* p. 177.

162. Pagel, *Harvey,* p. 208, refers to ideas of the "seething" of the blood initiating motion.

163. Lowe, p. 62.

CHAPTER V

1. See L.J. Rather, *Clio Medica,* 1968, *3*, pp. 337-347, and S. Jarcho, *Bull. Hist. Med.,* 1970, *44*, pp. 372-377. L. Lemnius (trans. T. Newton), *The Touchstone of Complexions,* London, 1576, Sig. F6^v, says "Galene calleth them causes conservatarie, because they serve and are able to keepe our bodies in good state, ... The Physitions of later time call them by the name of thinges not naturall." Of interest is J. Mackenzie, *The History of Health and the Art of Preserving it,* 1659, Part II, Chap. II, p. 367 and following.

2. Bullein, Sig. B6^r.

3. Referred to as such by Cogan, Sig. 994^r.

4. Elyot, Sig. B1^r.

5. Cogan, Sig. 4^r. See Hippocrates, *De morbis vulgaribus,* lib. 6 in *Opera Omnia* (ed. C.G. Kühn), Leipzig, 1825-27, Vol. III, p. 611.

6. Cogan, Sig. 993^v.

7. Examples of dictionaries are: T. Elyot, *The dictionary of syr T. Eliot* (Lat.-Eng.), London, 1538; T. Elyot, *Bibliotheca Eliotae: newly imprinted and inriched,* by T. Cooper, London, 1548; Robert Cawdrey, *A table alphabeticall, conteyning and teaching the true writing, and understanding of hard usuall English wordes,* London, 1604.

8. James Hart, KΛINIKH *or Diet of the Diseased,* London, 1633, p. 1.

9. Sixteenth century books on health give sections on purges and bloodletting related to Repletion. Detailed discussion of this type of treatment has been omitted from this study.

10. Langton, Sig. D5^v.

11. For a discussion of this see D. Fleming, "Galen on the Motions of the Blood," *Isis*, 1955, *46*, pp. 14-21.

12. Bullein, Sig. H2^r.

13. Elyot Sig. E2^r.

14. Cogan, p. 7.

15. Bullein, Sig. H1^v.

16. Boorde, p. 234.

17. Boorde, p. 238.

18. Hippocrates, *Airs Waters and Places*, p. 81. The characteristics of different winds are discussed in *Regimen II*, pp. 301-305.

19. Boorde, p. 239.

20. Sir John Harrington invented the water closet in 1594. See L.E. Pearson, *Elizabethans at Home*, 1957, p. 56.

21. Boorde, p. 236. Beware also of the "snoffe of candelles" and the smell of apples.

22. J. Lees-Milne, *Tudor Renaissance*, 1951, p. 56.

23. John Shute, *The first and chief groundes of architecture*, London, 1563, Sig. B3^v.

24. Lees-Milne, see plates 90 and 95.

25. Lees-Milne, p. 98.

26. Pearson, p. 11.

27. Erasmus was writing to Dr. Franciscus in 1515. See J. Jortin, *The Life of Erasmus*, London, 1758-60, Vol. I, p. 76 and Vol. II, pp. 341-342. To place this famous quotation in proper perspective see M. StC. Byrne, *Elizabethan Life in Town and Country*, 1961, p. 8.

28. L. Lemnius (trans. T. Newton), *The Touchstone of the Complexions*, London, 1576, Sig. F8^r. This view is supported in C. William's translation, *Thomas Platter's Travels in England, 1599*, 1937, p. 97.

29. Pearson, Chapter I, "Homes and Gardens" exemplifies this attitude.

30. Lees-Milne (p. 134) suggests that "The more-glass-than-wall façade is about the most moving and romantic contribution made to English architecture by the Tudors."

31. Thomas Tusser gives a list of "strewing herbs." See D. Hartley, *Thomas Tusser – 1577*, 1931, p. 152.

32. L. Lemery (trans. D. Hay), *A Treatise of all sorts of Foods*, London, 1745, p. 1. "... the Air ought to be look'd upon as real Food, ..."

33. F. Magendie (1783-1855) showed that nitrogenous foodstuffs were required: *Annales de Chimie et de Physique*, 1816, *3*, pp. 66-77; but the controversy about the nutritional value of atmospheric nitrogen continued.

34. Cogan, p. 231.

35. Langton, Sig. K8^r.

36. Cogan, p. 232.

37. Gratarolus, Sig. S4^r.

38. Cogan, p. 238. The subsequent information on sleep can be found between pages 231 and 239. See also Elyot, Sig. N3^r-N4^r; Langton, *Prin. parts*, Sig. F3^r-F5^r, and Bullein, Sig. F1^r-F2^v.

39. L. Fuchsius is quoted as saying that sleep after dinner should be either very

little or very much, so that the heat has hardly time to be drawn inward, or there is time for complete concoction.

40. Boorde, p. 246.

41. Cogan, p. 235.

42. The significance of different sorts of dreams is described in the Hippocratic *Regimen IV on Dreams*. Natural philosophers continued to produce treatises on the cause and interpretation of dreams. W. Vaughan (*Naturall and artificial directions for health,* London, 1600, Sig. C8^v) says "Dreames are either tokens of things past or significants of things to come." Langton (Sig. L6^v-M5^r) attributes dreams to an imagination during sleep when various spirits meet in the brain which, being the instrument of thought, makes images; at this time the "inner senses" are more at liberty than the "outer senses." There are four categories of dreams: (i) natural – people of different complexions were recognized as being susceptible to different types, (ii) dreams that foresee things; this is due to an individual natural talent, (iii) dreams that prophesy due to Divine power, and (iv) devilish dreams when the Devil provides terrible spectacles. Credit, says Langton, should be given only to dreams of Divine origin. The importance of dreams and their interpretation can be judged by the extensive dramatic use made of them by Chaucer and Shakespeare, for whom the basic premises about dreams were similar. Medievel dream lore is discussed in Chapters 8 and 9 of W.C. Curry's *Chaucer and the Medieval Sciences,* London, 1960.

43. Cogan, p. 235.

44. Hippocrates (Littré), *Des Epidémies*, Vol. V, p. 311.

45. Sleeping on the left side is approved of only after the first sleep.

46. Cogan, p. 237 gives no explanation of this. It is not stressed by other authors.

47. Elyot, Sig. N3^v.

48. A number of books on health provide guidance on the proper examination of the urine for diagnostic purposes. Detailed discussion of these sections has been omitted from this study.

49. *Regimen Sanitatis,* Sig. B3^r.

50. Elyot, Sig. O1^r. Rubbing is discussed further under "Exercise."

51. Bullein, Sig. D8^r. Washing with hot water "engendereth rheumes, wormes and corruption, in the stomacke."

52. Vaughan, Sig. F6^r, advocates retiring to one's chamber to clean the teeth after meals. Authors give advice on a wide range of materials suitable for cleaning the teeth, from a sage leaf to perfumed pastes. Comments are also made on the value of "[s]neesing and gargaling."

53. Boorde, p. 248.

54. Cogan, p. 1.

55. Langton, *Prin. parts,* Sig. F1^v.

56. Cogan, p. 1.

57. This theme – that those whose work is active are healthier than those who use their minds – goes right through the advice.

58. References to exercise are frequently found in advice on purges.

59. Hippocrates, *Regimen II,* p. 349. Elyot refers the reader to his *The Boke named the Governour,* London, 1531.

60. See Elyot, Sig. O2^r-P1^r; Langton, *Prin. parts,* Sig. F1^v-F3^r; Bullein, Sig. E7^v-F1^r; Gratarolus, Sig. C1^r-E3^r; Cogan, pp. 1-21.

61. Elyot, Sig. H2^v.

62. Cogan, p. 2.

63. F.G. Emmison, *Elizabethan Life: Disorder,* Chelmsford, 1970, p. 218. Set out in Act 33 Henry VIII c9 1541. Many of the games listed first appeared in Act 12 Richard II c6 1388. Penalties were severe for playing an unlawful game.

64. Byrne, p. 243.

65. Elyot, *The Governour,* Sig. N1^v. It is the remaining rancour and malice that matter most.

66. Cogan, p. 3.

67. Gratarolus, Sig. D1^v. Tennis could be played with the hand or with a racquet.

68. Gratarolus, Sig. D2^r.

69. Elyot, Sig. O2^v.

70. Elyot, Sig. O3^v.

71. Cogan, p. 3.

72. Elyot, Sig. O4^v.

73. Cogan, p. 21.

74. G. Finney, "Vocal Exercise in the Sixteenth Century Related to Theories of Physiology and Diseases," *Bull. Hist. Med.,* 1968, *42,* pp. 422- 429.

75. Walter Johnson, in *The Anatriptic Art,* London, 1866, makes detailed references to the advice of Hippocrates, Galen, and Celsus. Johnson, a physician, lived at Malvern (a spa) and treated his patients with massage combined sometimes with bathing.

76. Cogan, p. 5.

77. Gratarolus, Sig. E3^r.

78. See W. Turner, *A Booke of the nature, and properties, as well of the bathes in England. . .,* London, 1568; John Jones, *The Bathes of Bathes Ayde,* and *The Benefit of the Ancient Bathes of Buckstones,* both London, 1572.

79. Public baths were available, but the Bagnio which provided baths and sweating rooms had its greatest popularity in the eighteenth century. Turner has specific hygienic recommendations for communal bathing.

80. Gratarolus, Sig. E3^v.

81. Gratarolus, Sig. F1^r.

82. Vaughan, Sig. D3^r. Pearson (p. 445) describes bathing in the home.

83. Gratarolus, Sig. E1^v-E2^r.

84. Gratarolus, Sig. U1^r.

85. Bullein, Sig. F1^r.

86. This refers to cases where a localized infection might spread.

87. Cogan, p. 7.

88. Elyot, Sig. N4^v.

89. Cogan, p. 8. German scholars "never exercise but foorwith after meate, eyther leaping, or running."

90. Cogan, p. 9. The subsequent quotations come from the same section.

91. Langton, *Prin. parts,* Sig. F3^r.

92. Cogan (pp. 12-21) covers his chapter on exercise of the mind. C.D. O'Malley's "Jacobus Sylvius' Advice for Poor Medical Students," *Jour. Hist. Med.,* 1962, *17,* pp. 141-51, does not provide detailed information about methods of study.

93. Cogan, p. 14.

94. Some advocated a situation with a pleasant view of the countryside. Cogan considered this a distraction.

95. Cogan, p. 13.

96. Cogan, p. 20. The importance of music in Elizabethan life is obvious from the literature of the period. See also Pearson, p. 1.

97. Elyot, Sig. N4ʳ.

98. Elyot, Sig. K6ʳ.

99. Gratarolus, Sig. T4ʳ.

100. Batman, Sig. D2ʳ.

101. P. de la Primaudaye (trans. T.B.), *The French Academie,* London, 1586; P. Charron (trans. S. Lennard), *Of Wisdom, three bookes,* London, 1606; T. Wright, *The passions of the minde in generall,* London, 1604.

102. Wright, p. 7.

103. R.L. Anderson, *University of Iowa Humanistic Studies,* 1927, *3,* No. 4, p. 69.

104. Writers disagree on the actual number and classification of the passions, the two main groupings being concupiscent and irascible. See Anderson, p. 70.

105. Elyot, Sig. R4ᵛ. Vaughan (Sig. E2ᵛ) gives the alternative view that the cold and trembling is due to heat withdrawing into the heart. The pale cold anger was the most dangerous.

106. Langton, *Prin. parts,* Sig. H8ᵛ; C.T. Allbutt (*Greek Medicine in Rome,* 1921, p. 301) suggests that Praxagoras the Coan (c. 340-320 B.C.) was the first physician to give the pulse some place in diagnosis and therapeutics. His pupil Herophilius appears to have been the first to count the pulse by a water clock. Through the centuries a number of treatises were written on the pulses and information on them was included in the *Articella.* Langton (*Prin. parts,* Sig. M3ʳ) describes the pulse as "a sensible movynge of the hart and Arteries (that is to say vaynes, having two coates growing of the hart, and carriynge both blod and spirit) by the which they be lifted up and let done againe." He points out that though many physicians use the pulses diagnostically, ancient writers are not agreed on their use in diagnosis, saying that Celsus seemed to doubt whether "any thynge may certaynly be conjectured by them or no."

107. Like blasphemy, swearing or the use of profane language was considered a serious matter. Boorde (p. 243) tells the master of the household "specyally to punysshe swearers," for there is more swearing in England than anywhere else in the world.

108. Langton, Sig. K8ᵛ.

109. Bullein, Sig. F7ʳ and Langton, *Prin. parts,* Sig. H8ᵛ. Here perhaps the fear should be described as terror, for the initial reaction to fear is an increased secretion of adrenalin with a simultaneous increase in heartbeat.

110. For an anthology of the advice on madness given in this period see R. Hunter and I. MacAlpine, *Three Hundred Years of Psychiatry, 1535-1860,* 1963.

111. Gratarolus, Sig. T4ᵛ.

112. Elyot, Sig. S2ᵛ.

113. See T. Bright, *A Treatise of the Melancholie,* London, 1586, and Robert Burton, *The anatomy of melancholy, what it is. With all kindes etc.,* London, 1621.

114. Langton, *Prin. parts,* Sig. J1^r.
115. Elyot, Sig. T2^v.
116. Anderson, p. 73 and following.
117. Elyot, Sig. R4^v.
118. Elyot, Sig. S2^r-T1^v.
119. The heart-bone was considered good for a "trembling heart" (George Turberville [trans. Anon.], *The Noble Arte of Venerie or Hunting,* London, 1575, Sig. C4^r). See also O. Shepard, *The Horn of the Unicorn,* 1930.
120. Elyot, Sig. T2^r, includes emeralds, gold, and silver.
121. Cogan, p. 242.
122. Cogan, p. 240.
123. Langton, Sig. M5^r.
124. Cogan, p. 242. The information in the rest of this section comes from Cogan, pp. 239-254.
125. Cogan, p. 248.
126. Cogan, p. 245. No comment is made on the sexual needs of "good" women.
127. Cogan, p. 265.

CHAPTER VI

1. Bullein, Sig. C1^r-C1^v.
2. L.S. Goodman and A. Gilman (eds.), *The Pharmacological Basis of Therapeutics,* 1967, Section XVIII on vitamins, p. 1649. Paul Greengard differentiates between vitamins obtained in a normal manner in food for the healthy and the prescription of vitamins in their chemically pure form.
3. Jane O'Hara-May, "Foods or Medicines?" (A study in the relationship between foodstuffs and materia medica from the sixteenth to the nineteenth century), in *Transactions of the British Society for the History of Pharmacy,* 1971, *1* No. 2.
4. Cogan, p. 32 and p. 174.
5. Newton's *Approved Medicines* (see note 16 below) contains a number of foodstuffs of "low degree."
6. Gabriel Fernelius. Jean Fernel (1497-1558).
7. This refers to *Methodus Medendi,* sometimes called "Therapeutic," in a variety of sixteenth century spellings.
8. Jones, *Bucks Baths,* Sig. B4^v-C1^r.
9. Jean Fernel, *De abditis rerum causis,* Paris, 1560 (1st ed. 1548), Sig. 2Bs^r. I am grateful to Mr. H.J.M. Symons for his translation of this section.
10. In this context corn refers to wheat, barley, or rye. Maize or *zea mayse* is mentioned by sixteenth century writers as Turkey wheat, Chapter XI.
11. Langton, Sig. H8^v-J1^r.
12. H. Buttes, *Dyets Dry Dinner,* London, 1599.
13. Not everyone agreed about the benefits of tobacco. King James I produced his *A counter blaste to tobacco,* London, 1604.
14. This is the sequence used by Cogan.
15. Elyot, Sig. F2^r, F2^v.

16. T. Newton, *Approved Medicines and Cordiall Receipts, with the nature, qualities and operations of sundry Simples,* London, 1580.

17. O. Temkin, "Nutrition from Classical Antiquity to the Baroque," in *Human Nutrition Historic and Scientific,* Monograph III, ed. I. Galdston, New York, 1960, p. 87.

18. Marshall Clagett, *Osiris,* 1950, *9,* pp. 131-161 (Swineshead); M. McVaugh, *Isis,* 1967, *58,* pp. 56-64 (Bradwardine), *Bull. Hist. Med.,* 1969, *43,* pp. 397-413 (Arnald Villanova, Montpellier); J.M. Dureau-Lapeysonnie, *Médecin Humaine et Vétérinarie à la fin du moyen âge,* 1966 (Ricart); D. Skabelund and P. Thomas, *Isis,* 1969, *60,* pp. 331-349 (Walter of Oddington).

19; H. Billingsley, *The Elements of Geometrie of the most auncient Philosopher EUCLIDE of Megara,* London, 1570, Sig. *3r-*4v. See "Mathematical Praeface" by John Dee. Dee's calculation of the resulting degree of the hot qualitie of equal weights of H^4 and H^2 is 2½, i.e., in the middle of the third degree. Oddington's calculation (Skabelund and Thomas, p. 338) gives 3.5°.

20. Jones, *Bathes Ayde,* Sig. E4r. The following description of degrees in relation to the quality hot is taken from Dr. Parkins, *The English Physician an improvement on Culpeper's Herbal,* 1814, pp. ix and x. Here the "temperaments of the herbs" are described. Though this work was printed some two centuries later, it is similar in attitude to mid-seventeenth century vernacular writings and does not contradict sixteenth century advice. *1st degree* is equivalent to the heat of the body and only adds natural heat if required. *2nd degree* "as much exceeds that in first degree as our natural heat exceeds a temperature" (temperate heat). *3rd degree* is more powerful and able to inflame fevers. *4th degree* will burn the body if applied externally. Substances of this degree are used for raising blisters, corroding the skin, and causing inflammation. McVaugh, *Bull. Hist. Med.,* 1969, *43,* p. 399 describes the characteristics of different degrees of a quality in terms of their effects; temperate included those medicines which had no perceptible effect, though given repeatedly and in large quantities. "Those which acted insensibly over a long period were assigned to the first degree; and so on, up to those in the fourth degree, whose effect was immediate and violent, perhaps even fatal."

21. All are taken from Buttes, *Dyets Dry Dinner,* Sig. B4v, D8v, L1v, K1r, N2v, N7v, respectively.

22. Batman, Sig. 3H1v. See chapter XVI note 23.

23. Langton, *Prin. parts,* Sig. C6v. Buttes describes vinegar as cold and moist (Sig. 09v); Cogan says it is cooling and drying (p. 164).

24. Batman, Sig. E6r.

25. Scientific investigations into taste have been undertaken recently. Examples are *Principles of Sensory Evaluation of Food,* M.A. Amerine, R.M. Pangborne and E.B. Roessler, 1965. J.E. Amoore, G. Palmieri and E. Wanke, "Molecular Shape and Odour: Pattern Analysis by PAPA," *Nature,* Dec. 16, 1967, pp. 1084-1087.

26. Batman, Sig. E2r-E3r covers the information given here from Batman.

27. Modern physiology teaches that one of the functions of saliva is to dissolve food so that it can be tasted and then swallowed.

28. Sixteenth century writers do not refer to the Hippocratic thesis which says that when a sweet humour assumes another form by a self-caused change it will follow a set pattern and most easily become acid and that this must be taken into consideration when prescribing diets. Hippocrates, *Ancient Medicine,* Vol. I, p. 63.

29. See J. R. Partington, *A History of Chemistry,* 1970, Vol. I, p. 116.

30. Jones, *Bathes Ayde,* Sig. E2^r-E4^r.

31. Buttes, Sig. G5^v; Cogan, p. 79.

32. Batman, Sig. A36^r; Elyot, Sig. H3^r; Cogan, p. 99; Buttes, Sig. E1^v-E2^r.

33. Jones, *Bathes Ayde,* Sig. E2^r.

34. Batman, Sig. E2^v.

35. Elyot, Sig. F2^r, F2^v.

36. Clammy — soft, moist, sticky, tenacious, adhesive, viscid *(OED).* Clammy does not seem to be related in action to moist as might be expected from modern definitions. This characteristic might well be considered part of the "substance" of a food.

37. *Regimen Sanitatis,* Sig. K4^r.

38. W. Pagel, "Van Helmont's Ideas on Gastric Digestion and the Gastric Acid," *Bull. Hist. Med.,* 1956, *30,* p. 527.

39. Batman, Sig. L4^v

40. Boorde, P. 265.

41. J. Hester, *A compendium of the national secretes of the Worthie Knight and most excellent Doctor of Physick and chirurgerie L. Phioravante,* London, 1582, Bk. III, p. 39.

42. In this context neither "substance" nor "form" seem to have any Aristotelian philosophical connotation. See D. Ross, *Aristotle,* 1964, pp. 165-173.

43. Elyot, Sig. F1^r.

44. Lowe, Sig. D6^r.

45. Elyot, Sig. E1^v-E2^v.

46. The brains of hens were often referred to as being of value. Other brains were not usually recommended.

47. Langon, Sig. J5^r. Here a number of things making ill juice are listed.

48. Elyot, Sig. E2^r, E2^v.

49. Buttes, Sig. N6^v.

50. Langton, Sig. J3^r.

51. Elyot, Sig. E2^v, E3^r.

52. Buttes, Sig. D1^v.

53. Langton, Sig. K1^r and Sig. J8^v.

54. Langton, Sig. J8^r. Though many of Langton's lists of foods are quoted it is recognized that these are not comprehensive or in total agreement with other authors, but they do act as a good example of the advice given at that period.

55. Langton, Sig. J7^r.

56. Elyot, Sig. M1^r.

57. Elyot, Sig. D2^v.

58. Elyot, Sig. U1^v. This is also referred to under the Section on "diet for a choleric man," for abstinence causes adjusting of humours in the stomach, and then "fumosities and stynkeynge vapours ascendynge up to the head whereof is ingendered, duskynge of the eyes, head aches."

50. Boorde, p. 282.

60. Th. Meyer-Stiener and Karl Sudhoff (*Geschichte der Medizin im Uberblick mit Abfildungen,* 1928, p. 369) point out that parasites may arise from dead matter or from living material by the reduction of organic level, as in the case of sweat.

61. Langton, Sig. K1^v.
62. Buttes, Sig. O4^v, N1^v, D7^v, K6^v respectively.
63. Boorde, p. 285.
64. Cogan, p. 246.
65. Sir John Harrington, *The School of Salernum* (1607), ed. F.R. Packard and F.H. Garrison, 1930, p. 103.
66. Boorde, p. 284.
67. Harrington, p. 79.
68. Boorde, p. 283.
69. Elyot, Sig. D2^v-D4^r.
70. Boorde, p. 271.
71. Boorde, p. 277.

CHAPTER VII

1. J. Penkethman, *Authentic Accounts of the History and Price of Wheat, Breat Malt, etc.,* 1765, pp. 70-72.
2. See John Stow, *Annales, or a generall Chronicle of England* (Begun by John Stow, continued and augmented by Edmund Howes, Gent.), London, 1631.
3. Penkethman, p. 70.
4. P. Goubert, *Beauvais et les Beauvaises de 1600 à 1730,* 1960.
5. Fynes Moryson, *An itinerary written by F. Moryson Gent,* London, 1617, Part III, p. 150 and following.
6. Penkethman, pp. 71, 72. Other causes such as war, debasement of the coinage, and high rents are mentioned.
7. G. Botero (trans. R. Peterson), *A treatise concerning the causes of magnificencie and greatnes of cities,* London, 1606.
8. Harrison, p. 153.
9. Cogan, p. 28.
10. Cogan, p. 29.
11. P.H. McGrath, *The Marketing of Food and Fodder in the London Area in the Seventeenth Century,* unpublished M.A. Thesis, 1948.
12. Anon., *Here begynneth the boke named the assies of breade,* London [1580].
13. England, *Acts of the Privy Council* (1586-87), xiv, p. 338. See also *Orders devised by the especiall commandement of the Queenes Majestie, for the reliefe and stay of the present dearth of Graine within the Realme,* London, 1586.
14. N.S.B. Gras, *The Evolution of the English Corn Market from the Twelfth to the Eighteenth Century,* 1915, p. 229.
15. Gras, pp. 237-240.
16. E.M. Hampson, *The Treatment of Poverty in Cambridgeshire 1597-1834,* 1949, pp. 8-9.
17. H.P. Esq. (Sir Hugh Platt), *Sundrie new and artificiall remedies against Famine,* London, 1596. In this chapter "Platt" refers to this book, unless indicated otherwise.
18. Platt, Sig. A2^r-A3^v.
19. Platt, Sig. A4^r.

20. Platt, Sig. B3^r.

21. Hugh Platt, *The Jewell House of Art and Nature*, London, 1594, p.72.

22. Platt, Sig. B3^v.

23. H. Platt, *Certaine philosophical Preparations of Foode and Beverage for Seamen . . .*, London, 1607. Broadsheet, in the library of the Wellcome Institute of the History of Medicine.

24. Platt, Sig. B3^r.

25. The author of this book has not yet been traced.

26. Platt, Sig. D2^r.

27. Platt, Sig. B1^r-B2^r.

28. Platt, Sig. E1^v.

29. W. K. Lowther-Clarke (ed.), *Liturgy and Worship*, 1932. See "Fasting and Abstinence" by A.J. Maclean, pp. 245-256.

30. Boorde, p. 251.

31. Langton, *Prin. parts*, Sig. H1^r.

32. Gratarolus, Sig. R3^v.

33. Church of England, *The Second Tome of Homilies*, London, 1563, Sig. 2N^v.

34. *Homilies*, Sig. 2M7^v.

35. Anon., *A notable Treatyse wherin is shewed that by the word of god we may at al times. . .*, London, n.d. (Printed by R. Stoughton between 1548 and 1551), Sig. A3^r.

36. G. Harford and M. Stevenson (eds.), *The Prayer Book Dictionary*, 1925, p. 360.

37. Act 1548, 3 Ed. VI c.19.

38. Act 1552, 5 and 6 Ed. VI c.3, "For keeping Holidays and Fasting days." See O. Ruffhead, *Statutes at Large*, 1730, Vol. II, pp. 419 and 439.

39. Thomas Becon, *The Works of Thomas Becon*, London, 1563, Part II, "A Treatyse of Fastyng," Sig. 303^r.

40. *Homilies*, Sig. 2M3^v.

41. Cogan, p. 139.

42. *Homilies*, Sig. 2N2^v.

43. Cogan, p. 139. The order referred to was by Proclamation June 24, 1568.

44. *Homilies*, Sig. 2N2^v-2N3^r. Politicians were well aware that skilled fishermen help to provide a strong navy and that populated coastal areas are useful in times of threatened invasion.

45. Cogan, p. 139.

46. John Strype, *Annals of the Reformation*, 1724-5. Vol. I, Part II, pp. 273-4.

47. I. B., *A Treatise with a Kalendar*, n.p., 1608, Sig. A3^r (preface dated 1598). This is No. 61 in A.F. Allison and D.M. Rogers, *A Catalogue of Catholic Books in English printed abroad or secretly in England, 1558-1640*, 1956. It is said that the table was made up 26 years before [1572].

48. W. Wilkinson, *The Holie exercise of a true Fast, described out of God's word*, London, 1580, Sig. A2^v. This work has "seen and allowed" on the title page.

49. Lowther-Clarke, p. 248.

50. Becon, Sig. 303^r.

51. Individuals should also undertake "private" (or personal) fasts; these should be unostentatious.

52. *Liturgies, A Fourme to be used in Common prayer twyse a weke, and also an order of publique fast* . . . 30 July, 1563, Sig. C2^V-C3^r.

53. Lowther-Clarke, p. 248.

54. V. Staley, *Hierurgia Anglicana: or Documents and Extracts illustrative of the Ritual of the Church of England after the Reformation,* 1902-4, pp. 214 and 336 give examples of some seventeenth century licenses to eat flesh.

55. Elyot, Sig. P1^V.

56. Boorde, p. 250.

57. L. Lemnius (trans. T. Newton), *A Touchstone of the Complexions,* London, 1576, Sig. G4^V.

58. There are many forms of this saying, all indicating that fat people are less intelligent than thin people.

59. Cogan, p. 124. The list is given under the chapter headed "Of the Braine" and is taken from *Regimen Sanitatis.*

60. *Regimen Sanitatis,* Sig. G1^r-G3^V.

61. Batman, Sig. N2^r. The subsequent quotations come from this page. Refers to Constantine the African (d.1087 A.D.).

62. Batman, Sig. N2^V.

63. Batman, Sig. N2^r. The heat which destroyes fatness may be taken to mean when the body is hot as in a fever rather than simply the effects of external heat.

64. Batman, Sig. N2^r. In beasts, fatness in the male also inhibits conception.

65. Cogan, pp. 212, 213. Hippocrates, *Regimen III,* p. 373. It is good to vomit after drunkenness.

66. Platt, *The Jewell House,* p. 62. The theory today varies slightly in that the oil is said to coat the stomach wall and so delays the absorption of alcohol.

67. Gratarolus, Sig. L3^r.

68. Cogan, p. 211.

69. H. A. Monckton, *A History of English Ale and Beer,* 1966, p. 102.

70. *The Harleian Miscellany,* 1809, Vol. II, p. 262. The pamphlet quoted in *Bacchus' Bountie* by Philip Foulface of Alefoord. Student in good Fellowship. It is of note that spirits were not widely drunk in Tudor England.

71. A. Henderson, *The History of Ancient and Modern Wines,* 1824, p. 346; refers to W. Camden (trans. R. Norton), *The historie of the life and reigne of the most renowned and victorious Princesse Elizabeth, late Queen of England,* London, 1630, Book III, and Fynes Moryson, *Itinerary,* Part III, p. 152.

72. Philip Stubbs, *The Anatomie of Abuses,* London, 1585. Reference is to the reprinted edition (superintended by W.B.D.D. Turnbull), 1836, p. 113.

73. (Act of 1552), 5 and 6 Ed.VI c.25.

74. Monckton, p. 104.

75. (Act of 1603), 1 Jac.I C9 and (Act 1606) 4 Jac.I C5.

76. The record of menus and the costs of many banquets are available. See R. Warner, *Antiquitates Culinariae,* 1791, p. 107; J. C. Drummond and A. Wilbraham, *Englishman's Food,* 1939, p. 65, refers to an estimate of the food required for the great gathering at the Field of the Cloth of Gold (1520), given in *The Rutland Papers,* Camden Society Publication No. 21, 1842.

77. Warner, p. xviii.

78. Elyot, Sig. N^{r}1. The ordinances seem to be directed against extravagance rather than overeating.

79. A. Mizauld (1510-78), a French medical man and astrologer.

80. Elyot, Sig. b2^v-b4^v (signatures numbered incorrectly).

81. Boorde, p. 289.

82. According to C. Creighton (*History of Epidemics,* 1891-4, Vol. I, p. 236) the sweating sickness was not reported again in England after 1551.

83. Cogan, "Short Treatise," p. 255, "sickness at Oxford," p. 272 (*Haven of Health*). A recent study which touches on the late sixteenth century is A. B. Applebury, "Nutrition and Disease: The Case of London, 1550-1750," *Journal of Interdisciplinary History,* 1975, 6, pp. 1-22.

84. J.F.D. Shrewsbury, *A History of the Bubonic Plague in the British Isles,* 1970, pp. 163, 187, 310.

85. Simon Kellwaye, *A defensative against the plague,* London, 1593, chap. 11. Sig. E1^r-E2^r.

86. Kellwaye, Sig. E2^r. A connection between lack of food and epidemic diseases was recognized.

87. Cogan, pp. 257, 258.

88. Cogan, p. 259. Cogan does not make a specific reference to the theory of Hieronymus Fracastorius (c. 1478-1553) published in *De Contagione, Contagiosis Morbis et eorum Curatione,* 1546. See translation by W. Cave Wright, *Hieronymous Fracastorius, Contagion, Contagious Diseases and their Treatment,* 1930.

89. James Manning, *A new booke intituled, I am for you all, Complexion castle,* London, 1604, Sig. A1^v.

90. Elyot, Sig. b2^v.

91. See note 80 above.

92. Elyot, Sig. b3^r.

93. Cogan, p. 257. This advice is given generally by writers on the pestilence. Cogan discusses (pp. 2590260) whether it is proper to fly from the plague in terms of God's will over man's life. He concludes that God wishes man to follow the rules of physick that He has provided and to go from the plague is to follow the physician's advice.

CHAPTER VIII

1. With very few exceptions all foods are a mixture of nutrients, but in the rough rule of thumb classification Energy foods refer to predominantly carbohydrate or fatty foods. Body building foods refer to predominantly protein or mineral foods. Protective foods refer to foods providing a good source of vitamins. Vitamins regulate body processes and so help to protect the body against ill health.

2. In modern Recommended Intakes of Nutrients tables, people are grouped according to sex, age, sometimes height or weight, and activity.

3. Galen, p. 27.

4. The diseases listed are taken from Boorde and Elyot and are representative of the period. The order of listing is not significant.

5. R.L. Anderson, *University of Iowa Humanistic Studies,* 1927, *3*, No. 4, p. 31, note 10.

6. T. Bright, *A Treatise of the Melancholie,* London, 1586. Here reference is

made to the 1940 facsimile edition, with an introduction by Hardin Craig. A. Du Laurens (trans. R.C.), *A Discourse on the Preservation of the Sight; of Melancholike diseases; of Rheumes, and of Old Age,* London, 1599. Here the facsimile edition 1938, ed. S.V. Larkey, is referred to. See also R. Klibansky, E. Panofsky and F. Saxl, *Saturn and Melancholy,* 1964.

7. Bright, p. 97.

8. L. Lemnius (trans. T. Newton), *The Touchstone of Complexions,* London, 1576, Sig. D1^v.

9. Elyot, Sig. B2^r.

10. Langton, Sig. B5^v. "The nynth is neither hote, colde, drye, nor moyste, and is yet made of them all." Of the other eight "distemperate" temperatures four are simple and four are compound.

11. Langton, Sig. B6^r, "whyche is as muche for to saye, as a temperature measured accordynge to justice." See J.M. Dureau-Lapeysonnie in *Médecine Humaine et Vétérinaire à la fin du Moyen Âge* (Ed. G. Beaujouan), 1966, p. 247. Antoine Ricart's view of the proportion of the four humours gives *Temperatus ad justiciam* as the relationship of sanguine 4, phlegm 3, choler 2, melancholy 1.

12. Langton, Sig. B7^v-C1^r.

13. Lemnius, Sig. E5^v.

14. Du Laurens p. 84.

15. P. Lowe, *A Discourse of the Whole Art of Chyrurgerie,* London, 1612 (1st ed. 1596), p. 13. This idea can be found in Galen and Rhazes.

16. Lemnius, Sig. C2^r.

17. Lowe pp. 15, 16.

18. For an interesting analysis of "The Humor of Juliet's Nurse" by Angelino Guido, see *Bull. Hist. Med.,* 1945, *17*, pp. 290-303. This illustrates the complexity of determining the humour of an individual by observation of their behaviour.

19. Elyot, Sig. B2^r.

20. Lowe p. 17.

21. P.H. Kocher, *Science and Religion in Elizabethan England,* 1953, p. 284.

22. The question of whether the diet can affect the complexion is discussed by Anderson in her study, "Elizabethan Psychology and Shakespeare," *University of Iowa Humanistic Studies,* 1927, *3*, No. 4. On the premise that a complexion is derived from elemental qualities and is unaffected by alterations in the humours, then it is implied "that complexion, according to the exact usage of the term, is hardly subject to the influence of nourishment" (p 31, n. 11). Here Bright (p. 104) and J. Huarte (p. 301 – see note 68 below) are cited. Also the inexact use is illustrated by Anderson's quotation from John Davies of Hereford (*Microcosmos,* p. 30) ". . . Which we *complexion* cal; whereof are two, well and ill tempred; And the *Aliment* that feeds the *Body,* herein much can doe, For that can make and marre *Complexion* too."

23. Lemnius, Sig. A6^r.

24. Buttes, Sig. M8^v. The aphrodisiac characteristics of oysters are still referred to today.

25. W. Bullein, *The Government of Health,* London, 1595, Sig. C2^v.

26. Batman, Sig. N6^r.

27. Elyot, Sig. T3^r.

28. Laurence Babb (*The Elizabethan Malady,* 1951) states: "There is fairly general agreement that youth is sanguine and old age melancholic" (footnote 36, p.

11). This seems to me to be an oversimplification of the theory. I suggest that on the evidence available it is true that it was accepted that youth was hot:moist and age cold:dry, but this did not necessarily put every individual in each group into the class of a sanguine or melancholic complexion.

29. C. Sherrington, *The Endeavour of Jean Fernal*, 1946, p. 68.

30. H. Cuffe, *The differences of the ages of man's life*, London, 1607, pp. 113-114.

31. Elyot, Sig. T3^r.

32. Langton, Sig. B7^v and B8^r.

33. Elyot, Sig. T3^r.

34. T. Walkington, *The Optick Glasse of Humors*, London, 1607, gives a diagram (Sig. F.7^r).

35. Lemnius, Sig. N5^r.

36. Any excess of foods having predominantly heat or moisture would aggravate the humour. The inclusion of cold here is in the context of an excess.

37. Buttes, Sig. H8^v-L7^r. See also Chapter XIII.

38. Cogan, Sig. Q2^v.

39. Hippocrates, *Regimen II*, Vol. IV, p. 321.

40. Boorde, p. 287.

41. Elyot, Sig. U2^r.

42. Boorde, p. 288.

43. Lemnius, Sig. 07^v.

44. Elyot, Sig. U1^r.

45. Elyot, Sig. U1^v.

46. Elyot, Sig. Q4^r.

47. This is discussed by Hardin Craig in his introduction to the facsimile of Bright's *Treatise of the Melancholie*. There are many modern commentaries on the subject; those of Klibansky et al. (note 6) and Babb (note 28) have already been cited.

48. Du Laurens, pp. 105-106. Reference is also made here to air, emotions and music.

49. Bright, p. 260.

50. Bright, p. 258.

51. Elyot, Sig. U3^v.

52. Our present society places great emphasis on the needs of children, sometimes to the detriment of adults. In Elizabethan society their seniors (adults) took precedence over children in all things. However, the family was a closely knit unit (L.E. Pearson, *Elizabethans at Home*, 1957), and the fact that adults had first choice of the good things available did not indicate a lack of consideration or love on the part of the parents.

53. Richard Jonas, *The Byrth of Mankinde*, London, 1540. This is a translation of *De Partu Hominis* by Eucharius Roesslin. The earliest Latin edition of *De Partu* was 1532. The book used for reference in this study is J.W. Ballantyne's *The "Byrth of Mankynde." Its Author, Editions and Contents*, 1907. Ballantyne uses the 1560 edition of *The Byrth* by Thomas Raynalde, with some excerpts from other editions. All footnote references will be given under Ballantyne.

54. Ballantyne, p. 299.

55. The reference used is the 1965 reprint of Thomas Phaire, *The Boke of*

Chyldren, London, 1553, with Notes by A. V. Neale and H. R. E. Wallis.

56. T. Phaire, *The Regiment of Life,* London, 1544. There are many different ways of spelling the name Phaire.

57. Neale and Wallis, p. 7.

58. Phaire, *Boke of Chyldren,* p. 17.

59. Neale and Wallis, p. 73. Celsus, *De Medicina,* Vol. I, Book III, p. 263, says: "Indeed in general children ought not to be treated like adults."

60. Phaire, p. 17.

61. Lemnius, Sig. G1^V.

62. Lemnius, Sig. G2^V.

63. Batman, Sig. N5^r.

64. This is discussed by H.P. Adelmann, *Marcello Malpighi and the Evolution of Embryology,* 1966, pp. 744 and 745. A summary of Pre-Harveyan views can be found in Elizabeth Gasking's *Investigations into Generation, 1651-1828,* 1967, p. 19.

65. Batman, Sig. N5^V.

66. This idea was held by Galen. See J. Needman, *A History of Embryology,* 1959 (2nd edition), p. 73.

67. Batman, Sig. N6^r.

68. J. Huarte (trans. R.C.), *Examen de Ingenios. The examination of mens Wits,* London, 1594, p. 31. Also called *A triall of Wits* by later commentators. Modern superstitions regarding a pregnant woman's craving for a certain food, take other forms, such as the shape of a birthmark appearing on the child, similar to the shape of the food, if the craving is unsatisfied.

69. Ballantyne, p. 351.

70. Hippocrates, *Regimen I,* Vol. IV, p. 265. Jones, *Growing and Living,* Sig. C1^r, says "that evel life deformitie of body and disease of a principal parte, do discend from the graundfathers and parentes and are inherited."

71. Huarte, pp. 302-303.

72. Huarte, pp. 304-305 gives the information regarding children's characteristics.

73. There was an acknowledged relationship between the dominant qualities and intelligence. This added to the confusion over the humoural characteristics of individuals because melancholy men (cold:dry) could be found who had "good wits."

74. Ways of producing and improving a good memory were important in the sixteenth century and a good deal was written on the subject. An example is G. Gratarolus (trans. W. Fullwood), *The castel of memorie,* London, 1562.

73. Huarte, pp. 306-321. Owsei Temkin, *Soranus' Gynecology,* 1956, p. 37, footnote 71, says that Empedocles is credited with the idea that the embryo is shaped by the imagination of the mother during conception.

76. The Renaissance attitude of mind towards marvels in the realm of natural history is discussed by Madeleine Doran, in "On Elizabethan 'credulity' . . . .," *Journal of the History of Ideas,* 1940, *1*, pp. 151-76.

77. Huarte, p. 319.

78. Huarte, p. 322.

79. Examples are Boorde, *Breviary of Helth,* Elyot, and Cogan. Some authors' recommendations include plasters to be applied to the breasts.

80. Ballantyne, p. 362.

81. Phaire, p. 22.

82. Ballantyne, p. 343.

83. Cogan, p. 154. "The Earlie of Cumberlande was cured of a consumption by womans mylke."

84. Phaire, p. 18.

85. Phaire, p. 18.

86. G.F. Still, *The History of Paediatrics*, 1931, p. 29. See also Temkin, p. 95.

87. Jones, *Body and Soul*, choosing the nurse. See Sig. B2^v-F3^v.

88. Jones, *Body and Soul*, Sig. D2^r. There is disagreement among authors on this point.

89. Jones, *Body and Soul*, Sig. B2^v-B3^r.

90. Jones, *Body and Soul*, Sig. D1^r, gives examples of Roman emperors to whom this happened.

91. Jones, *Body and Soul*, Sig. D3^r-F3^v.

92. Jones, *Body and Soul*, Sig. F3^v.

93. Ballantyne, p. 326.

94. Jones, *Body and Soul*, Sig. H2^r.

95. Jones, *Body and Soul*, Sig. H3^r.

96. Jones, *Body and Soul*, Sig. H2^v.

97. Hippocrates, *Dentition*, Vol. II, p. 325.

98. Jones, *Body and Soul*, Sig. H4^r.

99. E. Hake, *A Touchestone for this time present*, London, 1574, Sig. G3^v-G4^r. The reference to the feeding of infants is given as an example of the similar care required in feeding the growing mind.

100. C. Hollyband, *The Frenche Littleton*, London, 1581, "the refreshing of scholars," pp. 151-213. Hollyband's books for teaching the French tongue give an insight into contemporary life.

101. Jones, *Body and Soul*, Sig. I3^r.

102. *NHB*. See also Chapter VI.

103. Elyot, Sig. L3^v.

104. T. Newton, *The Olde mans Dietarie*, London, 1586. Newton had previously translated *The Worthye book of Old age* by M.T. Cicero (London, 1569). This is quite different from the *Dietarie*, being a dialogue praising and defending old age. Gratarolus (Sig. C2^v) refers to a book on the subject by Antonius Fumanellus (*fl.* 1536) of Verona, but this has not been identified in his works.

105. Batman, Sig. N4^v. These are the groupings of Bartholomaeus Anglicus.

106. See *As You Like It*, Act II, Scene vii.

107. Newton, Sig. B1^v.

108. Lowe, p. 28.

109. Newton, Sig. B3^v.

110. Newton, Sig. C2^r.

111. Galen followed Aristotle (*De longitudine et brevitate vitae*, 466^a 24-25). Hippocrates (*Regimen I*, Vol. IV, p. 281) said that ageing produced a cold:moist condition.

112. Newton, Sig. B4^r.

113. Du Laurens, Sig. 2B1^r.

114. Newton, Sig. B2^r.

115. Newton, Sig. B6^v-B7^r.

116. Lowe, p. 34.

117. Newton, Sig. C3^r.

118. The quality and degrees quoted are those given by Buttes.

119. Lowe, pp. 33, 34.

120. Newton, Sig. D1^r.

121. Lowe, p. 35.

122. Gratarolus. The meaning of the word magistrate here is not clear. The usual meaning was (then as now) an officer of the law, but this specific meaning does not seem particularly relevant to Newton's title. Alternative meanings are that it referred in general to those who had supervisory positions, or it might here refer to "magister," which was still in use with the English meaning of master. The last two suggestions are applicable to Gratarolus' work.

123. The quotation is from the subtitle. Reference throughout is made to the edition of 1589 (B.M. shelf No. 7405-a-2).

124. Gratarolus, Sig. B3^r-B3^v.

125. Cogan, p. 9.

126. Cogan, p. 1 and p. 3.

127. Cogan, p. 29. The proverb referred to has not been traced and is not (in the form given) in *A Handbook of Proverbs* by H.G. Bohn, London, 1855. This includes the collection of J. Ray (1670).

128. Cogan, p. 28. As will become apparent the digestive powers varied with activity and social condition.

129. C.D. O'Malley, "Jacobus Sylvius' Advice for Poor Medical Students," *Journal of the History of Medicine*, 1962, *17*, pp. 141-151.

130. Cogan: see under sections on time and order of meals (pp. 180-193); also 1st edition (1584), p. 224.

131. Cogan, p. 99. Some "noble" students would have had their own servants.

132. Cogan, p. 1.

133. Cogan, p. 3.

134. In the next century one of the first things to be shown "arithmetically" in J. Graunt's important work, *Natural and political observations mentioned in a following index and made upon the bills of mortality,* London, 1662, was that life in the country was healthier than life in the city.

135. Cogan, p. 8.

136. Cogan, p. 43. This is written in reference to coriander which, despite the fact that Dioscorides says it produces madness, is said by Cogan to be wholesome if taken often, being steeped in vinegar or made into "confites."

137. Cogan, p. 33.

138. Cogan, p. 77.

139. Bernardino Ramazzini (trans. W.C. Wright), *Diseases of Workers from the Text of De Morbis Artificum,* 1940, p. 379. Translated from text of 1713. First Latin edition 1700. Ramazzini claims that Celsus said (Celsus, vol. I, p. 45) "But those who have weak stomachs, among whom are the majority of townspeople and nearly all who have a passion for letters. . . ." In fact, Ramazzini had added *stomacho.* See also the version "now done in English" anonymously 1705, p. 248.

140. Cogan, p. 20. Reference to this is made frequently in books on "Melancholy."

141. Cogan, p. 36.

142. Cogan, pp. 36, 37.

143. Cogan, p. 71, p. 69 and p. 80 respectively.

144. Cogan, p. 89. Saying not traced.

145. Cogan, p. 82.

146. Elyot, Sig. D2^v, D3^v, Q4^r.

147. Boorde, p. 300.

148. Elyot, Sig. Z2^r; Cogan, pp. 172 and 193; Jones, *Bucks Bathes,* Sig. B2^r.

149. Boorde, proheme to *Dyetary of Health.* This was dedicated to the Duke of Norfolk.

150. Gratarolus, Sig. B3^r.

151. Cogan, p. 31.

152. H.H.S. Croft (ed.), *The Boke named the governour (by Thomas Elyot, London, 1531),* 1880. Cranmer is quoted in a footnote on p. 33 of Vol. I.

153. Cogan, p. 174.

154. Elyot, Sig. F1^r.

155. Cogan, p. 175.

156. Cogan, p. 174.

157. Cogan, p. 176.

158. Lemnius, Sig. G2^v.

159. Cogan, p. 176.

160. *Fifth Report of the Medical Officer to the Privy Council,* 1862, Appendix V. The Cotton Famine. 3. Economics of diet, by Dr. E. Smith, p. 339.

161. Cogan, p. 176.

162. R.H. Chittenden, *Physiological Economy in Nutrition,* 1904, p. 470.

CHAPTER IX

1. Elyot, Sig. E1^v.

2. *Castel of Helth,* Sig. E2^v; *Haven of Health,* p. 168; *Discourse of the Whole art of Chyrygerie,* London, 1612, p. 47.

3. Great Britain, Dept. of Health and Social Security, *Recommended Intakes of Nutrients for the United Kingdom,* 1969, provides figures for ten nutrients, with additional advice (not tabulated) on more than fourteen others, related to people in twenty-one groups of the population.

4. Jane O'Hara-May, "Measuring Man's Needs," *Journal of the History of Biology,* 1971, *4*, pp. 249-273.

5. Cogan, p. 185.

6. M.S. Serjeantson, *Essays and Studies,* 1938, *23*, pp. 25-37.

7. *GHH,* Sig. G6^v.

8. *The Northumberland Household Book* (1512), edited by T. Percy in 1770, is one of the best of the records of large establishments available. Other records are listed by Conyers Read (ed.), *Bibliography of British History,* Tudor Period (1485-1603), 1959, pp. 345-346.

9. Examples of Livery are given in the *NHB* listed above and in Paul V.B. Jones, *The Household of a Tudor Nobleman,* 1917, p. 249.

10. A. Woodworth, "Purveyance for the Royal Household in the Reign of Queen Elizabeth," *Transactions of the American Philosophical Society,* 1946, N.S. *35*, 1, pp. 12, 84, 85.

11. John Nichols (for the Society of Antiquaries), *A Collection of Ordinances and Regulations for the Government of the Royal Household, made in divers reigns from King Edward III to King William and Queen Mary,* 1790, p. 162 and following, Henry VIII; p. 317 and following, Prince Henry (1610).

12. One "mutton" is subdivided into two shoulders, two loins, two breasts, two legs, and two rackes (necks). See "A Breviate touching the Order and governmente of a Nobleman's house," (1605), *Archaeologia,* 1800, *13,* p. 371. It should be remembered that the average size of sheep and cattle in sixteenth century England was smaller than now.

13. *OED.* The use in the military sense is the nearest among current usages to that of the sixteenth century.

14. J.O. Halliwell, *A Dictionary of Archaic and Provincial Words,* 1852. Sir Thomas More makes his Utopians sit four at a mess, as was the custom in Lincoln's Inn. *Utopia,* translated into English by Ralph Robinson, London, 1551, Sig. K1^v.

15. *NHB,* p. 83.

16. Anon., *The Booke of Carving and Sewing,* London, n.d., Sig. C1^v.

17. J.M. Osborn (ed.), *The Autobiography of Thomas Whythorne,* 1961, p. 81. Whytehorne is believed to have written his autobiography in 1576 (p. xiii).

18. Emmison, p. 241.

19. Woodworth, p. 12. William Cecil, who controlled the household while he was Principal Secretary (from 1558) and Lord Treasurer (1572-98), was known for his belief in strict economy.

20. See "Relicts and Fragments of Meat and Drinks," *Royal Household Ordinances,* p. 154.

21. Hippocrates, *Regimen III,* Vol. IV, p. 362.

22. Elyot, Sig. E3^v.

23. Cogan, p. 168.

24. Elyot, Sig. E3^v.

25. Cogan, pp. 169-170.

26. Cogan, p. 169.

27. Elyot, Sig. L2^r-M4^r.

28. In present day applications of nutritional theories climatic considerations are considered when formulating a dietary standard of recommended nutrients for groups of people. This is not related to each season of the year but to an average yearly temperature which is considered to influence significantly the Basal Metabolic Rate of individuals. *F.A.O. Nutritional Studies,* No. 15, 1957, uses $10°C$ as the reference temperature.

29. Elyot, Sig. L2^v; Cogan, p. 177.

30. Hippocrates, *Regimen in Health,* Vol. IV, p. 45.

31. Cogan, p. 178.

32. Elyot, Sig. L2^v.

33. Cogan, p. 177.

34. Elyot, Sig. L3^r and L3^v.

35. Elyot, Sig. L3^v. In later centuries, physicians in temperate climates noted the regularity with which symptoms, such as scurvy, appeared at the end of the winter.

36. Thomas Hill (trans.), *Treatise Intituled Naturall and Artificall Conclusions,*

written by sundry scholars of the University of Padua, London, 1586. See the section called "The profitable Arte of Gardening" (London, 1568), Sig. J1^r and J1^v.

37. Not in the *OED*. Its meaning here is likely to be candied.

38. For the effect of the moon on the movement of the natural humours see Chapter XIII, note 59.

39. Anthony Ascham (*f.* 1553) M.B. Cambridge, an astrologer and Vicar of Burneston, Yorkshire. H.M. Barlow in "Old English Herbals, 1525-1640," *Proc. Royal Society of Medicine,* 1913, *6,* pp. 108-149, suggests (p. 121) that Ascham may not be the author of the herbal usually attributed to him.

40. *[Bankes] Herball,* printed by Rycharde Banckes, London, 1525.

41. James Manning, *I am for you all Complexions Castle,* Cambridge, 1604.

42. Cogan, p. 193.

43. Hippocrates, *Regimen III,* Vol. IV, p. 369.

44. Celsus, Vol. I, p. 39.

45. O.C. Gruner, *A Treatise on the Canon of Medicine of Avicenna,* 1930, p. 395.

46. A.S. Way, *The Science of Dining (Mensa Philosophica),* 1936, p. 2. A translation of a mediaeval treatise on hygiene.

47. This refers to Book X of *Liber ad Almansorem*, which had been dedicated to the governor of Ray in A.D. 903. See C. Elgood, *A Medical History of Persia,* 1951, p. 201.

48. Way, pp. 3 and 4. On page four the text says, "if three meals be taken in two days." This should be reversed to two meals in three days to fit the timing of the rest of the context.

49. Harrison, p. 141.

50. Harrison, p. 162.

51. Examples are: records of King Edward IV's mother's household, quoted by R. Warner, *Antiquitates Culinaeiae,* 1791, p. xlvii. King Edward IV lived from 1442-83. See also *The Northumberland Household Book.*

52. F. Grose, *The Antiquarian Repertory,* 1809, Vol. IV, p. 648. The reference occurs in a report of Sir Richard Blunt on the duties of Gentlemen Ushers in the time of King Edward VI.

53. *NHB,* Notes p. 415, refers also to text p. 60.

54. Cogan, p. 182.

55. Langton, Sig. K5^v-K7^r, in his chapter on the time of meals.

56. Elyot, Sig. M3^r.

57. Cogan, p. 182. Cogan had pointed out that the "universities" (meaning Oxford) provide only dinner and supper for students. It was different at Cambridge: the statutes of Trinity College, quoted by J.B. Mullinger (*University of Cambridge from the Earliest Times* 1888, Vol. II, p. 143), show penalties for anyone who "shall either breakfast or sup out of hall" without the Master's permission. In the sixteenth century Oxford was well known for the meagreness of the meals it provided.

58. The item quoted is the Roxburghe Club publication of 1841, *Manners and Household Expenses in the Thirteenth and Fifteenth Centuries.*

59. See footnote 51 above.

60. Records of the fifth Early of Northumberland (1478-1527).

61. *NHB*, pp. 75-76.

62. G.R. Batho (ed.), *Household Papers of the Ninth Earl of Northumberland,* 1962.

63. Possibly food from supper was provided for breakfast (see below) and so was not itemized separately.

64. F.W. Hackwood, *Good Cheer,* 1911, p. 134.

65. D. Hartley, *Thomas Tusser – 1557,* 1931, p. 167.

66. Fynes Moryson, *An Itinerary written by Fynes Moryson, Gent,* London, 1617, Book III, Part III, Sig. 3R2^v.

67. Harrison, p. 141.

68. Emmison, pp. 308 and 309. These accounts give only the flesh and fish items. Omitted are the bread, sauces and herbs which would also have been served.

69. Haberden sometimes referred to barrelled or cured cod from Aberdeen; this was a "northern term." See *NHB*, p. 427.

70. Emmison, p. 141. According to other lists quoted by Emmison, fish days in the Petre household were usually on Fridays and Saturdays. This was the usual practice. See also Chapter X.

71. Emmison, p. 309.

72. Cogan, p. 185.

73. F.E. Eden, *The State of the Poor,* 1797, Vol. III, Appendix cxliii.

74. Hartley, *Tusser,* p. 172.

75. *Regimen Sanitatis,* Sig. C3^v.

76. L. Lemnius (trans. T. Newton), *The Touchstone of Complexions,* London, 1576, Sig. W3^v.

77. Cogan, pp. 188-191. The subsequent quotations are from this section.

78. Petrus de Albano (1250-1316), author of *Conciliator differentiarum philosophorum et medicorum conciliates Aristotle et Plato.*

79. Leonhard Fuchs (1501-66), German physician and botanist. Sir Thomas More gives this advice in his "Utopian Society" (Robinson, Sig. K2^v).

80. Cogan quotes (p. 190) the old proverb which says "after supper walk a mile," meaning do not go to sleep directly after supper.

81. Dr. J.A. Paris (*A Treatise on Diet:*, 1837) alters it to "for a rich man when he can get an appetite and for a poor one when he can get food," and uses it as an argument that in health appetite is regulated by habit.

82. Langton, Sig. K6^r.

83. Langton, Sig. K6^r.

84. Langton, Sig. K7^v.

85. E.M.W. Tillyard, *The Elizabethan World Picture,* 1948, p. 74, points out that brute beasts were believed to do instinctively what was best for them.

86. Elyot, Sig. M2^v.

87. Langton, Sig. K7^r.

88. Cogan, p. 190.

89. *NHB*, p. 310. The day was divided into two turns of duty. H.D. Traill and J.S. Mann (eds.), *Social England,* 1903, Vol. III, p. 218, suggests that the day started unusually late in this household.

90. Hartley, *Tusser,* p. 177.

91. Cogan, p. 197. The information that follows is from Cogan.

92. Langton, *Prin. Parts,* Sig. E8^r.

93. Cogan, p. 200.

94. Elyot, Sig. N2^v.

95. Cogan, p. 201.

96. Boorde, p. 265.

97. Cogan, p. 157.

98. J. Bannister, *The Historie of Man,* London, 1578, Sig. T4^r.

99. Quoted from J.S. Prendergast, "The Background of Galen's Life and Activities and its Influences on His Achievements," *Proceedings of the Royal Society of Medicine,* 1930, *23,* 1131-1148. (Prendergast is translating Kuhn's edition of Galen's works, Vol. II, p. 157). Galen did think the "fibres" of the stomach caused it to contract upon the food, but the movement of the stomach during vomiting was considered to be against nature.

100. Bannister, Sig. T4^r.

101. Bannister, Sig. U1^r.

102. Helkiah Crooke, ΜΙΚΡΟΚΟΣΜΟΓΡΑΦΙΑ *(Microsmographia), A description of the body of man,* London, 1615, Book III, pp. 161-166. The subject goes beyond the scope of this study. See also O. Temkin, "Vesalius on an Immanent Biological Force," *Bull. Hist. Med.,* 1965, *39,* pp. 277-280; translation is taken from *Fabrica,* 1543.

103. Translated by Eileen Power as *The Goodman of Paris,* 1928.

104. Elyot, Sig. N1^v.

105. Langton, *Prin. Parts,* Sig. E8^v.

106. Elyot, Sig. N2^r.

107. Boorde, p. 276.

108. Harrison, p. 166. The Scot he notes starts with the best foods, thereby leaving the worst for his servants.

109. The two cookery books quoted below give virtually the same information. They are: Anon., *A proper newe Booke of Cookery,* London, 1575, and Thomas Dawson, *The good huswifes Jewell,* London, 1596 (referred to elsewhere in notes as *GHJ*).

110. Cogan, p. 199. The lists of foods given in this table have been transcribed into modern English.

111. *Booke of Cookery,* Sig. A3^r.

112. *GHJ,* Sig. A2^v. In neither book is it made clear whether the fish dishes are for dinner or supper, but in both cases the list follows the flesh dishes suggested for dinner.

113. From a study of early recipes "soppes" seem usually to be pieces of toasted fine white bread soaked in an appropriate liquid, but the bread was not always toasted.

114. *Booke of Cookery,* Sig. A5^r.

115. *The Book of Carving,* Sig. A3^r.

116. Buttes, *Dyets Dry Dinner,* London, 1599, Sig. N7^v. (Book's signatures do not follow the correct sequence.) See also Chapter XVI.

117. Buttes, Sig. O3^v.

118. Cogan, p. 199.

119. Harrison, p. 142.

120. Harrison, p. 148.

121. James Woodforde (ed. J. Beresford), *The Diary of a Country Parson,* 1967, p. 210 (World Classics edition of five volumes, 1924-1931). Parson Woodforde had fewer dishes in his family meals. Woodforde lived 1740-1803.

122. In *GHJ* where under "service for fish daies" (Sig. A3^V) are included two pasties of fallow deer and a dish of leaches (sliced meat). Reference to the *Book of Cookery* shows that these lines have probably been transposed from elsewhere.

123. W.E. Mead, *The English Medieval Feast,* 1967 (1st ed. 1931), p. 154 and note 122, above.

124. Cogan, p. 199.

125. Harrison, p. 145.

126. Harrison, p. 145.

127. Cogan, p. 199. The argument that follows is taken from Cogan.

CHAPTER X

1. Cogan, p. 153; Buttes, Sig. C6^V, and others.

2. W. Langham, *The Garden of Health,* London, 1579. A simple is a medicinal herb or plant.

3. R.H. Tawney, *The Agrarian Problem in the Sixteenth Century,* 1912. R.E. Prothero (later Lord Ernle), *English Farming Past and Present,* 1st ed. 1912, 6th ed. 1961. J. Thirsk (ed.), *The Agrarian History of England and Wales (1500-1640),* 1967, Vol. IV. P.V. McGrath, *The Marketing of Food Fodder and Livestock in the London Area in the Seventeenth Century, with some References to the Sources of Supply,* unpublished M.A. Thesis, London University, 1948. R. Trow-Smith, *A History of British Livestock Husbandry to 1700,* 1957.

4. Thirsk, p. 173.

5. Thirsk, Chapter III, Sections B: Animal Husbandry, C: Grassland and stock, and D: Fruit and Market Gardening, pp. 163-199. This work is excellently documented, therefore the references cited are not repeated.

6. Enclosing and engrossing, two of the most controversial social topics in sixteenth century England are considered by J. Thirsk, pp. 200-240.

7. McGrath, p. 227.

8. Emmison, *Tudor Secretary,* 1961, and *Tudor Food and Pastimes,* 1964.

9. J. Dubravius (trans. G. Churchey), *A Newe Booke of good Husbandry, conteining the making of fish-pondes,* London, 1599.

10. McGrath, Part II, chapter on the marketing of vegetables and fruit.

11. N.F., *The Husbandmans fruitfull Orchard,* London, 1609, Sig. A2^r.

12. J. Gerard, *The Herbal or General History of Plants,* London, 1597, p. 325, from "Of Scurvie grasse, or Spoonewort," Gerard says it "groweth by the sea side at Hull, Boston and Lynne and many other places of Lincolneshire near unto the sea. . . ."

13. T.S. Willan (ed.), *A Tudor Book of Rates,* 1962, p. xii. In value, wine was the most important import into Elizabethan England.

14. J.E. Thorold Rogers, *A History of Agricultural Prices in England* (from 1259-1793), 1866-1903; *Six Centuries of Work and Wages,* 1884. E.H. Phelps Brown's price index from the thirteenth to twentieth century is based on wages-rates for building craftsmen measured against the price of consumables (E.H. Phelps Brown and Sheila V. Hopkins, "Seven Centuries of Building Wages,"

Economica New Series, 1955). This index is used by J. Burnett, *A History of the Cost of Living,* 1969.

15. Referred to by T.S. Willan, *Studies in Elizabethan Foreign Trade,* 1959, p. 331, n. 2.

16. A. Woodworth, *Transactions of the American Philosophical Society,* 1940, N.S. *35*, p. 66.

17. J.-J. Hémardinquer (ed.), *Pour une histoire de l'alimentation,* 1970, pp. 35-42: Frank Spooner, "Régimes alimentaires: proportions et calculs en calories."

CHAPTER XI

1. William Ashley, *The Bread of Our Forefathers,* 1928, p. 149. Other authors give the dates of the *Assize of Bread* as 1266.

2. R. Sheppard and E. Newton, *The Story of Bread,* 1957, p. 48.

3. J. Burnett, *A History of the Cost of Living,* 1969, pp. 207-209, shows the variation in the price of wheat and comments on the effect of the Repeal of the Corn Laws. The basic controversy was over free trade or protection.

4. Anon., *Here begynneth the boke named the assise of breade,* London [1580].

5. Ashley, p. 150.

6. R.A. McCance and E.M. Widdowson (*Breads White and Brown,* 1956, p. 12) maintain that the Assize was clearly drawn up to protect the influential and the vociferous townsmen and "Gentilitie" rather than the poor. Therefore the act was framed upon the price of wheat, which gave wheat an importance unrelated to the acreage cultivated.

7. N.S.B. Gras, *The Evolution of the English Corn Market,* 1915, p. 38.

8. Cogan, p. 24 and following.

9. A. Edlin, *A Treatise on the Art of Bread-making,* 1805, p. 166.

10. J. Powell, *The Assise of Bread,* London, 1600.

11. The *OED* refers to "cocket" as a seal or customhouse document and says that the term cocket-bread was obsolete by 1500, though the word cocket retained a connection with the Assize of Bread and baking. Edlin *(A Treatise on the Art of Breadmaking)* in the nineteenth century, refers to forms related to flour meal being returned to the Cocket Office of the Royal Exchange in London.

12. Powell, Sig. B1r.

13. The changing meaning of these terms is referred to by Ashley, p. 153.

14. The entry in the *OED* under *Treat, treet*; in section 2, "Bread of trete," this point is illustrated; eighteenth century authorities are quoted as not knowing what the term really means.

15. Water mills were used in England in Roman times. Windmills were introduced in the twelfth century. See J. Storck and W.D. Teague, *Flour for Man's Bread,* 1952, Chap. VIII.

16. J.B. Drummond and A. Wilbraham, *The Englishman's Food,* 1939, p. 351.

17. The term extraction rate refers to that percentage of the whole grain that has been extracted. The higher the extraction rate the darker the flour will appear, as it will contain more of the coarse material in proportion to the starch present.

18. A mechanical bolting maching had been invented by Boller in 1502 but was

not universally accepted. See C. Singer, E.J. Holmyard, A.R. Hall and T.I. Williams, *A History of Technology,* 1957, Vol. III.

19. "The making of manchets after my Ladie Graies way. Take two pecks of fine flower, which must be twise boulted. . ." (from undated *GHH,* Sig. G4^v).

20. Harrison, p. 153.

21. Powell's version of 1600.

22. Boorde, p. 258 and following.

23. Emmison, pp. 134, 135.

24. André L. Simon, *The Star Chamber Dinner Accounts,* 1959, p. 31.

25. Anon., *The Booke of Carving and Sewing,* London, n.d., Sig. A5^r. This work is derived from earlier manuscripts.

26. *NHB,* p. 58.

27. Harrison, p. 154.

28. Boorde, p. 259.

29. Edward Smith, *Foods,* 1883 (8th ed.), p. 196.

30. Harrison, p. 153.

31. Sheppard and Newton, p. 70. All the references in the following paragraph are from this source.

32. Harrison, p. 153.

33. McCance and Widdowson, p. 21, give a general discussion of this point.

34. Harrison, p. 153.

35. Jones, *Bucks baths,* Sig. C1^v.

36. This use of the term grains should not be confused with "grains" (of paradise) or cardamon (see Chap. XVI). Cogan includes beans and peas between oats and rice (pp. 28-33).

37. Wheat has from ancient times generally been considered the best and most nutritious of the grains. See Francis Adams, *The Seven Books of Paulus Aegineta,* 1844, Vol. I, pp. 120-125.

38. Cogan, p. 23.

39. John Gerard, *The Herball or General Historie of Plantes,* 1597 (Chaps. 40-56). Included is information on a number of varieties of wheat, barlie, oats, darnell, Italian millet, maize, "panick," including "Indian panick" or sorghum. Panicum is a very extensive genus; "panick" is frequently applied to Italian millet *(OED).*

40. Boorde, p. 258.

41. Gerard's *Herball* of 1597 (p. 74) suggests this. The error was corrected in the 1636 edition, edited by T. Johnson. Further reference can be made to A.P. De Candolle, *The Origin of Cultivated Plants,* 1884, and to Vol. III of *A History of Technology.*

42. Cogan, p. 26.

43. Frumenty can also be made with other grains, e.g. barley (see Buttes, Sig. F1^r), but was more usually made with wheat.

44. *GHH,* Sig. G3^r-G6^v.

45. Cogan, p. 24.

46. Cogan, p. 26.

47. See note 1.

48. See note 7.

49. Cogan, p. 27.

50. Gerard, p. 61 (numbered as 63). Gerard also points out that Belgian physicians (whose patients presumably ate more rye than did Englishmen) believed rye bread to have advantages over wheaten bread.

51. Cogan, p. 27.

52. Anon., *A proper newe Booke of Cookery,* London, 1575, Sig. A8^v.

53. Cogan, pp. 27 and 28.

54. Hippocrates, *Regimen II,* Vol. IV, p. 307, and *Regimen in Acute Diseases,* Vol. III, p. 69.

55. Gerard, p. 65.

56. Cogan, p. 27.

57. Gerard, p. 69.

58. Cogan, p. 29.

59. *A proper newe Booke of Cookery,* Sig. G4^r.

60. Gerard, p. 1035.

61. Gerard, p. 1054.

62. Scientific name *Lathyrus montanus.* Put by William Turner (1548) under the heading *Astragalus.* He says it should not be confused with *Apios.*

63. Cogan, pp. 29 and 30.

64. Pulses are good sources of protein and make a valuable addition to the diet of those existing on subsistence-agricultural levels. Giving such advice today one still meets the problem of the quantity to recommend because of the difficulty of digesting pulses of poor quality, badly cooked. Many people who need protein will reject large quantities of pulses because they "cause the wind."

65. Cogan, p. 29 and Buttes, Sig. E8^r.

66. Hippocrates, *Regimen II,* Vol. IV, p. 315.

67. In cooking pulses, the soaking of the dried variety before cooking improves the digestibility. No reference has been found to the pre-soaking of beans or peas. Overcooking can harden the skin of the seed. One sixteenth century recipe (*GHJ,* Sig. C1^v) says that the "husks" (or skins) which come to the top should be removed.

68. Buttes, Sig. E8^v and Cogan, p. 29.

69. Cogan, p. 29.

70. Cogan, p. 29.

71. Buttes, Sig. E6^r.

72. Buttes, Sig. E6^v.

73. Cogan, p. 31.

74. Cogan, p. 30 and J. Jones, *Bucks baths,* Sig. C1^v.

75. Gerard, p. 72. Imports of rice are referred to by T.S. Willan, *Studies in Elizabethan Foreign Trade,* 1959, p. 70.

76. Buttes, Sig. E8^v.

77. Bullein, Sig. L6^v.

78. Gerard, p. 73.

79. Gratarolus, Sig. G1^r.

80. Cogan, p. 25.

81. Galen (Kühn), *De Alimentorium Facultatibus,* Vol. VI, p. 494.

82. Celsus, *De Medicina,* Vol. I, p. 203. Unleavened bread is best for the stomach.

83. Boorde, p. 258. Boorde agrees with the Hippocratic advice; see Hippocrates, *Regimen II,* Vol. IV, p. 313.

84. Cogan, p. 23.

85. *GHH*, Sig. G5^r, G5^v, and G6^v.

86. Bullein, Sig. L5^v.

87. *GHH*, Sig. G4^v. This is likely to be in the order of 2 oz.

88. *Regimen Sanitatis,* Sig. M2^v.

89. Only baking is considered here. Boiled breads, such as simnels and cracknels were dismissed as "unwholesome." They would have had too great a degree of moistness.

90. Cogan, p. 25. This is derived from Boorde (p. 261), who says virtually what is said in Hippocrates, *Regimen II,* Vol. IV, p. 313.

91. Bullein, Sig. L5^v.

92. Cogan, p. 25.

93. Bullein, Sig. L6^r.

94. John Russell's *Boke of Nurture* (in F.J. Furnivall's *Early English Meals and Manners,* 1868, p. 4).

95. Bullein, Sig. L6^r.

96. These ideas are put forward by a number of authors at different times in this period; from Boorde (1542) who quotes *Regimen Sanitatis Salerni,* to Bullein (1595) and can, of course, be found also well before and after this time.

97. Gratarolus, Sig. V3^v.

98. Boorde (p. 261) asks bakers to shake out their flour sacks properly and not to "sophystycate" the bread made of pure wheat.

CHAPTER XII

1. Boorde, p. 252.

2. Cogan, p. 204.

3. Bullein, Sig. K7^r.

4. W. Vaughan, *Naturall and artificiall directions for health,* London, 1600, Sig. B3^r.

5. Cogan, p. 206. The advice is ascribed to Jean Fernal.

6. Jones, *Bucks baths,* Sig. C2^r.

7. Boorde, p. 252.

8. Cogan, p. 205.

9. John Coke, *A Debate between the Heralds of England and France,* 1550, Sig. L3^v.

10. William Turner, *A new Boke of the natures and properties of all wines. . .,* London, 1568. Reference is made to the facsimile edition, with notes by S.V. Larkey and P.M. Wagner, 1946, p. 6.

11. 7 Ed. VI C.5. Quoted by A. Henderson, *The History of Ancient and Modern Wines,* 1824, p. 294.

12. Henderson, p. 295.

13. Henderson, p. 296.

14. Henderson, p. 268.

15. D. Hartley, *Thomas Tusser – 1557,* 1931, p. 133.

16. Boorde, p. 255. T.S. Willan, *Studies in Elizabethan Foreign Trade,* 1959, makes many references to the import of wine at provincial ports as well as through London.

17. Boorde, p. 254.

18. Cogan, p. 209.

19. Hippocrates, *Regimen II,* Vol. IV, p. 327.

20. Cogan, p. 207.

21. The title of Turner's book is self-explanatory, namely: *A new Boke of the natures and properties of all Wines that are commonlye used here in England, with a confutation of an errour of some men, that holde, that Rhennish and other small white wines ought not to be drunken of them that either have, or are in daunger of the stone...* He believed that besides a natural inherited disposition to the stone, "the matter or materiall cause of the stone is a grosse or thicke humor, and that the worker or efficient cause of the same is a greate heate in or about the kidneyes or bladder." (p. 18)

22. The main authorities referred to are: Aetius, Anguillara, Aristotle, Dioscorides, Galen, Mundella, Pliny.

23. Cogan, p. 207.

24. *OED.* After about 1600 claret was used to refer to red wines generally.

25. Cogan, p. 213.

26. Boorde, p. 254.

27. A comparison of calorie values of sweet and dry sherries gives: 135 Cal. (sweet) and 114 Cal. (dry) per 100 ml. R.A. McCance and E.M. Widdowson, *The Composition of Foods,* 1967.

28. D.C. Browning, *Dictionary of Quotations and Proverbs,* 1959. There are many variations of this saying, which was familiar to Henry Buttes who quotes it in his *Dyets Dry Dinner,* 1599.

29. J. Bickerdyke, *The Curiosities of Ale and Beer,* 1886, Chapter IV.

30. Boorde, p. 256.

31. J.C. Drummond and A. Wilbraham. *The Englishman's Food,* 1939, p. 44; also Boorde (p. 239) refers to a brew house when discussing the way in which a man should build his house.

32. Harrison, p. 159. *Note: OED* gives 1 hogshead = 63 old wine gallons or 52½ Imperial gallons. *NHB* gives a hogshead of wine equal to 48 gallons. The size of a gallon was set by statute but did vary in different parts of the country.

33. Cogan, p. 217.

34. P. Hentzer (trans. R. Bently), *A Journey into England in the year 1598,* 1757, p. 87 (edited by Horace Walpole).

35. Drummond and Wilbraham, p. 45.

36. Hartley, p. 89.

37. Boorde, p. 256. This is a well known symptom of inflammation in the urinary path, and would be associated with the idea of fluid intake.

38. Boorde, p. 256.

39. Cogan, pp. 217 and 218.

40. Boorde, p. 256.

41. Elyot, Sig. K4[r].

42. Cogan, p. 217. See also H.A. Monckton, *A History of English Ale and Beer,* 1966, p. 26, where he refers to Dioscorides as saying "koumi made from barley" was often drunk instead of wine and that a similar drink from wheat may be produced in Britain.

43. *Regimen Sanitatis,* Sig. R2[r].

44. *Lolium Temulentum,* a deleterious grass found among wheat *(OED).* See also E. Lieber, *Bulletin of the History of Medicine,* 1970, Vol. 44, p. 337.

45. A. MacDonell (ed.), *The Closet of Sir Kenelm Digby Knight Opened,* 1910, p. 105. This book was originally published in 1669 by permission of Sir Kenelm's son.

46. Compare William Hogarth's view of "Beer Street" and "Gin Lane" in the eighteenth century.

47. Most beers, ale and stout contain from three to seven per cent of ethanol. Their caloric value is usually between thirty and sixty Cal./100 ml. They contain no protein, fat, or useful amounts of calcium. The only vitamins present in significant amounts are nicotinic acid and riboflavin. S. Davidson and R. Passmore, *Human Nutrition and Dietetics,* 1966, pp. 313, 314.

48. Cogan, p. 221.

49. *Hayden's Dictionary of Dates,* revised by B. Vincent, 1881.

50. Cogan (edition of 1584), p. 224.

51. Cogan, p. 220.

52. The early history of mead is described in *Wassail! in Mazers of Mead,* by G. R. Gayre, 1948.

53. Cogan (edition of 1584), p. 226. Cogan refers to the complaints at Sig. 994^r.

54. Cogan, p. 222.

55. Mcdonnell, e.g. "Sir William Paston's Meathe," p. 41; "White Metheglin of my Lady Hungerfords which is exceedingly praised," p. 6.

56. Cogan, p. 222.

57. Cogan, p. 222.

58. Cogan, p. 223.

59. R. V. French, *Nineteen Centuries of Drink in England* (2nd ed.), c.1891, p. 133.

CHAPTER XIII

1. F. Moryson, *An itinerary written by F. Moryson, Gent.,* London, 1617, Part III, p. 150.

2. Cogan, p. 113.

3. C. Skeel, "The Cattle Trade between Wales and England from the Fifteenth to the Nineteenth Centuries," *Trans. Roy. Hist. Soc.,* 1926, 4th series, *9,* pp. 135-158.

4. P.V. McGrath, *The Marketing of Food, Fodder and Livestock in the London Area,* unpublished M.A. Thesis 1948 (London University), p. 167. The Act of 1550 was 5 and 6, Ed. 6, c.25.

5. Lawrence Stone, *The Crisis of the Aristocracy 1558-1641,* 1965, Appendix XXIV, p. 783.

6. J. Burnett, *A History of the Cost of Living,* 1969, p. 60.

7. Cogan, p. 122.

8. F.G. Emmison, *Elizabethan Life: Disorder,* 1970, p. 234.

9. Boorde, p. 286.

10. McGrath, p. 180.

11. H. Buttes, *Dyets Dry Dinner,* London, 1599.

12. Cogan, p. 115.

13. Cogan, chapter on Beef, pp. 113-115.

14. Cogan, on Mutton, pp. 115-116.

15. Gratarolus, Sig. H3^r.

16. Cogan, on Swine's flesh, pp. 116-119.

17. Pigs were one of the animals that Galen observed and dissected.

18. Brawn is commonly found as the first course to meals. See "brawn and mustard," Anon., *A proper new Booke of Cookery,* London, 1575, Sig. A3^v.

19. Cogan, on Goat, p. 119.

20. Cogan, on Hare, p. 121.

21. Cogan, on Rabbits, p. 121. Readers should beware that some "conie catching" referred to conies caught for the stews of Southwark rather than the stewpot. See Robert Greene, *A notable discovery of coosenage* (The art of coney-catching), London, 1591.

22. C. Estienne and J. Liebault (trans. R. Surphlet), *Maison Rustique, or the Countrie Farme,* London, 1600, pp. 151-152.

23. Cogan, on Venison, pp. 122-123.

24. J. Thirsk (ed.), *The Agrarian History of England and Wales (1500-1640),* Vol. IV, 1967, p. 195. See Chap. VII.

25. Cogan, on Strange Beasts, p. 123.

26. Cogan, on Parts of Animals, pp. 124-130.

27. Cogan, on Birds, pp. 131-138.

28. *Regimen Sanitatis,* Sig. N2^v-N4^v.

29. F.G. Emmison, *Tudor Food and Pastimes,* 1964, pp. 40-44.

30. Cogan, on Chickens, pp. 131-133.

31. Cogan, on Pheasant, p. 133.

32. Cogan, on Partridge, pp. 133-134.

33. Cogan, on Woodcocks, p. 134.

34. Cogan, on Pigeons, pp. 134-135.

35. Cogan, on Quaile, p. 135.

36. Cogan, on Blackbirds, pp. 135-136.

37. Cogan, on other birds, pp. 136-138.

38. Boorde, p. 270.

39. Cogan, on Parts of Birds, p. 138.

40. Cogan, on Fish, pp. 139-150.

41. The breeding of freshwater fish in ponds and dams was encouraged by writers on husbandry; see J. Taverner, *Certaine experiments concerning fish and fruite,* London, 1600.

42. Hippocrates, *Regimen II,* Vol. IV, p. 321. William Cullen, *A Treatise of the Materia Medica,* 1789, p. 387, makes the point that unlike some writers he is not going to differentiate between fish which come from different environments.

43. Bullein, Sig. K6^r.

44. Cogan, pp. 142-143.

45. Tench is commonly called the physician of other fishes because when they are hurt they are healed by touching the tench.

46. Cogan, pp. 144-145.

47. Cogan, p. 144.

48. Cogan, on Lampreys, p. 144.

49. Cogan, on Conger, p. 145.

50. Cogan, on Salmon, p. 145.

51. Cogan, on Raie and Thornback, p. 145.

52. Cogan, on Porpoise and Sturgeon, p. 146.

53. Cogan, on Herring and Pilchards, p. 147.

54. Cogan, on Shellfish, pp. 147-148.

55. Cogan, on the Puffin, p. 148.

56. Cogan, pp. 149-150.

57. Cogan, p. 115. Martilmas refers to Martinmas, November 11.

58. Boorde, p. 271.

59. Estienne and Liebault, p. 41. It was recognized that the moon reflected the light of the sun and the degree of brightness of the moon influenced the movement of natural humours. As the light increased so did the movement of moisture towards the outer parts. It was therefore of importance for the farmer to recognize the effects of the moon as well as the sun on his plants and animals at different times.

60. Estienne and Liebault, p. 152.

61. D. Hartley, *Food in England*, 1954, pp. 319-347. Only part of this section refers to sixteenth century methods.

62. Hartley, p. 343.

63. Thirsk, "Grassland and Stock," pp. 179-197; Emmison, *Tudor Foods,* p. 40.

64. D. Hartley, *Thomas Tusser,* 1931, p. 139.

65. Cogan, p. 149. The "red" herring was cured, the "white" was eaten fresh.

66. Cogan, p. 150.

67. The anonymous manuscript (1605) of "A Breviate Touching the Order and Government of a Nobleman's House, etc." *Archaeologia,* 1807-1809, *13,* pp. 315-373.

68. John Nichols, *Illustrations of the Manners and Expences of Antient Times in England,* London, 1797, p. 34. F.M. Eden, *The State of the Poor,* London, 1797, Vol. III, Appendix, pp. lix and lxi.

CHAPTER XIV

1. Cogan, p. 150. Because they are neither flesh nor fish they can be eaten on fish days.

2. Buttes, Sig. L6^v.

3. W. Cullen, *The Treatise of Materia Medica,* 1789, Vol. I, p. 342.

4. Harrison, pp. 143, 144.

5. J. Thirsk (ed.), *The Agrarian History of England and Wales,* 1967, Vol. IV, particularly Chapters II, VII, VIII.

6. C. Estienne and J. Liebault (trans. R. Surphlet), *Maison Rustique, or the Countrie Farme,* London, 1600, p. 102.

7. Boorde, p. 264.

8. Gratarolus, Sig. I4^r.

9. Cogan, p. 152. This view was held by Aristotle and Albertus Magnus. See J. Needham, *A History of Embryology,* 1959, pp. 52 and 86.

10. Estienne and Liebault, p. 98.

11. *Book of Thrifte,* 1589. See F.H. Cripps-Day, *The Manor Farm,* 1931, p. 9 (facsimile of the *Booke of Thrifte,* 1589).

12. L. Mascall, *The Husbandlye ordring of Poultrie,* London, 1581, Sig. C4^r, C4^v. Boorde (p. 265) refers to a Turkish method of pickling hard boiled eggs.

13. Bright, *A Treatise of the Melancholie,* London, 1586, Sig. R4^r, allows roasted eggs for those suffering from melancholy.

14. Cogan, p. 151.

15. Cogan, p. 150.

16. Estienne and Liebault, p. 105.

17. 1552, Emmison, p. 242; 1567/68 and 1590, André L. Simon, *The Star Chamber Dinner Accounts,* 1959, p. 33; 1594-96, T.S. Willan, *Studies in Elizabethan Foreign Trade,* 1959, p. 331.

18. Cogan, p. 152. Alexandra Aphrodisseaus was a Greek philosopher of Athens (*fl.* 200 A.D.).

19. Estienne and Liebault, p. 102.

20. Cogan, p. 153.

21. Barnabe Googe, *Four books of husbandry,* London, 1577, Sig. T2^v.

22. Googe, Sig. T2^r.

23. Cogan, p. 154.

24. This advice also applies to the first milk after childbirth.

25. Estienne and Liebault, p. 90.

26. Estienne and Liebault, p. 90.

27. Cogan, p. 153. Cogan says he is quoting Dioscorides. See R.T. Gunther, *The Greek Herbal of Dioscorides,* 1934, p. 109.

28. Buttes, Sig. N3^r.

29. Buttes, Sig. N2^v. This is the usual description of the parts.

30. Cogan, p. 155.

31. Boorde, p. 296.

32. Cogan, p. 158.

33. Cogan, p. 158.

34. Willan, p. 331.

35. Estienne and Liebault, p. 90.

36. Emmison, p. 136.

37. Cogan, p. 158. He is saying this in relation to the importance of May butter.

38. F.G. Emmison, *Tudor Food and Pastimes,* 1964, p. 39.

39. 1552, Emmison, p. 241. Dishes of butter are computed in various ways; Emmison (p. 136) refers to 24 oz. and 2½ lb.; 1589, Hubert Hall, *Society in the Elizabethan Age,* 1886, p. 216; 1594/96, Willan, p. 331.

40. Cogan, p. 157.

41. Cogan, p. 158.

42. Cogan, p. 156.

43. Boorde, p. 267.

44. Buttes, Sig. N4^v.

45. Cogan, p. 156.

46. Islington had a reputation for good milk: P.H. McGrath, *The Marketing of Food, Fodder and Livestock in the London Area in the Seventeenth Century,* unpublished M.A. Thesis, 1948.

47. All prices are from Simon, pp. 31, 32.

48. D. Hartley, *Food in England,* 1954, p. 475.

49. Val Cheke, *The Story of Cheese-making in England,* 1959, Chapter I, particularly pp. 3 and 4.

50. Estienne and Liebault, p. 90.

51. Cogan, p. 155.

52. *GHH,* Sig. F4^v.

53. Buttes, Sig. N5^v. Milk was one of Cogan's vaporous foods: see "Sleep and Watch."

54. D. Hartley, *Thomas Tusser – 1577,* 1931, pp. 71, 72.

55. Emmison, p. 136, follows Walter of Henley and refers to ten milking sheep being equivalent to one cow.

56. Cheke, p. 89.

57. Hartley, *Tusser,* p. 72. Local rhyme on Suffolk cheese.

58. Googe, Sig. T3^r.

59. Estienne and Liebault, p. 91. Cheke (pp. 65-75) discusses rennets and plant coagulants used in the period.

60. Boorde, p. 266.

61. Cheke, p. 96, suggests it means a full-cream cheese. It could also be derived from the obsolete work "ruen," meaning rennet, or could be related to cows being fed on the second growth of grass in a season.

62. Boorde, p. 267.

63. Cogan, p. 160.

64. Buttes, Sig. N6^v.

65. Cogan, p. 159.

66. Cogan, p. 161. The first edition is 1584.

67. The following information about cheese is all from Googe, Sig. T3^r.

68. McGrath, p. 216.

69. Hartley, *Tusser,* p. 161.

70. H. Platt, *Sundrie new and artificiall remedies against Famine,* London, 1596, Sig. D4^r.

CHAPTER XV

1. John Evelyn in *Acetaria: a Discourse of Sallets,* London, 1699, p. 17.

2. Quoted by D. Hartley, *Food in England,* 1954, p. 380, as being from "A gardeners book of 1699."

3. Great Britain, *Sixth Report of the Medical Officer of Health to the Privy Council,* 1864, p. 29.

4. See A. Arber, *Herbals, Their Origin and Evolution,* 1938.

5. See F. Adams, *The Seven Books of Paulus Aegineta,* 1844, Vol. II, p. 5. Charles Alston, *Lectures on the Materia Medica* (published from manuscripts by John Hope), 1770, Vol. I, p. 15.

6. W. Turner, *A new herball,* London, 1551; J. Gerard, *The herball,* London, 1597.

7. H. Barlow, "Old English Herbals, 1525-1640," *Proc. Roy. Soc. Med.,* 1913, *6,* pp. 132 and 144. Thomas Johnson's edition was 1633.

8. T. Bright, *A Treatise wherin is declared the sufficiencie of English medicines. . .,* London, 1580.

9. A. Amherst, *A History of Gardening in England,* 1896 (2nd ed.), p. 136.

10. Harrison, p. 329.

11. See C. Welch, *The History of the Worshipful Company of Gardiners. . .,* 1900 (2nd ed.).

12. Richard Gardiner of Shrewesbury, *Profitable instructions for the Manuring, sowing and Planting of Kitchen Gardens,* London, 1603.

13. Buttes, Sig. F2^v-H8^r.

14. Cogan, pp. 32-84. Many herbs are discussed in detail by Colin Clair, *Of Herbs and Spices,* 1961.

15. Cogan, p. 85.

16. Cogan, p. 107. See Chapter XVI.

17. W. Langham, *The Garden of Health,* London, 1579. Sage (pp. 574-581) has 131 recipes; Coleworts (pp. 150-156) 102; Cresses (pp. 170-173) 59.

18. Cogan, p. 32.

19. Cogan, pp. 32-33.

20. *Regimen Sanitatis,* Sig. U1^r.

21. Cogan, p. 84.

22. Cogan, p. 64.

23. Cogan, pp. 57-59.

24. Galen (Kühn), Vol. VI, pp. 756, 792, 793, and Vol. XVII, part II, p. 577.

25. Cogan, p. 88.

26. J. Taverner, *Certaine Experiments concerning fish and fruit,* London, 1600, Sig. E3^r.

27. Cogan, pp. 88-90.

28. Cogan, p. 104.

29. Cogan, pp. 105-107.

30. Cogan, p. 107.

31. Cogan, pp. 99-100. Almonds are placed between figs and dates, not amongst the other nuts.

32. One of the group of gourds (Cucurbita). The name vegetable marrow was introduced in the nineteenth century *(OED).*

33. J. Gerard, *The Herbal or General History of Plants,* London, 1597, p. 948.

34. A.P. de Candolle, *Origin of Cultivated Plants,* 1884, p. 83.

35. *OED.*

36. Buttes, Sig. H8^r; Gerard, Cole Florie, p. 243.

37. Gardiner, Sig. C2^r.

38. C. Estienne and J. Liebault (trans. R. Surphlet), *Maison Rustique, or the Countrie Farme,* London, 1600, p. 214.

39. Buttes, Sig. H2^v.

40. Gerard, pp. 872-876.

41. Gerard, p. 876. The stinking and deadly carrots belong to the family *Thapsia.*

42. Gardiner, Sig. A4^v.

43. Gardiner, Sig. D2^v.

44. John Coke, *A debate between the heralds of England and France,* London, 1550, Sig. L4^r.

45. John Taverner, writing fifty years later (Sig. E3^r).

46. Boorde puts capers with olives (p. 285).

47. M.W. Labarge, *A Baronial Household of the Thirteenth Century,* 1965.

48. Clair, p. 113.

49. T.S. Willan, *Studies in Elizabethan Trade,* 1959. See pp. 27 and 85 for references to imports of oranges. Shakespeare uses the pun "civil as an orange" in several plays: see *Twelfth Night* or *Much Ado About Nothing* (Act II, Sc. i).

50. Langton, Sig. J1^r.

51. Elyot, Sig. M1^r.

52. T. Hill (trans.), *Arte of Gardening,* London [1563], Sig. 2C5^r.

53. D. Hartley, *Thomas Tusser – 1577,* 1931, p. 151.

54. *GHJ* (second part), Sig. C2^v.

55. André L. Simon, *The Star Chamber Dinner Accounts,* 1959, p. 26.

56. Gerard, "Of Potatoes" and "Of Potatoes of Virginia," pp. 780, 781.

57. See R.N. Salaman, *The History and Social Influence of the Potato,* 1949, and R.J. Forbes, "The Rise of Food Technology (1500-1900)," *Janus,* 1958, *47,* pp. 101-105. C. Clair, *Kitchens and Table,* 1964, p. 111 and pp. 119-129.

58. I. Beeton (ed.), *Beeton's Book of Household Management,* 1861.

59. Henry Thompson, *Food and Feeding,* 1894 (8th ed.).

60. Forbes, p. 107.

61. See B. Lillywhite, *London Coffee House,* 1963.

62. King James I (of England), *A counter blaste to tobacco,* London, 1604. For further references on tobacco see Jerome E. Brooks, *Tobacco,* Vol. I (1507-1615), 1937.

63. N.F., *The Husbandman's fruitfull Orchard,* London, 1608, Sig. B2^v-C3^v. The information about carriage and storage is taken from this source.

64. H. Platt, *The Jewell House of Art and Nature,* London, 1594, p. 4.

65. T. Tasso (trans. T.K.), *The Householders Philosophie,* London, 1588, Sig. E4^r.

66. Platt, p. 71.

67. Buttes, Sig. C5^v.

68. Cogan, p. 95. Detailed instructions are given.

69. Cogan, p. 94.

70. H. Platt, *Floraes Paradise,* London, 1608, p. 30.

71. The main sources of vitamin A are fatty fish and their liver-oils, dairy produce, "vitaminised" margarine and liver. The vitamin can be stored in the human liver for future use.

72. The differences in the amounts of ascorbic acid recommended by various nutritional authorities are based on whether or not it is believed desirable to keep the tissues "saturated" with the vitamin.

73. J. Lind, *A Treatise of the Scurvy,* 1753. Reference is made here to *Lind's Treatise on Scurvy* (eds. C.P. Stewart and D. Guthrie), 1953, pp. 262-282. This bicentenary volume contains a reprint of the first edition.

74. Gerard, p. 325.

75. Gerard, p. 195.

76. Gerard, pp. 189-201.

77. Parsley is one example of a plant, rich in ascorbic acid, which is likely to have been eaten as a herb and not used simply as a garnish in the way it is used today.

78. *The Fruitful Orchard,* Sig. A2^v.

CHAPTER XVI

1. See S. Pegge, *The Forme of Cury*, 1780, from a fourteenth century manuscript. Thomas Austin, *Two Fifteenth Century Cookery Books*, 1888; also Anon., *The good Huswives handmaid*, n.p., n.d., and Thomas Dawson, *The good huswives handmaid*, n.p., n.d.

2. Prices are indicated by R. Roberts in "The Early History of the Import of Drugs into Britain," *The Evolution of Pharmacy in Britain*, 1965 (ed. F.N.L. Poynter), where extracts from the customs valuations of the 1604 "Rate Book" are given. Also Gerard Malynes, *The Centre of the circle of Commerce*, 1623, indicates some comparative prices of spices in the East Indies and London. J. Burnett's *A History of the Cost of Living*, 1969, gives prices of necessities rather than such luxuries as spices.

3. Cogan, *Haven of Health*; Buttes, *Dyets Dry Dinner*; Bullein, *The Government of Health*; Boorde, *Dyetary of Health*; Gratarolus, *A Direction for Health of Magistrates and students.*

4. Both galingale and saffron are put with "herbs" by Cogan.

5. Treacle and Methridatum had special uses against poison and are discussed below.

6. Theophrastus (trans. A. Hart), *Enquiry into Plants*, 1916, Vol. II, pp. 315 and 428.

7. Dioscorides (ed. R.T. Gunther), *The Greek Herbal of Dioscorides*, 1934, p. 189.

8. C. Clair, *Of Herbs and Spices*, 1961, p. 68.

9. Margaret Wade Labarge, *A Baronial Household of the Thirteenth Century*, 1965, pp. 90 and 76.

10. Walter Bailey, *A short Discourse on three kinds of PEPPERS in common use*, London, 1588, Sig. A4[r].

11. This uncertainty was also referred to by other writers, e.g. Cogan, p. 107.

12. As regards black and white pepper, the ancients were nearer the truth than were some later theorists. The production of black or white pepper depends on the state of ripeness at harvesting and the treatment of the fruit afterwards.

13. Bartholomaeus Anglicus gives a description of this: see Batman, Sig. 3Hl[r].

14. J. Gerard, *The Herbal or General History of Plants*, London, 1597, p. 1355.

15. Bailey, Sig. A7[r].

16. Gerard, p. 1355.

17. Bailey, Sig. A8[r]. Bailey also gives information in his treatise about other types of "pepper" (e.g. pimentos) besides those considered in this study.

18. Cogan, p. 108. See Galen (Kühn), Vol. VI, p. 270.

19. Bullein, Sig. L7[v].

20. Besides referring to the ancient sect of physicians who relied upon observation and experience, rather than theory, in their practice of medicine, the word "Empericke" could also mean a charlatan. This connotation is also found in sixteenth century references.

21. Gerard, p. 1356. This reference to the beliefs of Indian physicians has not been followed up for this study.

22. *Regimen Sanitatis*, Sig. Y1[v].

23. Batman, Sig. 3Hl[v].

24. Buttes, Sig. N7^V says "hot and dry in the third [degree] and almost in the beginning of the fourth."

25. Batman, Sig. 3Hl^V.

26. The headings are taken, basically, from Cogan, p. 108. Boorde (p. 286) says black pepper makes a man lean.

27. Buttes, Sig. N7^V.

28. *GHJ*, Sig. A4^r, B1^r, and D6^V respectively. This recipe to make peascods was for "fish days"; peascods made for Lent had sweeter spices.

29. Cogan, p. 107. Bailey also refers to this at length, giving two recipes (Sig. B7^r).

30. *WT*, London, 1595, Sig. A3^r. This book contains some cookery recipes but mostly advice on home medicines. Diatrion pipereon recipes have not been found in "true" cookery books of the period.

31. Bailey, Sig. B7^r.

32. Gerard, p. 1348.

33. F. Adams, *The Seven Books of Paulus Aegineta*, 1884, Vol. III, p. 161. Adams' commentary refers to the opinion of Salmasius [Claude de Saumaise (1588-1653)].

34. Cogan, p. 111. "Maths." here would refer to P.A. Matthiolus, Italian doctor and botanist, 1500-1577. An alternative possible reference, namely Mathias L'Obel, a distinguished contemporary botanist, was of too late a date (1559-1616) to be quoted by Cogan; also L'Obel's work was followed closely by Gerard, who does not confuse the two plants.

35. Buttes, Sig. N8^V.

36. Gerard, p. 1242 (incorrectly numbered 1234). Bullein (Sig. L8^V) writes of *Cassia fistula* in its own right.

37. Bullein, Sig. L8^V.

38. Cogan, p. 111.

39. Cogan, p. 111.

40. Gerard, p. 1349.

41. Cogan, p. 111.

42. *GHH*. The references for the recipes are: (i) Sig. A4^r, (ii) Sig. A4^V, (iii) Sig. B3^r, (iv) Sig. C4^r, (v) Sig. C5^r, (vi) Sig. E5^r, (vii) Sig. F7^r, (viii) Sig. G1^r, (ix) Sig. G3^V. The recipes quoted have been chosen to illustrate their wide range.

43. Labarge, p. 91.

44. Buttes, Sig. P1^V. It is usually considered that the name is derived from the resemblance of the dried buds to a nail *(clou de girofle) OED*.

45. Cogan, p. 109.

46. Gerard, p. 1352.

47. Buttes, Sig. P1^V.

48. *GHH*, (i) Sig. A7^V, (ii) Sig. B8^r, (iii) Sig. D2^r. This includes veal, kidney and suet; (iv) Sig. D3^r, (v) Sig. D6^r, (vi) Sig. E3^r, (vii) Sig. E3^V.

49. Gerard, p. 1353.

50. Gerard, p. 1353. A recipe from W.L. Dawson, *A Leech Book or Collection of Medicinal Recipes of the Fifteenth Century*, 1934, p. 159 suggests the eye drops contained a rather high concentration of cloves.

51. Gerard, p. 1352, follows Galen in this idea: Galen (Kühn), XIV, p. 462. A seventeenth century translation of Dioscorides (Gunther, *The Greek Herbal of*

Dioscorides, 1934) does not include cloves. It is estimated they reached Europe in the second century A.D.

52. Clair, p. 152.

53. Labarge, p. 92.

54. Malynes, Sig. O4^r.

55. *GHH,* Sig. F4^r.

56. Here "turnsall" is likely to refer to colouring matter rather than the inclusion of the plant Tornesol *(Heliotropium)* as an ingredient.

57. Nell Heaton, in her collection of recipes (*The Complete Cook,* undated, revised 1947 edition), gives an even more highly spiced drink in "The Low Countries Night Cap" (p. 402).

58. Clair, p. 61.

59. Wilfred Bonser, *The Medical Background of Anglo-Saxon England,* 1963, p. 46. Here pepper, galingale, ginger, and (possibly) cinnamon are referred to.

60. E. Power, *The Goodman of Paris,* 1938, p. 286.

61. Gerard, p. 55. Gerard owed much more than this to L'Obel's work.

62. Buttes, Sig. O2^v.

63. Cogan, p. 110.

64. Gerard, p. 55.

65. Gunther, *Dioscorides,* Bk. II, p. 200.

66. Cogan, p. 110.

67. A. Du Laurens (trans R. Surphlet), *The Preservation of Sight,* London, 1599. (Facsimile edition with notes by Sanford V. Larkey, 1938, p. 62.)

68. *GHH* (i) Sig. B7^r, (ii) Sig. C6^r, (iii) Sig. D1^r, (iv) Sig. D7^r, (v) Sig. E3^r, (vi) Sig. E5^r, (vii) Sig. E6^v.

69. Bullein, Sig. L7^r.

70. Cogan, p. 74.

71. Gerard, p. 28.

72. Cogan, p. 75.

73. Galingale appears frequently in medical recipes in fifteenth century leechbooks, see Dawson, *A Leech book.*

74. Gerard, p. 1353.

75. Cogan, p. 109.

76. Cogan, p. 109.

77. Malynes, Sig. O4^r.

78. *GHH,* (i) Sig. C1^r, (ii) Sig. C2^r, (iii) Sig. D1^r, (iv) Sig. E3^r, (v) Sig. E3^v, (vi) Sig. E5^r, (vii) Sig. E5^r.

79. Gerard, p. 1354.

80. Gerard p. 1354.

81. Cogan, p. 110.

82. A caudel is a mixture of eggs, cereal and malt (D. Hartley, *Food in England,* 1954 p. 558).

83. Cogan did recognise that hempseed taken by man "extinguished nature" in contrast to making those hens who ate it lay more frequently (p. 152).

84. *GHH,* Sig. C3^r and Sig. F7^r respectively.

85. Harrison, p. 50. Later (p. 59) he says it was not "commonly planted" until the time of Richard II (i.e., last part of the fourteenth century).

86. Labarge, p. 93, refers to saffron as the most important and most costly of

herbs. In the thirteenth century it was imported from Spain and cost the Countess of Leicester between 10/- and 14/- a pound.

87. Gerard, (i) p. 123, (ii) p. 126, (iii) p. 1006, (iv) p. 1008.

88. Gerard, p. 124.

89. Cogan, p. 69.

90. Here it might appear that the connection between the yellow of saffron and jaundice followed the doctrine of "signatures," whereby the value of a plant was based on shape and colour rather than effect. However, this doctrine is referred to very little by genuine herbalists in England before the seventeenth century. Boorde (p. 286) thinks that saffron is too hot for the liver.

91. St. Anthony's fire in this context is ergotism; it later came to be used to refer to erysipelas.

92. Cogan, p. 96.

93. *GHH,* (i) Sig. D5^r, (ii) Sig. E3^r, (iii) Sig. E4^v, (iv) Sig. F6^v, (v) Sig. G2^v.

94. Harrison, p. 60.

95. Emmison p. 316.

96. J.C. Drummond and A. Wilbraham, *The Englishman's Food,* 1939, p. 34.

97. Harrison, p. 54.

98. Labarge, p. 93.

99. *A Profitable and necessarie Discourse for the meeting with the bad garbelling of spices used in these days,* London, [1592], by "divers grocers" of the Grocers Company.

100. Harrison, p. 57.

101. Gerard, p. 1358.

102. Gerard, p. 1358.

103. Cogan, p. 112. He discussed them under the heading of "Graines."

104. Boorde p. 287.

105. This type was also called "sweet root." According to Gerard (p. 1120) it was unknown to the apothecaries and ordinary people in England.

106. Gerard, p. 1120.

107. William Langham, *The Garden of Health,* London, 1579. Liquorice, p. 362; pepper, p. 485; onion p. 444.

108. Lists of sauces and their constituents are given on pages 77 and 108 of Austin's *Two Fifteenth-Century Cookery Books.*

109. Anon., *The Booke of Carving and Sewing,* London, n.d. This is derived from earlier manuscripts.

110. *Book of Carving,* Sig. B2^v, also Sig. B1^r and B7^v.

111. André L. Simon, *The Star Chamber Dinner Accounts,* 1959.

112. Cogan, p. 162.

113. Cogan, p. 163.

114. Cogan's explanation of the importance of salt is interesting in that it is physiological. Many other explanations are based more on tradition and superstition.

115. Cogan, p. 163. Examples are Northwich, Nantwich, and Middlewich. See also Harrison, p. 183. Rock salt was discovered in Cheshire in 1690 (see [C. Tomlinson] , *A Natural History of Common Salt,* 1850, p. 36).

116. Emmison, p. 242.

117. Bullein, Sig. K8^r.

118. Cogan, p. 164.

119. Bullein, Sig. K8^r.

120. Cogan, p. 165.

121. J. Bickerdyke, *The Curiosities of Ale and Beer,* 1889, p. 404.

122. Simon, p. 35; *NHB* (p. 15) quotes 4d. per gallon (variety unspecified).

123. *Regimen Sanitatis,* Sig. R3^v. Cogan, p. 164. Buttes, Sig. O8^v. See also Chapter III.

124. See Chapter VI.

125. *Regimen Sanitatis,* Sig. R3^v, quoted also by other authors.

126. Philemon Holland, *Regimen Sanitatis Salerni,* London, 1617, Sig. P4^r.

127. Cogan, p. 164.

128. The steam produced by vinegar thrown on hot stones should be breathed up the nose to clear the head.

129. Cogan, p. 165.

130. This reference is given by D. Hartley, *Food in England,* 1954, p. 653. Basically, corn, wheat or rye is pounded to a paste in a mortar with the strongest vinegar. The paste is made into little balls and sun dried. To make vinegar, some of this dried paste should be dissolved in wine or water.

131. Buttes, Sig. P1^r.

132. *NHB,* p. 15.

133. Gerard, pp. 189, 190, 206, 211, 212; also pp. 140, 159.

134. Cogan, p. 165.

135. *Regimen Sanitatis,* Sig. W4^v.

136. Bullein, Sig. H3^r. Bullein implies that mustard was commonly used for the eyes.

137. A. MacDonell (ed.), *The Closet of Sir Kenelm Digby Knight Opened,* 1910, p. 194.

138. It should be realized that there was likely to be only one size of spoon at that time, with no gradation from teaspoon to tablespoon.

139. As given in *Regimen Sanitatis,* Sig. L4^r.

140. Buttes, Sig. P2^v. He relates it to an Italian sauce. This connection is taken up by E.B. Aresty in *The Delectable Past,* 1965, p. 50.

142. Austin, pp. 12, 96, 115.

143. Boorde, p. 265.

144. Bullein, Sig. K5^r.

145. Bullein, Sig. K6^v.

146. T.S. Willan, *Studies in Elizabethan Foreign Trade,* 1965.

147. Cogan, p. 130. See also Boorde, p. 276.

148. *GHH,* Sig. B5^v. The recipes all seem to come from the nobility.

149. See past and current work of Prof. J. Yudkin and others at Queen Elizabeth College, London University.

150. See W.R. Aykroyd, *Sweet Malefactor,* 1967, Chapter I. The main part of this interesting book deals with sugar and slavery and is concerned with a period later than this study.

151. Galen, p. 191.

152. Buttes, Sig. O5^v.

153. Bullein, Sig. K8^v. Here again (like vinegar) there is a contradiction of ideas regarding moistness and dryness; apparently viscosity was not directly related to ideas of moisture.

154. Galen makes a number of references to honey being altered or transmuted into bile. See Galen, pp. 179, 191.

155. Thomas Hill, *A pleasaunt Instruction of the parfit orderinge of Bees*, London, 1568. Tusser advises on honey and bee-keeping (see D. Hartley, *Thomas Tusser – 1557*, 1931, pp. 62, 68, 70, 97, 121). This collection of "Englished" sayings of the ancients is attached to Hill's *The proffitable Arte of Gardening* (4th ed.), London, 1568.

156. Willan, p. 331. Reference is also made here to 12d. worth of treacle.

157. *NHB*, p. 3.

158. Willan. See Chapter V, "Sugar and the Elizabethans," pp. 313-332.

159. Paul Hentzer (trans. R. Bently), *A Journey into England in the year 1598*, 1757, p. 48.

160. Macdonnel, pp. 5-96.

161. See R. Warner, *Antiquitates Culinariae*, 1791, pp. 4-35.

162. *GHH*, (i) Sig. A4^r, (ii) Sig. E1^r, (iii) Sig. F6^r, (iv) Sig. G3^r.

163. There are a large number of different ways of spelling both these words.

164. Drummond and Wilbraham, p. 34.

165. W.E. Mead, *The English Medieval Feast*, 1931, p. 77. Details of a number of dishes using spices are given.

166. François Pierre de La Varenne, *Le Cuisinier François*, Paris, 1651. La Varenne's influence was revolutionary in developing the famous French cuisine. See also R. Barber, *Cooking and Recipes from Rome to the Renaissance*, 1973, pp. 111-112.

POSTSCRIPT

1. The variety of opinions held are referred to by E.H. Ackernecht, "The End of Greek Diet," *Bull. Hist. Med.*, 1971, *45*, pp. 242-249.

2. O. Temkin, *Galenism, the Rise and Fall of a Medical Philosophy*, 1973, p. 134.

3. W. Cullen, *First Lines of the Practice of Physic*, 1786, Vol. I, p. xvi. The first edition (1776-84) does not contain this reference.

4. Temkin, p. 135.

5. Lester H. King, "Medicine 1695; Friedrich Hoffmann's *Fundamenta Medicinae*," *Bull. Hist. Med.*, 1969, *43*, p. 28.

6. Louis Lémery, *Traité des Alimentes*, Paris, 1702. Translated anonymously into English 1702. D. Hay's (acknowledged) translation as *A Treatise of all Sorts of Food* appeared in 1745.

7. Cullen, *First Lines*, Vol. I, p. xxxii.

8. W. Cullen, *Treatise of Materia Medica*, 1789, was based on teaching notes that had been prepared over a period of more than twenty years.

9. Cullen, *Materia Medica*, Vol. I, p. 59.

10. The animal mixt was also called "gluten." This was the name given to the "coaguable lymph" part of blood. Gluten is the modern name for wheat protein; the word originally had the meaning of a "gluey substance," and referred to a number of substances apparently similar to coaguable lymph. The discovery by Beccari (in 1728) of gluten in wheat showed that the important substance could be found in vegetable as well as animal matter. See E.F. Beach, "Beccari of Bologna, the Discoverer of Vegetable Protein," *J. Hist. Med.*, 1961, *16*, pp. 345-373.

11. W. Cullen, *Institutions of Medicine,* 1785, Part I: Physiology, Section IV, "Of the Natural Functions," p. 231. (First edition 1772.)

12. Cullen would have been familiar with dry distillation methods, but was too near the end of his life to be able to visualize the significance of the newer methods called by F.L. Holmes the second stage of analytical development. See "Elementary Analysis and the Origins of Physiological Chemistry," *Isis,* 1963, *54,* pp. 50-81.

13. Cullen, *Materia Medica,* Vol. I, p. vii.

14. J. Hart, in ΚΛΙΝΙΚΗ *or the Diet of the Diseased,* 1633, had extended the use of diet in disease to the whole second part of his book. On the other hand J.B. Van Helmont had said (*Oriatrike or Physick Refined,* 1662) that "Curing is not subject to the dietary part of medicine," p. 450.

15. John Quincy, *Pharmacopoeia Officinalis and Extemporanea,* 1718, p. 618.

16. For a discussion of the relationship between aliments and medicaments see Jane O'Hara-May, "Foods or Medicines," *Transactions of the British Society for the History of Pharmacy,* 1971, Vol. I, No. 2.

17. Cullen, *Materia Medica,* Vol. I (pp. 217-432) devoted to aliments; medicines fill Vol. II (pp. 1-590).

18. Cullen, *Materia Medica,* Vol. II, pp. 1-2.

19. Antoine Lavoisier (trans. Robert Kerr), *Elements of Chemistry,* Edinburgh, 1790; facsimile Dover Edition, 1965, with an introduction by Douglas McKie. Reference at p. xxx.

20. Lavoisier, *Elements,* p. 175. Referring to the term *calorie* Lavoisier says (p. 4): "This substance, whatever it is being the cause of heat, or, in other words, the sensation which we call warmth being caused by the accumulation of this substance, we cannot, in strict language distinguish it by the term *heat;* because the same name would then very improperly express both cause and effect. For this reason, in the memoir which I published in 1777, I gave it the names of *igneous fluid* and *matter of heat.*" With the reformation of nomenclature these words were replaced by the term caloric.

21. A. Lavoisier and P.S. de Laplace, "Mémoire sur la Chaleur," *Mémoires de l'Académie Royale des Sciences,* 1870 (published 1784), pp. 355-408. See also E. Mendelsohn, *Heat and Life,* 1964, pp. 147-154.

22. J.A. Paris, *Elements of Medical Chemistry,* 1825. Author of *A Treatise on Diet,* 1826.

23. William Prout (1785-1850), *Philosophical Transactions,* 1827, Part 2, pp. 355-388.

24. J. von Liebig (1803-73), *Animal Chemistry or Organic Chemistry in its Application to Physiology and Pathology,* trans. William Gregory (Facsimile Edition, 1964). See Introduction by F.L. Holmes. The original German edition was published in Giessen in the same year.

25. A. Fick and F.J. Wislicenus, *Philosophical Magazine* (4th series), 1866, *31,* p. 159. Analysis of urine for nitrogen indicated that muscular work expended must have been sustained by non-nitrogenous food.

26. J.R. Mayer (1814-87), put forward the theory of the conservation of energy in 1843. He had previously announced the equivalence of heat and work, which was proved in 1847 by H. von Helmholtz (1821-94). J.P. Joule also postulated the equivalence of thermal and mechanical energy, and has given his name to the unit

of energy now being introduced into nutrition to replace the Kilocalorie. *1 Kilocalorie = 4.19 Kilojoule.*

27. J. Pereira (1804-53), *Treatise on Food and Diet,* 1843.

28. Pereira, *Treatise,* p. 2.

29. Pereira, *Treatise,* p. 4.

30. J. Moleschott (1822-93), included in the *second* edition of *Physiologie der Nahrungsmittel: ein Handbuch der Diätetik,* 1859, Section VIII.

31. Moleschott used the term *Feltbildner* for carbohydrates.

32. Jane O'Hara-May, "Measuring Man's Needs," *Journal of the History of Biology,* 1971, *4,* pp. 249-273.

33. A. Quetelet, *Sur l'homme et le développpment de ses facultés,* 1855. English translation ("under superintendence of Dr. R. Knox"), 1842. Quetelet was an astronomer and mathematician. He drew together the main statistical developments and tendencies of his time.

34. J. Moleschott, *Lehre der Nahrungsmittel fur das Volk,* 1850, p. 116. This book has Erlangen as the place of publication; some bibliographies give Stuttgart.

35. Great Britain (Dep't. of Health and Social Security), *Recommended Intakes of Nutrients for the United Kingdom,* 1969.

36. Moleschott used twenty-one reported dietaries collected by seven workers. Included were: Dutch, English, French, Bavarian and Hessian soldiers, English sailors, agricultural labourers. Of particular interest is Anselm Payen's (1795-1871) reference to the fact that English railway workers on the Rouen railway did much more work than their French counterparts, the explanation being that they had a larger daily ration of meat. This comparison was frequently quoted by later writers to illustrate the importance of meat in the diet when doing hard work.

37. The French Revolution and the impact of such writings as Tom Paine's *The Rights of Man* contributed to a climate of awareness about the ordinary man.

38. Naval ration scales were altered in 1825 and 1844. W.B. Carpenter (1813-44), the noted physiologist, said of the latter scale that there could be no "complaint of an insufficiency of food, although the allowance [31-35 oz. of nutritious matter daily] cannot be regarded as superfluous." Carpenter, *Principles of Human Physiology,* 5th ed., 1855, pp. 45, 47 (First edition, 1843).

39. Great Britain, Poor Law Commissioners, *Second Annual Report,* 1836, p. 63. The Poor Law Commissioners suggested six general dietaries (based on past usage) for able-bodied men and women in workhouses.

40. Pereira, *Treatise,* p. 462.

41. Pereira, *Treatise,* p. 497.

42. Pereira, *Treatise,* p. 450.

43. F.W. Pavey, *A Treatise on Food and Dietetics,* 1875, pp. 500-505 (First edition, 1874).

44. Pavey, *Treatise,* p. 501; see also p. 452.

45. Pavey, *Treatise,* pp. 503, 504. The energy needs are described in terms of force-production and measured in foot-pounds or foot-tons of work. The Continental system was a kilogrammètre (p. 103).

46. Max Rubner, *Die Gesetze des Energieverbrauchs bei der Ernährung,* 1902. *The Laws of Energy Consumption in Nutrition,* 1968, translated and reprinted by the U.S. Army.

47. W.O. Atwater, "Chemistry and Economy of Food," *Bulletin No. 21 U.S. Dept. of Agriculture,* 1895.

48. R.H. Chittenden, *Physiological Economy in Nutrition,* with special reference to the minimal protein requirement of the healthy man (1904).

49. Claude Bernard, *Introduction à l'étude de la médecine expérimentale,* 1865. Trans. H.C. Greene, *An Introduction to the Study of Experimental Medicine,* Life of Science Library Series, 1949.

50. W.B. Cannon, *The Wisdom of the Human Body,* 1932, p. 24.

51. George Budd (1808-82), *The London Medical Gazette,* NS 2, pp. 632 and following.

52. N. Lunin, "Ueber die Bedeutung der anorganischen Salze für die Ernährung des Thieres " *Z. f. Physiol. Chem.* 1881, 5, p. 31; originally presented in a Dissertation at Dorpat, 1880.

53. G. Bunge (trans. L.C. Woodridge), *Textbook of Physiological and Pathological Chemistry,* 1890, Lecture VII, p. 118.

54. F.G. Hopkins, *Journal of Physiology,* 1912, *44,* p. 425.

55. A.J. Ihde and S.L. Becker, *Journal of the History of Biology,* 1971, *4,* pp. 1-33. Concepts referred to include: 1. The germ theory; 2. Toxins as a cause of disease; 3. The Liebig-Vort views on nutrition; 4. The Schmidt-Bunge views on minerals in nutrition; 5. Proximate principles in Food Analysis. The article provides an excellent survey of the thought in the period.

56. Great Britain, Dept. of Health and Social Security, *Recommended Intakes of Nutrients for the United Kingdom,* 1969. Thiamine was previously called vitamin B_1. The amount of thiamine recommended as the daily intake for a moderately active man on a diet providing 3000 Kcal is 1.2 milligrams.

57. Great Britain, Medical Research Council, *Report on the Present State of Knowledge of Accessory Food Factors (Vitamins),* 1924; Preface to the second edition.

58. Great Britain, Medical Research Council, *Vitamins: A Survey of Present Knowledge,* 1932, Preface (p. 3).

59. C.A. Elvehjem (1901-62), distinguished nutrition research worker and President of the University of Wisconsin: *Essays on the History of Nutrition and Diet,* 1967, pp. 54-57 (published by the American Dietetic Association).

60. E.F. Du Bois, *Essays on the History of Nutrition and Diet,* pp. 252-257.

61. League of Nations, *The Relation of Nutrition to Health, Agriculture and Economic Policy,* 1937.

62. An important example is: Ancel Keys et al., *The Biology of Human Starvation,* 2 Vols., 1950.

63. U.S. Food and Nutrition Board, National Research Council, *Recommended Dietary Allowances,* 1943. See also Lydia J. Roberts, "Beginnings of the Recommended Dietary Allowances," *Essays on the History of Nutrition and Diet,* pp. 107-112.

64. For Recommended Allowances in other countries see: G.H. Beaton and E.W. McHenry (eds.), *Nutrition,* 1964, Vol. II, pp. 299-350 (E. Gordon Young, "Dietary Standards").

65. R. Schoenkeimer, *The Dynamic State of Body Constituents,* 1942.

66. Great Britain; Ministry of Agriculture Fisheries and Food, *Household Food Consumption and Expenditure: 1970 and 1971,* 1973.

67. See: A.N. Exton-Smith, "Nutrition Surveys and the Problems of Detection of Malnutrition in the Elderly," *Nutrition,* 1970, *24,* pp. 218-223. Also: Great

Britain, Dept. of Health and Social Security, *First Report by the Sub-Committee on Nutritional Surveillance,* 1973.

68. Examples in the U.K. are: All margarine sold by retail shops is required by law to contain on average the equivalent of 900 micrograms per 100 g of retinol (vitamin A) and 8 micrograms of vitamin D per 100 g. All flours must contain the following minimum quantities of nutrients per 100 g: Iron 1.65 mg, Thiamine 0.24 mg, Nicotinic acid 1.6 mg.

69. R.A. McCance and E.M. Widdowson, *The Composition of Foods,* 1967 (first edition 1939). Many countries have prepared sets of food tables appropriate to their own foods.

70. S. Davidson, R. Passmore and J.F. Brock, *Human Nutrition and Dietetics,* 1972.

71. Davidson and Passmore, p. 315.

72. World Health Organisation: W.R. Aykroyd, *Conquest of Deficiency Diseases,* FFHC Basic Study No. 24, 1970.

73. H.M. Sinclair and D.F. Hollingsworth, *Hutchison's Food and the Principles of Nutrition,* 1969, p. v.

74. Quoted in *Conquest of Deficiency Diseases,* p. 7.

BOOK LIST
PRIMARY SOURCES: CHRONOLOGICAL LIST

One of the diseases of this age is the multitude of books that doth
so overcharge the world that it is not able to digest the abundance
of idle matter that is every day hatched and brought into the
world...

Barnaby Rich (1610)

THE FOLLOWING LIST of sixteenth and seventeenth century English
books constitutes the primary sources consulted for this study and includes all the books of that period referred to in the text. The list is
intended as no more than a guide for those who are interested in the
material. Titles are given in chronological order of the first English edition, according to the *Short-title Catalogue of English Books,
1475-1640*. The numbers of the editions printed (also from the S.T.C.)
are given in brackets as an indication of the demand for the book. The
editions consulted are marked with an asterisk. For ease of reference an
alphabetical list of authors with the date of the first editions of their
works follows this book list. Brief notes are included on authors and
translators in order to illustrate the general background of the writers
on the dietary of health. No attempt was made to trace obscure individuals and inconsistencies in the spelling of names, and book titles
have been left unchanged.

The full reference to the S.T.C. is: A.W. Pollard and G.R. Redgrave, *A
Short-title Catalogue of Books Printed in England, Scotland and Ireland
and of English Books Printed Abroad 1475-1640,* 1946. Alterations in
S.T.C. datings have been made here only where the information came
to hand.

"Watt" refers to Robert Watt, *Bibliotheca Britannica: or a General
Index of British and Foreign Literature,* 1824.

"Ferguson" refers to John Ferguson, *Bibliotheca Chemica,* 1906.

"Duff" refers to E. Gordon Duff, *Fifteenth Century English Books,*
1917.

The main works consulted for authors and translators were: Leslie Stephen (ed.), *Dictionary of National Biography,* 1855; Pierre Larousse, *Grande Dictionnaire Universel du XIXe siècle,* 1866; William Smith, *Dictionary of Greek and Roman Biography and Mythology by Various Writers,* 2 vols., 1880.

1500
ANON. *This is the boke of cokerye.* London. First edition 1500.
Cookery book for "a pryncis household or any other estates." NOT SEEN. See 1545 and 1575 below.

1508
ANON. *The boke of keruynge.* London.
This book, printed by Wynkyn de Worde, was developed from earlier manuscripts and was printed in many editions under the title *The Book of Carving* and also *The Booke of Carving and Sewing.* The edition used for this study is the undated edition bound with other late sixteenth century books (B.M. shelf no. 1037.e.l).* F.J. Furnivall, editor of *Early English Meals and Manners,* 1868,* includes the 1513 edition. The book gives instructions for the carving and serving of food in noble households.

[1510]
WALTER OF HENLEY. *Boke of husbandry.* London. Translation ascribed to Robert Grosseteste. First edition 1510.
First edition was printed by Wynkyn de Worde. NOT SEEN. This work is an English translation of a tract on husbandry which was incorporated into a number of later works by a variety of authors. Modern editions are: *Walter of Henley's Husbandry,* transcribed and translated by E. Lamond, 1890,* and F.H. Cripps-Day, *The Manor Farm,* 1931.* This contains a facsimile of the [1510] edition. Walter of Henley (*fl.* 1250), was a writer on agriculture said to have become a Dominican friar. Robert Grosseteste (d. 1253) was Bishop of Lincoln.

1521
ANON. *Here begynneth a devoute treatyse named the Dyetary of ghostly helthe.* London. First edition 1521.*
A devout book with 24 "considerations" on subjects such as patience and obedience.

[1523]
JOHN FITZHERBERT. *The Boke of husbandry. Here begynneth a newe tract or treatyse moost profytable for all husbande men.* London. First edition 1523.* (10).
The first book in English on husbandry. See also W.W. Skeat (ed.), *Book of Husbandry,* 1882.* Title indicates content. John Fitzherbert (1460-1531?), was Lord of the Manor of Norbury in Derbyshire, elder brother to the Judge, Sir Anthony Fitzherbert who was at one time credited with the authorship of the book on husbandry.

1524
LEONARD COX. *The arte or crafte of rhethoryke.* London. First edition 1524.*
Title indicates content. Leonard Cox (*fl.* 1572), incorporated B.A., Oxford,
1529-30, died 1599, was a schoolmaster, according to the D.N.B. A Leonard Cox
appears in the list of examiners of the Surgeon's College at an appropriate time
for Thomas Newton's reference in 1586.

1525
ANON. (W.C. Walter Cary). *Here begynneth a new mater: the which is called an
Herball.* London. First edition 1525.* (10)
Title indicates content. The identity of "W.C." and Walter Cary are discussed by
H.M. Barlow, "Old English Herbals," *Proc. Roy. Soc. Medicine,* 1913-14, pp.
116-118. See under 1583.

1526
ANON. *The grete herball.* London. First edition 1526.* (2).
A translation of *Le Gran Herbier*. Printed by Peter Treveris.

[1526]
ANON. *Here begynneth a newe boke of medecynes intytuled the treasure of pore
men.* London. First ed. [1526] (9), 1539.*
A book of medical treatments. Later called "a good book of medicines."

1527
HIERONYMUS VON BRAUNSCHWEIG. *The vertuose boke of distyllatyon.* Lon-
don. First edition 1527.*
Translated by L. Andrewe: Laurence Andrew (*fl.* 1510-1537), was also a printer.
Hieronymus von Braunschweig (? -1534?), was a German surgeon famous for his
writings on gunshot wounds. Title indicates content.

[1528]
ANON. *Here begynneth the Boke named the Assyse of breade.* London.
The title is taken from the [1528]* edition. The first edition given in the S.T.C. is
undated. There were 10 editions between the first and the edition of 1600.*

1528
ARISTOTLE. *Secreta Secretorum. Thus endeth the secretes of Arystotle.* London. First edition 1528.
Translated by R. Copeland. A large number of pseudo-Aristotelian works of a similar kind were printed in the period. The edition consulted was that of 1702*
based on the 1572 edition. Contains advice on government followed by that on
the preservation of health. Aristotle (384-323 B.C.). Robert Copeland, the translator, flourished 1508-1547; he was an author, translator, and printer.
*Schola Salernitana. Regimen Sanitatis Salerni. This boke techying al people to
governe them in helthe.* London. First (English) edition 1528.*
Translated by Thomas Paynell (*fl.* 1528-1567), Augustinian friar, Canon of Mer-

ton Abbey, translator of a large number and variety of works. There were at least
14 editions up to 1624. See also the modernised version of J. Harrington's *The
Englishmans doctor* (1607), with a note by F.R. Packard, 1920; also see Philemon
Holland, *Regimen Sanitatis Salerni,* London, 1617, and J. Ordronaux (ed.), *The
Code of Health of the School of Salernum,* 1870. Paynell retains the poem in
Latin and translates Villanova's commentary.

[1530]
ROGER BACON. *This boke doth treate all of the beste waters artyfycialles.* Lon-
don. First edition [1530].*
It is doubtful that Roger Bacon was the author of this work. The book explains
the value of 24 different waters made by infusion of herbs, vegetables, and fruits.
Roger Bacon's dates are c.1214-1292.
PLUTARCH. *The governaunce of good helthe, Erasmus being interpretoure.* Lon-
don. First edition [1530].
A later edition appeared in 1543,* translated by J. Hales, and entitled *The pre-
cepts of Plutarch for the preservacion of good healthe.* Title indicates contents.
Plutarch (46-120 A.D.); John Hales (d. 1571), was a writer of miscellany, one
time clerk in the Court and member of Parliament.

1531
THOMAS ELYOT. *The boke named The Gouernour.* London. First edition
1531.* (8).
Deals with the proper behaviour of men. Thomas Elyot (1490?-1546) was a diplomat, courtier, and author.

[1534]
A moche profitable treatise against the pestilence. London. First edition [1534].
Original author not given. The translation was by T. Paynell. There is one later
undated edition* (B.M. shelf No. 1167-d-7). Title indicates content. Elyot based
his advice on the same sort of material as is given here.

[1535]
ANON. *The boke of Knowledge whether a sycke person shall lyve or dye.* London. First ed. [1535].*
There is another issue with different spelling in the title. Places strong emphasis
on moral aspects.
J. DE VIGO. *This lytell practyce of J. de Vigo is translated for the helthe of the
body of man.* London. First edition [1535]. (3).
Translation by B. Traheron. The edition used here is that of 1564.* A book of
medical receipts for the treatment of various diseases. Giovanni da Vigo (*fl.* 1514)
was an Italian surgeon. Bartholomew Traheron (1410?-1558?), was a Protestant
writer on theological subjects.

1536-1539
THOMAS ELYOT. *The castel of helth.* London. First edition 1536-39. (15).
The edition of 1541* is used here. Deals with health and diet. Thomas Elyot
(1490?-1546) was a diplomatist, courtier, and author.

1538
THOMAS ELYOT. *The dictionary of syr T. Elyot.* London. First edition 1538.*
Later editions were entitled *Bibliotheca Eliotae* (6) 1548.* This is a Latin-English
dictionary.

1539.
ANON. *Treasurie of pore men.*
See above [1526].

[1539]
THOMAS MOULTON. *This is the myrrour or glasse of helth.* London. First edition [1539].* (10).
This is a medical book which refers to the influence of the planets. Reference is
made to a number of diseases, including the pestilence. Thomas Moulton (*fl.*
1540) was a Dominican friar who called himself "Doctor of Divinity of the Order
of Friar Preachers." His influence was felt well into the seventeenth century.

1540
ARNALDUS DE VILLANOVA. *Here is a newe boke called The defence of age
and recovery of youth.* London. First edition (from a manuscript) undated,
1540.*
A small book of eight leaves with some reference to diet for the preservation of
youth and delay of old age. Translated by Jonas Druumde (Drummond), who is
not in the DNB. Arnald of Villanova (1235-1312).

[1540]
ANDREW BOORDE. *The boke for to lerne a man to be wyse in buyldyng of his
howse for the helth of body.* London. First edition 1540.*
Title indicates content. See also F.J. Furnivall (ed.), *The Fyrst Boke of the Introduction of knowledge made by A. Borde. . . .* 1870. Andrew Boorde, or Borde
(c.1490-1549), a one time Carthusian monk, was a physician; he studied medicine
at Montpellier.

1540
EUCHARIUS ROESSLIN. *The byrthe of mankynde.* London. First edition
1540.* (13). Translated by Richard Jonas, believed to be a "studius and diligente
clarke." Later editions were translated by Thomas Raynalde (*fl.* 1546), a physician of London. Eucharius Roesslin (d. 1526) was a physician of Frankfurt-
on-Main.
JOANNES LUDOVICUS VIVES. *An introduction to wysedome.* London. First
edition 1540.* (5). Title indicates contents. Translated by R. Morysine – Richard
Morysine, Morison (d. 1556), a diplomat and ambassador. Later editions also include T. Elyot's *Banket of sapience,* and the *Precepts of Agapetus,* translated by
T. Paynell. Juan Luis Vives (1492-1540), a Spanish philosopher and humanist,
held a chair at Oxford under the protection of Catherine of Aragon. He was a
friend of Wolsey and Thomas More.

1541
T. ELYOT. *Castel of Helth.*
See above, 1536.

1542
ANDREW BOORDE. *Here foloweth a compendyous regyment or a dyetary of helth made in Mountpyllor.* London. First edition 1542.* (4).
See also J. Furnivall, *The Fyrste Boke of the Introduction of Knowledge,* 1870.*
Boorde's work is on diet, and is to be read in conjunction with his *Breviary of Health.*

1543
J. DE VIGO. *The most excellent workes of chirurgerye made by M.J. Vignon.* London. First edition 1543.* (4).
Translated by B. Traheron. Title indicates content.

1544
JEHAN GOEUROT. *The Regiment of Life.* London. First edition 1544. (6).
Translated from Goeurot's French version of *Regimen Sanitatis Salerni.* Thomas Phaer, who made the translation into English, was a lawyer and physician (1510?-1560). J. Goeurot (d. 1551?) was physician to Francis I of France.(1550*)

[1545]
ANON. *A Proper Newe Booke of Cokerye.* London.
There is great variation in the titles and considerable confusion as to which books are referred to. See A.W. Oxford, *Bibliography of English Cookery Books to the Year 1850,* 1913. Books with this sort of title appear through the centuries. The [1545] version was edited with additional notes by C.F. Frere, *A Proper New Booke of Cokerye,* 1913.* Another edition referred to in this study is that of 1575 (B.M. shelf no. C.31.a.14).* Early cookery books are frequently catalogued under "Book."
SAINT BERNARD. *A compendius and a moche fruytefull treatyse of well livynge.* First edition [1545].* Translated by Thomas Paynell.
The book deals with the moral aspects of living well. Saint Bernard (1091-1153).
HUGH RHODES. *The boke of nurture for men servants and children.* London. First edition [1545].* (6).
A book on good manners and behaviour. Hugh Rhodes (*fl.* 1550), was a Gentleman of the King's Chapel. See also F.J. Furnivall (ed.), *The Babees Book,* 1887.*

1547
ANDREW BOORDE. *The breviary of healthe (The second boke named Extravagantes).* London. First edition 1547. (6).
Medical receipts with cross references to *Dyetary of Helth.* The 1557* edition is used in this study.
CHRISTOPHER LANGTON. *A very brefe treatise, ordrely declaring the principal partes of phisick.* London. First edition 1547.*
This deals with the factors of health and includes sections on meat and drink and identification of diseases. Christopher Langton (1521-1578) was a physician of considerable professional ability.

ROBERT RECORDE. *The Urinall of Physick.* London. First edition 1547. (4).
The 1567* edition is used here. A work explaining the importance of the study of urine in medicine. Robert Recorde (1510?-1558) was a practising physician and famous as a mathematician. He was one of the first in England to adopt the Copernican system.

1548

T. ELYOT, revised by T. COOPER. *Bibliotheca Eliotae: newly imprinted and inriched.* London. First edition 1548. See also 1538 above.
JEAN FERNEL. *De abditis rerum causis.* Paris. First edition 1548.
1560.* Latin editions only. Jean Fernel (1485-1557) was a physician and philosopher of great influence.

[1548]

WILLIAM TURNER. *The names of herbes in Greke, Latin, Englishe, Duche and Frenche.* London. First edition [1548].*
William Turner (d. 1568) was Dean of Wells, a physician and botanist, and writer of many works. His books were prohibited as heretical in 1555.

[1549]

ALBERTUS MAGNUS [pseudo]. *Secretes of the vertues of herbes.* London. First edition [1549].* (10).
Later called *The secretes of Albertus Magnus.* See M.R. Best and F.H. Brightman (eds.), *The Book of Secrets of Albertus Magnus,* 1973. The *Book of Secrets* is an anthology rather than a single work. It has sections on herbs, stones, beasts, and planets. Albertus Magnus (1193-1280) has been described as "great in magic, greater in philosophy, greatest in theology."

1550

ANTHONY ASCHAM. *A little Herball of all the properties of Herbes . . . declaring what Herbes hath influence of certain sterres.* London. First edition 1550.* (2).
Refer to H.M. Barlow in *Proc. Royal Soc. Med.,* 1913, *6,* pp. 108-149. Contains no astrological law. Anthony Ascham, or Askham (*fl.* 1553), was a Bachelor of Medicine (Cambridge), astrologer, and Vicar of Burneston, Yorks.
JOHN COKE. *A debate between the heralds of England and France.* London. First edition 1550.*
Two heralds describe the virtues of their own country.
CHRISTOPHER LANGTON. *An introduction into phisycke with an universal dyet.* London. First edition 1550.*
Deals with diet and gives a considerable amount of theory.

1551

PETRUS HISPANUS (POPE JOHN XXI). *The treasurie of helth.* London. First edition 1551.* (3).
Translated by Humphrey Lloyd. Deals with diet in the widest sense. Pope John XXI (d. 1277), is identified with Petrus Hispanus, a Portuguese physician. Humphrey Lloyd, Hufre Lhoyd, Humfre Lloyde or Lhwy or Lhuyd (1527-1568), was a physician and antiquary, author of a number of works. He lived in Denbigh.
THOMAS MORE. *A fruteful and pleasaunt worke of the beste state of a publyque weale, and the newe yle called Utopia.* London. First edition 1551.* (5).

Translated by Ralphe Robinson (b. 1521), citizen and goldsmith of London, possibly clerk to Sir William Cecil. Thomas More (1478-1535) was Lord Chancellor of England, beatified by Pope Leo XIII in 1886.

WILLIAM TURNER. *A new herball.* London. First edition 1551* (S.T.C.).
Agnes Arber says the first Latin edition was 1538 and the first English edition 1548 (see above, [1548]). See also Facsimiles, with introductory material by James Britten, B. Daydon Jackson and W.T. Stearn, *William Turner* (Royal Society), 1965. Title indicates content.

WILLIAM TURNER. *A preservative, or triacle agaynst the poyson of Pelagius.* London. First edition 1551.*
This is a religious treatise.

[1551]
HENRY WINGFIELD. *A compendious treatise conteynynge preceptes necessary to the preservacion of healthe.* London. First edition [1551].* (2).
Deals mainly with diet, rather than medicine. Henry Wingfield is not listed in the DNB.

1552
ANTHONY ASCHAM. *A little Treatise of Astronomy very necessary for physick and surgery.* London. First edition 1552.
This work is rare and has not been examined.

JOHN CAIUS. *A boke, or counseill against the disease called the sweate, or sweatyng sicknesse.* London. First edition 1552.*
This work is a simplified version of an earlier Latin work. John Caius (1510-1573) was Royal Physician, one time President of the College of Physicians, translated some of Galen into Latin.

1553
THOMAS GEMINUS. *Compendiosa totius anatomie delineatio.* London. First edition 1553.* (2), and one later edition with additions.
A book of anatomy. Thomas Geminus, Gemynous, Gemine, Gemyny: actual name was Lambritt (?-1562). He was an engraver, but practised medicine and surgery illegally. Translation by Nicholas Udall, Uvedale (1505-1556), dramatist and scholar, one time Headmaster of Eton College.

1557
A. BOORDE. *Breviary of Health.*
See above, 1548.

THOMAS TUSSER. *A hundreth good pointes of husbandrie.* London. First edition 1557.* (12).
After the first few editions it was increased to "500 points." Modern versions are: *Tusser Redivivus,* by W. Mavor, 1812; *A Hundred good pointes of Husbandrie,* by W. Payne and S.J. Heritage, 1878; *Thomas Tusser, 1557,* by D. Hartley, 1931.*
The latter draws on a number of editions of Tusser's works. Title indicates contents. Thomas Tusser (?1524-1580), an agricultural writer, farmer, and poet of Essex, died a prisoner for debt.

[1558]
WILLIAM BULLEIN. *A new boke entituled the government of healthe.* London.
First edition [1558]. (2).
The 1595* edition was used here. A general guide on the diet and regimen, given
in the form of a dialogue. William Bullein (?1500-1576), physician, was a one
time Rector of Blaxall in Suffolk.

1558
ALEXIS OF PIEMONT. *The secretes of Alexis of Piemont containing remedies
against diseases.* London. First edition 1558.* (9).
Translated from the French by William Ward (1534-?1604), a Cambridge professor and physician. This is a medical book. Alexis of Piemont is a pseudonym,
probably for Hieronymo Rosello or Girolamo Ruscelli.

1559
CONRAD GESNER. *The treasure of Euonymus: conteyninge the hid secretes of
nature.* First edition 1559,* 1565.* (2)
Translated by Peter Morwyng, Morwent, Morwen (1530?-1573), Fellow of Magdalen College, Oxford and a rigid Protestant, who became chaplain to the Bishop
of Lichfield. A collection of "secret" remedies. Author Conrad Gesner
(1516-1565) was a Swiss physician and naturalist.

1561
HIERONYMUS VON BRAUNSCHWEIG, *A most excellent and perfecte homish
apothecarne or homely physick booke for all the grefes and diseases of the bodye.*
Collen [Cologne]. First edition 1561.*
Translated by John Hollybush, not in *DNB*. Title indicates content.

[1562]
LEONARD FUCHS. *A most worthie practise of L. Fuchsius.* London. First edi-
tion [1562], 1575.*
Translated anonymously. Gives advice on the plague. Leonhard Fuchs
(1501-1566) was a German physician and botanist.
G. GRATAROLUS. *The castel of memorie.* London. First edition 1562.* (3).
Translated by William Fullwood (*fl.* 1562), author and member of the Merchant
Taylors' Company. Diet, medicines, and exercises for the memory. Gulielmus
Gratarolus (1510-1568) was a famous Italian physician.
WILLIAM TURNER. *A Booke of the nature, and properties, as well of the bathes
in England* . . . London. First edition 1562. (2).
1568* edition used here. Title indicates content.

1563
THOMAS BECON. *The Works of Thomas Becon.* London. First edition 1563.*
Influential theological works. Thomas Becon (1512-1567), influential Protestant
theological writer, was chaplain to Archbishop Cranmer, and Prebendary of Canterbury.
CHURCH OF ENGLAND. *The Second Tome of Homilies.* London. First edition
1563.* (16)
Contains the Homilie on Fasting. The first collection of Homilies without the Second Book appeared in 1547. (24).

THOMAS GALE. *Certain workes of chirurgerie.* London. First edition 1563.* (2). Title indicates content. Thomas Gale (1507-?), English surgeon, served in the armies of Henry VIII and King Philip, then settled in London. Author and translator.
served in the armies of King Henry VIII and King Philip, then settled in London.
[1563]
THOMAS HILL. *The proffitable Arte of Gardening* . . . To this are annexed two treatises *The marveilous government* . . . *of the Bees* and *The yerely conjectures for meet husbandmen to knowe.* London.
Englished by T. Hill. It is difficult to disentangle the editions of these works. It is thought that the first edition of the *Arte of Gardening* was [1563], (7) 1568.* Titles indicate contents. Thomas Hill was an English compiler and translator. His works also included material on divinations, astrological predictions, and the interpretation of dreams. He is believed also to have used the pseudonym of D. Mountain.

1563
LITURGIES. *Liturgies, A fourme to be used in Common prayer twyse a weke, and also an order of publique fast* . . . 30th July.
Includes a description of those who should fast.
JOHN SHUTE. *The first and chief groundes of architecture.* London. First edition 1563.* (2).
Facsimile of first edition, with a note by Lawrence Weaver, 1912.* Title indicates contents, the emphasis being on building. John Shute (d. 1563) was a self-described "peynter and archytecte."

1564
WILLIAM BULLEIN. *A dialogue bothe pleasaunt and pietifull against the fever pestilence.* London. First edition 1564. (5).
The 1578* edition used here. See also M.W. and A.H. Buller (eds.), *A dialogue Against the Fever Pestilence,* 1888.* This is a dialogue among twelve people concerning the plague, with much reference to the religious, logical, and philosophical aspects.
WILLIAM CUNINGHAM. *A new almanack and prognostication.* London. First edition 1564.*
Title indicates contents. William Cunningham flourished around 1565. He was a physician and astronomer, and translated for Thomas Gale (see above, 1563).

1565
JOHN HALL. *A most excellent . . . woorke of chirurgerie* . . . London. First edition 1565.*
This is an "Epitome," rather than a verbatim translation of *Chirurgia parma Lanfranci* – i.e. Lanfrancus Mediolanesis (d. 1315?). John Hall, or Halle (1529-1568) was a surgeon of Maidstone, Kent.
LEVINUS LEMNIUS. *The touchstone of complexions.* London. First edition 1565. (5).
1576* edition used here. Translation is by Thomas Newton (?1542-1607), a Latin poet, schoolmaster, divine and physician, as well as Rector of Little Ilford, Essex. Most of Newton's publications were translations. Levinus Lemnius (1505-1568) was an eminent physician of Zeeland who gave up medicine to enter the ministry of the Church.

PHILIP MOORE. *The hope of health (a table for xxx yeres to come).* London. First edition 1565* (preface dated 1564).
Advice on a "goodlie regimen of life" related to medicine, diet, and herbs. The calendar of instruction regarding the moon and planets is not connected with dietary advice. Philip Moore (*fl.* 1573) was a medical writer who practised physick and surgery in Suffolk and aimed to disseminate a knowledge of medicinal herbs among the poor.

1566

JOHN SECURIS. *A detection and querimonie of the daily enormities committed in physick.* London. First edition 1566.*
Title indicates content. John Securis (*fl.* 1566) was a medical writer licensed by the Bishop of Salisbury to practice physick. Securis is the latinized form of Hatchett.

1568

HUMPHREY BAKER. *The well-spryng of sciences.* London. First edition 1568.* (10).
Concerned with arithmetic, Baker's book gives some measures and weights of different places in Europe. Humphrey Baker (*fl.* 1502-1587) wrote on arithmetic and astrology, including "Judiciall Astrology."
THOMAS HILL (Englished by). *A pleasaunt Instruction of the parfit orderinge of Bees.* London. First edition 1568.*
(See above, 1563). These are collected sayings and writings from ancient authors.
WILLIAM TURNER. *A new Boke of the natures and properties of all wines. . . .* London. First edition 1568.*
Title indicates contents. See also S.V. Larkey and P.M. Wagner (eds.), *A Book of Wines,* 1941.*

1569

H.C. AGRIPPA. *Henrie Cornelius Agrippa of the vanitie of artes and sciences.* London. First edition 1569.* (5).
Translated by Ja. San. gent. (James Sanford). Deals with a wide variety of subjects, touching on housekeeping and husbandry, but not on diet. H. Cornelius Agrippa (1486-1535) was born in Cologne, and died in Grenoble. He wrote popular works and was a man of considerable learning as well as a reputable magician. James Sanford, or Sandford (*fl.* 1567), born in Somerset, was well read and worked laboriously as a translator. He is described as "gent."
M.T. CICERO. *The worthye booke of old age.* London. First edition 1569.*
Translated by Thomas Newton, who says it had previously been translated "about xxx yeares agone." See also W.H.D. Rouse (ed.), *Cicero's "Friendship," "Old Age" and "Scipio's Dream,"* 1906.* The work consists of a dialogue praising and defending old age. Marcus Tullius Cicero (106-43 B.C.).
P. BOAISTUAU. *Certain secrete wonders of nature.* London. First edition 1569.*
Translated by E. Fenton (not in *DNB*) from *Histoires prodigieuses,* giving descriptions of "sundry strange things." Pierre Boaistuau, Boistuau or Boaistuau de Launay lived from 1520 to 1566.

1570
EUCLID. *The elements of geometrie.* London. First edition 1570.*
Translated by H. Billingsley (d. 1606), Lord Mayor of London and the first translator of Euclid into English. Contains a "Mathematical Preface" by Dr. John Dee
(1527-1608), a mathematician and astrologer held in high esteem by Queen Elizabeth. Euclid flourished around 300 B.C.

1572
JOHN JONES. *Bathes of the Bathes ayde.* London. First edition 1572.*
Discusses the benefits to health of the spas in the south of England. John Jones
(*fl.* 1579), was a physician who practised mostly in the Midlands but visited Bath
and Buxton in the season. He advocated the value of mineral baths.
JOHN JONES. *The benefit of the auncient bathes of Buckstones.* London. First
edition 1572.*
Refers to the benefits to health from these baths.

[1572]
LEONARD MASCALL. *A booke of the arte and maner, how to plant and graffe
sortes of trees.* London. First edition [1572].* (6).
Title indicates content. Leonard Mascall (d. 1589), author and translator, was
clerk of the kitchen in the household of Matthew Parker, Archbishop of Canterbury.

1573
HUMPHREY LLOYD. *The Breviary of Britayne.* London. First edition 1573.*
Translated by Thomas Twyne (1543-1613), a physician with a large practice in
Lewes, Sussex. History, with geographical description of Britain. Includes a short
glossary of Welsh/English words.
JOHN PARTRIDGE. *The treasurie of commodius conceites and hidden secrets.*
London. First edition 1573. (16).
Title later changed to *The widdowes treasure plentifully furnished with sundry
secrets.* John Partridge, translator and poet, flourished 1566.

1574
GEORGE BAKER. *The composition or making of the oil called Oleum Magistrale.* London. First edition 1574.*
Includes a declaration of weights in surgery, also the third book of Galen, "of the
curing of pricks and wounds of the sinews." George Baker (1540-1600), was a
barber-surgeon with a wide practice in London.
W. BOURNE. *A regiment for the sea.* London. First edition 1574. (11).
1577.* This is a book on navigation and makes no reference to a dietary regimen.
William Bourne (d. 1583) was a mathematician and one time innkeeper of Graves-
end, Kent, described in DNB as a "self-taught genius."
GULIELMUS GRATAROLUS. *A direction for the health of magistrates and
studentes.* London. First edition 1574.*
Title indicates contents, when Gratarolus' definition of student is noted. Translated by Thomas Newton.
EDWARD HAKE. *A touchestone for this time present.* London. First edition
1574.*

(Edward Hake, *cont'd.*)
A reference to the feeding of infants is made as an example of the similar care required in feeding the growing mind. Edward Hake (*fl.* 1579) was a satirist and translator, concerned with the education of children.

JOHN JONES. *A briefe, excellent and profitable discourse of the beginning of all growing and living things, etc.* London. First edition 1574.*
Title indicates contents.

JOHN JONES. *Galenes Bookes of Elementes, as they be in the Epitome. . . .* London. First edition 1574.*
Title indicates contents.

REYNOLDE SCOT. *A perfite platforme of a hoppe garden.* London. First edition 1574.* (3).
Title indicates contents. Reynolde (Reginald) Scot (c.1538-1599) was a Kentish farmer at a time when hops must have been a lucrative crop.

1575

ANON. *A proper new book of cookery.* London.
See above, 1545.

GEORGE TURBERVILLE. *The noble arte of venerie or hunting.* London. First edition 1575.* (2)
Translated anon. [Christopher Barker]. Title indicates content. George Turberville, Turvervile (1540?-1610?) was a poet and translator. Christopher Barker, Barkar (1529?-1599), was Queen's printer.

1576

CONRAD GESNER. *The newe jewell of health.* London. First edition 1576.*
Translated by T. Hill and G. Baker. According to Ferguson the second edition (1599) was entitled *The Practice of New and Old Phisicke.* Gives secrets of physick and philosophy, including preparations and distillations. Conrad Gesner (1516-1565) was a Swiss physician and naturalist.

CLAUDE HOLYBAND. *The French Littelton; a most easie way to learne the french tongue.* London. First edition 1576. (10).
1581.* This method of teaching French by everyday dialogue gives good descriptions of English life, including references to meals. Claude Holyband, Claude de Sainliens (*fl.* c.1576). was a Huguenot refugee who taught French in London. See M. St. Clare Byrne (ed.), *The Elizabethan Home,* 1949.

L. LEMNIUS. *Touchstone of the complexions.*
See above, 1565.

THOMAS TWYNE. *The schoolemaster, or teacher of table philosophie.* London. First edition 1576. (2).
This work and a number of others by different authors are based on the Latin original of Michael Scotus (see below, 1609). A modern translation of a medieval treatise is Arthur S. Way (trans.), *The Science of Dining,* 1936.* Twyne's book contains information about food and drink, and manner of eating.

1577

WILLIAM HARRISON. *Description of England.* London. First edition 1577.*
This is part of the Holingshed Chronicles given below. Copy used for reference in

this study is F.J. Furnivall (ed.), *Harrison's Description of England in Shakespeare's Youth*, 1877-1909.* William Harrison (1534-1593) was Canon of Windsor.
CONRADUS HERESBACHIUS. *Four bookes of husbandry, newely Englished by B. Googe.* London. First edition 1577.* (5).
Title indicates contents. This translation of Heresbachius' work has been "increased" by Googe. Conrad Heresbach (?1496-1576) was a scholar, writer and translator. Barnabe Googe (1540-1594), highly esteemed by his contemporaries, was a poet, and translated a number of works.
RAPHAEL HOLINGSHED. *The firste volume of the Chronicles of England, Scotlande and Irelande.* London. First edition 1577.*
There are many other editions, with added volumes. Title indicates contents. Raphael Holingshed (d. 1580?) was originally employed as a translator in the printing office of Reginald Wolfe.
CHRISTOPHER JOHNSON. *Counsel against the plague, or any other infectious disease.* London. First edition 1577.*
Title indicates contents. Christopher Johnson, Jonson (1536?-1597) was a Latin poet and philosopher. After being Headmaster at Winchester College, he became a physician and practised in London.
NICHOLAS MONARDES. *Joyfull newes out of the newe founde worlde.* London. First edition 1577.* (5).
Translated by John Frampton. A reprint of the 1577 edition with an introduction by Stephen Gaselee was published in 1925.* Gives much information about foods and herbs in the new world. Nicholas Monardes (1493-1588) was a successful physician in Seville, and writer of botanical dissertations. John Frampton, (from Moreton in Dorset?) was a merchant adventurer, who also made translations of the travels in China of Marco Polo and Bernardino de Escalante.
THOMAS VICARY. *A profitable treatise of the anatomie of mans body.* London. First edition 1577.*
Title indicates content. Thomas Vicary (d. 1561), was Sergeant Surgeon to Henry VIII, Edward VI, Mary, and Elizabeth, as well as Chief surgeon at St. Bartholomew's Hospital.

1578
JOHN BANISTER. *The historie of man, sucked from the sappe of the most approved anathomistes.* London. First edition 1578.*
A comprehensive book on anatomy with references to the changes in contemporary man compared to man in the past. John Banester (1533-1610) was a well known London surgeon in the reign of Queen Elizabeth; he previously practised in Nottingham.
THOMAS BRASBRIDGE. *The poore mans jewel, that is to say a treatise of the pestilence.* London. First edition 1578.* (4).
A treatise on the pestilence. Thomas Brasbridge (*fl.* 1590) was a vicar, schoolmaster, and physician at Banbury. In 1588 he was assaulted by certain parishioners who liked dancing and other pastimes. The case went to the Privy Council.
W. BULLEIN. *Against the fever pestilence.*
See above, 1564.

1578
REMBERT DODOENS. *A niewe herball or historie of plantes.* First edition 1578, 1586.* (4).
Translated by Henry Lyte. English version from a French translation of the original published in Antwerp in 1554. Title indicates content. Rembert Dodoens (1517-1585) was a Dutch botanist. Henry Lyte (1529?-1607) was a botanist, antiquary, and translator.

1579
WILLIAM CLOWES. *A short and profitable treatise touching the cure of the morbus gallicus by unctions.* London. First edition 1579.*
Title indicates content. William Clowes (1540?-1604) was a naval surgeon, later surgeon at St. Bartholomew's Hospital. He wrote only in English. His works are considered to be the best surgical writings of the Elizabethan age.
GATHERED BY T.C. *An hospitall for the diseased.* London. First edition 1579.* (7).
Contains medicines, plasters, potions or drinks and "receptes bothe for the Restitution and the Preservation of bodily healthe."
JOHN JONES. *The arte and science of preserving bodie and soul in healthe, wisedome, and Catholike Religion.* London. First edition 1579.*
Title indicates content.
WILLIAM LANGHAM. *The garden of health.* London. First edition 1579.* (2).
Refers to the virtues and properties of simples and plants. (William Langham (not in DNB) describes himself as a "practicioner in physicke."

[1579]
LEONARDO FIORAVANTI. *A joyfull jewell.* London. First edition [1579].*
Translated by T. H[ill]. Contains directions and preservatives against the plague. Leonardo Fioravanti (d. 1588) was a physician of Bologna, and author of a wide variety of works, many concerned with aspects of alchemy.
THOMAS LUPTON. *A thousand notable things of sundrie sorts.* London. First edition [1579].* (15).
The 1720 edition was written by G. Johnson. The last edition appeared in 1815. A collection of miscellaneous pieces of information, both fact and myth. The British Museum Catalogue suggests 1579 for the first edition, but this would appear too early, as the book quotes from Thomas Hyll, *Natural and Artificial conclusions of the Scholars of Padua,* which was probably not published before 1581 (S.T.C. gives 1586 and Watt 1581). Thomas Lupton (*fl.* 1583) was a miscellaneous writer whose works include a comedy and a "moral work."

[1580]
ANON. *Here begynneth the boke named the assise of breade.* London.
See above, 1528.

1580.
THEODORE DE BEZE. *A shorte learned and pithie treatize of the plague.* London. First edition 1580.*
Title indicates content. Théodore de Bèze (1519-1605) was a celebrated Protestant theologian. John Stockwood, who made the translation into English (d. 1610) was a schoolmaster and vicar of Tunbridge, Kent.

T[IMOTHY] B[RIGHT]. *A treatise wherein is declared the sufficiencie of English medicines.* London. First edition 1580. (3).
1615* edition used here. Aims to show that local plants can be used for medicines in England. Timothy Bright (1551?-1615) was a Doctor of medicine and the inventor of modern shorthand. He took Holy Orders and abandoned medicine.

PRUDENS CHOISELAT. *A Discourse of Housebandrie.* London. First edition 1580.*
Translated by R.E. See also *Discours Oeconomique of Prudent Choyselat*, facsimile with notes by H.A.D. Neville, 1951.* Advice on how to make money by keeping hens. Includes a table of French/English money equivalents. Neville says Prudent Le Choyselat was "Procureur du Roy à Sezanne." In any case, he was certainly not a professional poultry farmer. R.E. is possibly Richard Eden.

LEONARDO FIORAVANTI. *A short discourse upon chirurgerie.* London. First edition 1580.* (2).
Translated by John Hester (d. 1593), a surgeon of London, translator of a number of works, and a self-styled "Practioner in the Spagericall Arte."

THOMAS NEWTON. *Approved Medicines and Cordiall Receiptes, with the natures, qualities and operations of sundry Simples.* London. First edition 1580.*
Discusses medicines under the grouping of their qualities and degrees, e.g. "temperate heat," or "cold and dry in the second degree." Also gives medicines appropriate for various symptoms.

WILLIAM WILKINSON. *The holie exercise of a true fast, described out of God's word.* London. First edition 1580.* (2).
Title indicates content. William Wilkinson (d. 1613) was a theological writer and schoolmaster.

1581
CLAUDE HOLYBAND. *The Frenche Littelton; a most easie way to learne the french tongue.* London.
See above, 1576.

LEONARD MASCALL. *The Husbandlye Ordring and Governmente of Poultrie.* London. First edition 1581.*
Title indicates content.

RICHARD MULCASTER. *Positions wherin those circumstances be examined necessarie for the training up of children.* London. First edition 1581.*
Another issue appeared in 1581. Modern commentary: Robert H. Quick, *Positions: by Richard Mulcaster*, 1888.* Contains comments on many aspects of children's training, including health. Richard Mulcaster (1530 or 1531-1568), was Headmaster of Merchant Taylors' School.

W.S. [commonly attributed to]. *A Discourse of the Common Weal of this Realm of England.* London.
First printed in 1581, the Dialogue clearly took place in 1549. Information about this book can be found in the work, edited from the MSS, by E. Lamond, 1893.*

1582
BARTHOLOMAEUS ANGLICUS. *Batman uppon Bartholome his booke De proprietatibus rerum, enlarged and amended.* London. First edition 1582.*
The original English translation was by J. Trevisa in 1495. However, Stephen Batman, translator of the 1582 edition here, not only enlarged upon the original but

clearly indicated his additions. This is an encyclopaedic type of work. Bartholomaeus Anglicus (*fl.* 1230-1250) was an English Franciscan friar, professor of theology in Paris. Stephen Batman (?-1584), was Doctor of Divinity, Parson of Newington Butts, Surrey, a poet, translator, and author.

LEONARDO FIORAVANTI. *A compendium of the rationall secretes of L. Phioravante.* London. First edition 1582,* 1652.

Translated by John Hester. Contains receipts for the treatment of symptoms, includes herbs, metals and stones and instructions on how to make "Petra Philosophalle." Ferguson says that this translation differs in several details from the original Italian and deals only with the medical section of the original.

1583

PHILIP BARROUGH. *The method of phisicke.* London. First edition 1583.* (9).

A popular medical book. Philip Barrough (*fl.* 1590) was a medical writer, licensed to practice surgery and physic.

WALTER CARY. *A briefe treatise called Caries farewell to physicke.* London. First edition 1583.* (3).

Said to provide "diverse rare and speciall helps" for many ordinary diseases. See 1525, above. Barlow suggests the author of this work is Walter Cary of High Wycombe, M.A. of Magdalen. Not in DNB.

PHILIP STUBBES. *The anatomie of abuses.* London. First edition 1583.* (4).

Facsimile editions are those edited by W.B.D.D. Turnbull, 1836, and by F.J. Furnivall, 1877-79.* (This study uses the 1583 edition, collated with other editions.) Description of some manners and customs in England through the eyes of a relentless Puritan. Philip Stubbes (*fl.* 1581-1593) was a Puritan pamphleteer.

1584

THOMAS COGAN. *The haven of health.* London. First edition 1584.* (7).

1589* edition used here. A book on health which follows closely Elyot's work. Thomas Cogan, Coghan (1545?-1607), doctor and schoolmaster, practised in Manchester, and published a number of works, including an introduction to Latin.

A.W. *A booke of cookry. Now newly enlarged.* London. First edition 1584.* (4).

See reference above [1545].

1585

ANON. *A discourse of the medicine called Mithridatium.* London. First edition 1585.*

Title indicates content.

R.B. ESQ. (ROBERT BOSTOCK). *The difference between the auncient phisicke and the latter phisicke.* London. First edition 1585.*

Attempts to show that Aristotelian philosophy differs from the truth of God's word and is injurious to Christianity. Robert Bostock is not in DNB.

HORATIUS MORUS. *Tables of surgerie.* London. First edition 1585.*

First Latin edition 1569. The Latin and English texts are given on opposite pages. Horatius Morus, flourished 1569, was a Florentine physician. Richard Caldwall (1505?-1584), who made the English translation, was a physician born in Staffordshire and a member of the College of Physicians.

THOMAS VICARY. *The Englishmans treasure. With the true anatomye of mans*

body. London. First edition 1585. (8).
The 1586* edition used here, was also edited by F. J. Furnivall in 1888.* Deals
with anatomy, remedies for travellers, and some domestic medicine.

[1585]
THOMAS DAWSON. *The good huswives jewell.* London. First edition with this
title [1585].
Edition consulted 1596* (British Museum shelf no. 1037-e-1). See also reference
above, [1545]. A cookery book with some recipes based on French and Italian
cookery. Thomas Dawson is not in the DNB.

1586
WALTER BAILEY. *A briefe treatise touching the preservation of the eiesight.*
London. First edition 1586 (6) 1616).*
Edition consulted here is 1616.* This (1616) edition contains two treatises con-
cerning the Preservation of Eie-sight, one by Bailey, the other "collected out of
those two famous physicians Fernelius and Riolanus." Printed in Oxford. Relates
the preservation of sight to good diet. Walter Bailey is not in the DNB. Jean
Riolan (1539-1606) was a French anatomist and botanist.
TIMOTHY BRIGHT. *A treatise of melancholie, containing the causes thereof.*
London. First edition 1586.* (3).
Facsimile of the 1586 edition with an introduction by Hardin Craig, 1939.* The
book is written to a friend suffering from melancholy. A much respected work in
its time.
ENGLAND. *Acts of the Privy Council,* xiv, p. 338 (1586-87).
See also *Orders devised by the especiall commandement of the Queenes Majestie,
for the reliefe and stay of the present dearth of Graine within the Realme.* Lon-
don.
GALEN. *Certain works of Galen called Methodus Medendi.* London. First edition
1586.*
Translated by Thomas Gale.
[SCHOLARS OF PADUA]. *A briefe and pleasaunt treatise intituled: Natural and
artificial conclusions.* London. First edition 1586.*
Translated by Thomas Hill. This work was said to be written by sundry scholars at
the University of Padua at the request of Bartholomew, a Tuscan. Title indicates
content.
THOMAS NEWTON. *The old mans dietarie.* London. First edition 1586.*
Translated from the work of an unknown Latin author. There is no copy of this
work in the British Museum. A xerox copy of the book is in the Chester Public
Library was used. It is believed that this is the only copy of the book in the
United Kingdom. Deals with the health and diet of old men, with particular refer-
ence to food and drink.
P. DE LA PRIMAUDAY. *The French academie.* London. First edition 1586.* (9).
Translated by T.B. [T. Bowes or Beard]. The last four editions were derived from
parts or all of the previous editions of the original translation and appeared be-
tween 1594 and 1618. A treatise of moral philosophy. Pierre de la Primaudaye,
Primayday (c. 1545-1584), was a French moralist.

1587

ANDREAS BERTHOLDUS. *The wonderfull and strange effect and virtues of a new terra sigillata lately found out in Germanie.* London. First edition 1587.*
Description of how the "earth" from Silesian gold mines can cure and preserve health when taken internally or applied externally. Of interest because of the references to poisons, diseases, and wounds. Andreas Bertholdus of Oschatz.
LEONARD MASCALL. *The first Booke of Cattell.* London. First edition 1587.* (8).
Later title was *The government of cattell.* Title indicates content.

1588

ANON. *The good hous-wives treasurie.* London. First edition 1588.*
Contains about forty three recipes plus about ten with "medicines." Emphasis is on the dressing of meats.
ANON. *The good huswives handmaid for cookerie.* London. First edition 1588.*
Also called *The good huswives handmaid in her kitchen.* Title indicates content.
WALTER BAILEY. *A short discourse of the three kindes of peppers in common use.* First edition 1588.* (2).
Title indicates contents.
TORQUATO TASSO. *The householders philosophie: whereunto is anexed a dairie booke.* London. First edition 1588.*
Translated by T.K. (unknown). Book on how to organise and run a household. The section of dairy work is omitted from the British Museum copy (shelf no. 1037-d-41). Torquato Tasso (1544-1595) was a distinguished Italian poet.

1589

C. COOPER. *A notable and prodigious historie of a mayden (C. Cooper) who for sundry yeeres neither eateth, drinketh nor sleepeth.* First edition 1589.*
Possibly translated by T. Bright. The Commissioners investigating this matter met at Schmidweiler on Tuesday, 24 November 1584.
T. COGAN. *Haven of health.*
See above, 1584.
J. BELLOT. *The booke of thrift.* London. First edition 1589.
Original edition not available. Facsimile reprint in F.H. Cripps-Day, *The Manor Farm,* 1931.* Advice on economic farming; includes references to yields to be aimed for from farm livestock; reproduces *Walter of Henley's husbandry.* James Bellott (?) was a Gentleman of Caen.

1590

WILLIAM CLEVER. *The flower of phisicke.* London. First edition 1590.*
Includes theory of physic supported by Greek, Arabic and contemporary references, including Paracelsus. William Clever is not in the DNB.
LEONARD MASCALL. *A booke of fishing with hooke and line.* London. First edition 1590.* (2).
Modern edition (based on the 1606 edition) with a preface and glossary by Thomas Satchell, 1884.* This book is taken from a treatise on "fishing with an angle" in *Maison Rustique* of 1496. See reference below, 1600.

1591
ROBERT GREENE. *A notable discovery of coosenage.* London. First edition
1591.*
Also, the three parts of "the art of conny-catching" were published as tracts. One
of a series of exposés of the Elizabethan underworld. Portrays the deceptions of
thieves, presented in a form more likely to entertain than reform. Robert Greene
(1558?-1592) was born in Norwich, held degrees from Oxford and Cambridge,
was a professional pamphleteer and dramatist. By his own admission he led a dissolute life.

[1592]
DIVERS GROCERS OF LONDON. *A Profitable and necessarie Discourse, for the
meeting with bad Garbelling of Spices, used in these daies.* London. First edition
[1592].*
Title indicates content.

1592
NICHOLAS GYER. *The English phlebotomy.* London. First edition 1592.*
A small treatise on blood and blood-letting. Nicholas Gyer (*fl.* 1592) was a "Min-
ister of the Word."
JOHN STOW. *Annales, or a generall chronicle of England.* London. First edition
1592. (7).
1631* edition used here. Title indicates content. Begun by John Stow, continued
and augmented by Edmund Howes, Gent. John Stow (1525?-1605) was one of
the most accurate and businesslike of English annalists and chroniclers of the sixteenth century. Edmund Howes (*fl.*) 1607-1631) was a chronicler, and self-
designated "Gent."

1593
THOMAS CHURCHYARD. *Churchyards challenge.* London. First edition 1593.*
Includes short pieces on a variety of subjects, one being a poem on the "hospital-
ity and consuming of time and wealth in London." Thomas Churchyard
(1520?-1604) was a soldier and poet.
SIMON KELLWAYE. *A defensative against the plague.* London. First edition
1593.*
Title indicates content. Simon Kellwaye is not in the DNB.
EDMUND SOUTHERNE. *A treatise concerning the right use and ordering of
bees.* London. First edition 1593.*
Title indicates content. Edmund Southerne is not in the DNB.

1594
JOHN HESTER. *The pearle of practise or practisers pearle for phisicke and
chirurgerie.* London. First edition 1594.*
This is a collection of works put together after Hester's death by James Four-
estier. Contains a number of sections including much material from L. Fioravanti
and a part called "The Flowers of Celsus." James Fourestier is not in the DNB.
JUAN HUARTE. *Examen de ingenios, the examination of mens wits.* London.
First edition 1594.* (6).

JUAN HUARTE *(cont'd.)*
Translated by R.C. Esq. (Richard Carew). This is an attempt to show that by dis-
covering the nature of a person his aptitudes may be estimated. Juan de Dios
Huarte Navarro (c. 1535-1600) was a Spanish physician and philosopher. Richard
Carew (1555-1620) was translator of a number of books. He lived in Cornwall.
HUGH PLATT. *Diverse new sorts of soyle.* London. First edition 1594.*
Title indicates content. Hugh Platt (1552-1611?), an inventor and writer on agri-
culture, did experimental work in horticulture and agriculture. He was knighted
for his inventions.
HUGH PLATT. *The jewell house of art and nature.* London. First edition 1594.*
(3).
Includes a collection of pieces of information concerning such things as manuring
and chemical distillation.

1595
ANON. *The widdowes treasure plentifully furnished with sundry secrets.* London.
First edition 1595.* (5).
Contains a confused sequence of recipes and medicines, including some suitable
for cattle.
W. BULLEIN. *The Government of health.*
See above, 1558.

1596
THOMAS DAWSON. *The good huswifes jewell: rare devises for conseites in cookerie.* London. First edition 1596.* (5).
Cookery book along traditional lines. See also [1585], above, page 374.
PETER LOWE. *A discourse of the whole art of chyrurgerie.* London. First edition
1596. (5)
1612* edition used here. Besides surgery this contains sections on the theory of
physick. Peter Lowe (1550?-1612) was founder of the Faculty of physicians and
surgeons in Glasgow.
THOMAS PHAER. *A treatise on the pestilence.* London.
The first edition of this was an added part to Phaer's translation of Goeurot's
Regiment of Life with the Boke of Children in 1545 or 1550. Separate version
1596.* Title indicates content.
HUGH PLATT. *Sundrie new and artificiall remedies against famine.* London. First
edition 1596.* Title indicates content.
A.T. *A Rich Store-house or Treasury for the Diseased.* London. First edition
1596.* (8).
Gives receipts for various ills, "Now set forth for the great benefit and comfort of
the poorer sort of people that are not of abillitie to go to the Physitions." A.T.
was a "Practitioner in physick."

1597
ARISTOTLE (pseudo). *The problemes of Aristotle with other philosophers and
phisitions.* London. First edition 1597.*
Also 25th edition dated 1702* consulted. Title indicates contents.
JOHN GERARD. *The herball.* London. First edition 1597.* (3).

JOHN GERARD *(cont'd.)*
Extracts from the 1636 edition of T. Johnson have been collected together in
Gerard's Herball by Marcus Woodward, 1927.* A complete facsimile edition of
the 1633 revision of this work by Thomas Johnson is available from Dover Publications, Inc. (1975). Title indicates contents. John Gerard (1545) was a barber-
surgeon, superintendent of the gardens of Lord Burghley.

1598

J.B. *A treatise with a Kalendar, and the proofes thereof, concerning the Holy-
daies and Fasting-dais in England.* N.P. First edition 1598.*
The table was prepared 26 years earlier [1572]. See A.F. Allison and D.M.
Rogers, *A Catalogue of Catholic Books in English Printed Abroad or Secretly in
England 1558-1640.* "Biographical Studies" (Bognor Regis), 1956, *3*, nos. 3 & 4.
J.B. was a Catholic priest exiled from England.
CHRISTOPHER WIRTZUNG. *Praxis medicinae universalis, or a generall practise
of physicke.* London. First edition 1598.* (4).
Translated by J. Mosan (Jacob Mosan, James Mose), a German doctor of the
faculty of Heidelberg. A purely medical work. Christopher Wirsung (1500-1571)
was a German physician and teacher at Heidelberg.

1599

T. BLUNDEVILLE. *The arte of logike plainely taught according to the doctrine
of Aristotle.* London. First edition 1599.* (3).
Title indicates content. Thomas Blundeville (*fl.* 1561) was a writer on horseman-
ship and author of a variety of educational and historical works.
HENRY BUTTES. *Dyets dry dinner.* London. First edition 1599.*
Deals with "dry foods," but does include milk. Gives qualities and degrees and
other information about foods. Henry Buttes (?-1632) was a Fellow of Corpus
Christi College Cambridge, Vice-Chancellor in 1629.
JANUS DUBRAVIUS. *A newe booke of good husbandry, conteining the making
of fish-pondes.* London. First edition 1599.*
Translated at the request of George Churchey. Discusses a variety of types of fish-
ponds. Janus Dubravius (d. 1553) was a German historian, Bishop of Olmutz.
ANDRE DU LAURENS. *A discourse of the preservation of the sight ... of
Melancholike diseases ... of Rheumes, and of old age.* London. First edition
1599.*
Translated by Richard Surphlet. See also the reprint edition of 1938, edited by
S.V. Larkey. Contains four treatises on sight, melancholy, rheumes and old age.
André Du Laurens (c. 1558-1609) was Professor of Medicine at Montpellier, and
author of a number of publications. He was much admired by his contemporaries.
Richard Surphlet, Surphet, Surflet, is not in the DNB.
OSWALDUS GABELHOUER. *The Book of Physicke.* Dorte [Dordrecht]. First
edition 1599.*
Translated by Charles Battus, "Ordinarye Physitione of the Citye of Dorte." Contains recipes or prescriptions for a number of diseases with a glossary for the common and vulgar people. Oswaldus Gabelhouer (1538-1616), was a physician and
historical writer.

1600

CHARLES ESTIENNE [STEVENS] and JEAN LIEBAULT. *Maison Rustique or the Countrie Farme*. London. First edition 1600.*

Translated by Richard Surflet. Also published by Gervase Markham in 1616. Contains a large amount of information about many aspects of farming. Charles Estienne (1504-1564), was a physician and printer to the king of France. Jean Liebault (c. 1535-1596) was a physician and agronomist.

JOHN POWELL. *The assize of bread: newly corrected*. London. First edition 1600.*

See also under 1528. John Powell is not in the DNB.

SAMUEL ROWLANDS. *The letting of humours blood*. London. First edition 1600.* (5).

Entertaining, satirical work on the abuses of contemporary society. Samuel Rowlands (1570?-1630) was a voluminous writer of tracts in prose and verse.

JOHN TAVERNER. *Certaine experiments concerning fish and fruite*. London. First edition 1600.*

Gives a description of making a dam and references to counties which grow fruit and the use made of fruit by the poor. John Taverner is not in the DNB.

WILLIAM VAUGHAN. *Naturall and artificial directions for health*. London. First edition 1600.* (7).

Title indicates contents. William Vaughan (1577-1641) was not a physician. He is known for his promotion of settlements in Newfoundland.

1601

THOMAS WRIGHT. *The passiones of the minde*. London. First edition 1601. (5). The 1604* edition is used here. Title indicates content, which includes reference to both moral and physical effects of passions. Thomas Wright (*fl.* 1604), is described by the DNB as a protege of the 3rd Earl of Southampton. This Thomas Wright should not be confused with two other well known Thomas Wrights of the period.

1603

RICHARD GARDINER. *Profitable instructions for manuring, sowing and planting of kitchin gardens*. London. First edition 1603.*

The author intended this work to be "greatly for the help and comfort of poore people." Richard Gardiner is not in the DNB.

1604

ROBERT CAWDREY. *A table alphabeticall, conteyning, and teaching the true writing, and understanding of hard usuall English words*. First edition 1604.* (4).

Title indicates content. Listed as the first English dictionary by R.C. Alston, *Bibliography of the English Language*, Vol. V, 1966. Robert Cawdrey is not in the DNB.

KING JAMES I (of England). *A counter blaste to tobacco*. London. 1604.*

A number of editions were published with *The Essayes of a Prentise, in the Divine Art of Poesie*. King James I (1566-1625).

JAMES MANNING. *A new booke, intituled, I am for you all, Complexions castle*. Cambridge. First edition 1604.*

JAMES MANNING *(cont'd.)*
Gives advice about the complexions, including proper diet. Relates the time of
feeling pain to the planet in ascendency together with tables to show the cause.
James Manning is not in the DNB.
THOMAS WRIGHT. *The passions of the minde in generall.*
See above, 1601.
THOMAS WRIGHT. *Treatise occasioned by the death of Q. Elizabeth.* London.
First edition 1604.*
Title indicates content.

1605
PIERRE ERONDELL. *The French garden, being an instruction for attayning the
French tongue.* London. First edition 1605.* (2).
Title indicates content. Pierre Erondelle is referred to in the discussion of San-
lien's works by M. St. Clare Byrne, *The French Littleton,* 1953.

1606
G. BOTERO. *A treatise concerning the causes of magnificencie and greatnes of
cities.* London. First edition 1606.*
Translated by R. Peterson (*fl.* 1600), translator and member of Lincoln's Inn.
Giovanni Botero (1540-1617) was an Italian Jesuit political writer. Title indicates
content.
PIERRE CHARRON. *Of wisdom, three bookes.* London. First edition 1606.* (5).
Translated by Samson Lennard. Book I considers the natural parts of man; Book
II contains instruction and general rules for wisdom; Book III enumerates the
duties related to the four moral virtues of prudence, justice, fortitude, and tem-
perance. Pierre Charron (1541-1603) was a French author and moral sceptic.
Samson Lennard (d. 1633) was a genealogist and translator.
WILLIAM RAM. *Ram's little Dodoen.* London. First edition 1606.*
This is called a "briefe epitome of the new Herbal abbridged by W. Ram." Dodoens' work was earlier translated by Henry Lyte (see above, 1578). William Ram is
not in the DNB.

1607
HENRY CUFFE. *The differences of the ages of mans life.* London. First edition
1607.* (3).
Written in 1600. A general and philosophical discussion of the beginning and end-
ing of man's life. Henry Cuffe (1563-1601), author and politician, was executed
at Tyburn, a "base fellow by birth but a great scholar."
J. HARRINGTON. *The Englishmans doctor. Or the Schoole of Salerne.* London
1607.
This is Harrington's translation of *Regimen Sanitatis.* John Harrington,
Harington (1561-1612), a poet and miscellaneous writer, was godson to Queen
Elizabeth.
HUGH PLATT. *Certaine philosophical Preparations of Foode and Beverage for
Sea-men . . .*
Broadsheet; unique to the Library of the Wellcome Institute of the History of
Medicine. Advice intended for long voyages.

THOMAS WALKINGTON. *The opticke glasse of humours.* London. First edition 1607.* (3).
The subtitle of this work is "the touchstone of a golden temperature, or the Philosophers stone to make a golden temper." Thomas Walkington (d. 1621) was Vicar of Fulham in Middlesex, and author of religious works.

1608
N.F. *The husbandmans fruitfull Orchard.* London. First edition 1608. (2).
The 1608* edition is used here. On the gathering and keeping of fruit.
HUGH PLATT. *The Garden of Eden.* London. First edition 1608. (2).
The 1653* edition is used here. Also referred to as *Floraes Paradise.* Not in S.T.C.; is in Watt. Description of flowers and fruits then growing in England. A few vegetables are mentioned.

1609
SIMION GRAHAME. *The anatomie of humours.* London. First edition 1609.*
This work is severe, sarcastic, and melancholy. Chiefly occupied with the delineation of vice in all its varieties. See also R. Jameson, *The Anatomie of Humours,* Bannatyne Club, Edinburgh, 1830. Simion Grahame (c. 1570-?1614), little known, is described by Thomas Urquhart as a "great traveller and very good scholar," who became a Franciscan in the last years of his life.
MICHAEL SCOTUS. *The philosophers banquet.* London.
Translated by W.B. No copy of the first edition has been traced. The S.T.C. quotes the second edition of 1614.* Other authors have used parts of this work (see above, Thomas Twyne, 1538). Material taken from the works of the Arabs. Michael Scotus, Scott (1175?-1234?) was a mathematician, scholar, and physician attached to the court of Frederic II.

1610
WILLIAM CAMDEN. *Britain, or a chorographical description of England, Scotland and Ireland.* London. First edition 1610.* (4).
Translated by P. Holland. The 1630* edition is also used here. Title indicates content. William Camden (1551-1623), antiquary and historian, at one time held the office of Clarenceux king-of-arms. Philemon Holland, translator (1552-1637) studied at Cambridge and Oxford, obtaining his M.D. from another college. He settled in Coventry with a small medical practice, and chiefly translated the classics.

1612
JAMES GUILLIMEAU. *Child-birth or the Happy Delivery of Women.* London. First edition 1612.* (2).
Translator unknown. Bound in the British Museum edition (shelf no. 117-d-40) with *The Nursing of Children* also by Guillimeau. Jacques Guillemeau (d. 1609) was a celebrated medical man, surgeon to the king of France.
P. LOWE. *A discourse on chyrurgerie.*
See above, 1596.

1615
HELKIAH CROOKE. *Microsmographia, A description of the body of man.* London. First edition 1615. (2).
Title indicates content: Book III deals with nutrition. Helkiah Crooke (1576-1635) was Physician to James I.

1617
Regimen Sanitatis Salerni. London. First edition 1617.*
Translated by Philemon Holland. This edition gives the poem and commentary in English. See above, 1528.
WILLIAM LAWSON. *The Countrie Housewifes Garden.* London. First edition 1617.* (3).
Later published with *A new garden and orchard* (see below, 1618). This is an original work on the subject. William Lawson was a Yorkshireman, not in DNB.
FYNES MORYSON. *An itinerary written by F. Moryson, Gent.* London. First edition 1617.*
Descriptions of travels in twelve countries including England, Scotland and Ireland. Travels started in 1591. First written in Latin and then translated by Moryson. Fynes Morison (1566-1630), Gent. and traveller, gives truthful but unimaginative descriptions, and delights in listing distances and the value of coins.

1618
WILLIAM LAWSON. *A new orchard and garden.* London. First edition 1618. (10).
Title indicates content. See also E.S. Rohde, *A New Orchard and Garden*, 1927.

1621
ROBERT BURTON. *The anatomy of melancholy, what is is. With all the kindes etc.* First edition 1621.*
Twelve editions listed up to 1800. Modern edition consulted, Everyman Library, 1932, Nos. 886-888, introduction by Holbrook Jackson. Robert Burton (1577-1640), Vicar of St. Thomas', Oxford and then Rector of Seagrave.

1623
GERARD MALYNES. *The center of the circle of commerce.* London. First edition 1623.*
Concerned with the balance of trade and written as a refutation of a treatise written by Edward Musseldon. Gerard de Malynes (1586-1641) was a merchant and writer on economics.

1633
JAMES HART. ΚΛΙΝΙΚΗ *or the diet of the diseased.* London. First edition 1633.*
Title indicates content. James Hart (*fl.* 1633) was a physician, who also wrote on the Urines and denounced the "intrusion of parsons . . . upon the profession of phisicke."

NEMESIUS OF EMESA. *The nature of man.* London. First edition 1636.*
Translated by George Wither. This is the earliest English version, though there is a translation from Greek into Latin in 1564. For a discussion of the whole work see W. Telfer (ed.), *Cyril of Jerusalem and Nemesius of Emesa,* 1955. The book deals with the philosophy of the body and soul relationship. Nemesius of Emesa flourished 400 A.D. George Wither (1588-1667), a poet and pamphleteer, is given 20 columns in the DNB.

1652

NICHOLAS CULPEPER. *The English Physitian: or an Astrologo-physical Discourse of the Vulgar Herbs of this Nation.* London. First edition 1652.*
More than 100 editions printed. See also *The English Physician, enlarged . . . .* by Dr. Parkins, 1814.* Title indicates contents. N. Culpeper (1616-1654) was an astrological herbalist. Dr. Parkins is not in the DNB.

1655

THOMAS MOFFETT. *Health's Improvement: or the Rules Comprizing and Discovering the Nature, Method and Manner of Preparing all sorts of Food used in this Nation.* Corrected and enlarged by Christopher Bennett. London. First edition 1655 [probably compiled about 1595].
There is another edition (1746) with a preface by Mr. Oldys and an introduction by R. James M.D. Title indicates contents. Thomas Moffett (Moffat, Moufet, Muffet), 1553-1604, was a physician who studied at Cambridge, travelled and studied in Europe, obtaining his M.D. at Basle. He practised in Ipswich and London, and was one-time Physician to the Forces. He was a member of the College of Physicians, defender of Paracelsus, and a member of Parliament. His Latin works include a digest of Hippocrates. Christopher Bennett (1617-1655) was also a physician, and was Censor of the College of Physicians. He studied at Oxford and Cambridge and was the author of *Theatri Tabidorum Vestibulum,* in which he relied on observed cases and dissections rather than the authorities.

1659

EDMUND GAYTON. *The Art of Longevity or a Diateticall Institution.* London. First edition 1659.*
In verse. Title indicates content. Edmund Gayton (1608-1666), a writer and actor, once studied medicine.

1662

J. GRAUNT. *Natural and political observations mentioned in a following index and made upon the bills of mortality.* London. First edition 1662.* (6).
Title indicates content. This is the first work of its kind. J. Graunt (1620-1674) was a shopkeeper and Fellow of the Royal Society.
J.B. VAN HELMONT. *Oriatricke or Physick Refined.* London. First edition 1662.*
Translated by J. C[handler], who is not in the DNB. The book puts forward new theories in physick. John Baptista van Helmont (1577-1644).

1669
KENELM DIGBY. *The Closet of the Eminently Learned Sir Kenelme Digbie K^t opened.* London. First edition 1669.* (2).
Published by his son's consent. See also A. Macdonell (ed.), *The Closet of Sir Kenelm Digby Knight Opened,* 1910. Contains cookery recipes gathered up from his friends. Main interest is meade. Sir Kenelm Digby (1603-1665) was an author, naval commander, diplomatist, student of astrology and alchemy.

1699
J[OHN] E[VELYN]. *Acetaria. A discourse of Sallets.* London. First edition 1699.* Title indicates contents. John Evelyn (1620-1706) was a diarist and author of a celebrated work on sylviculture.

BOOK LIST
PRIMARY SOURCES: ALPHABETICAL LIST

The following alphabetical list of authors and translators, is intended as a supplement to the preceding section on primary source materials of the sixteenth and seventeenth century materials used in this study. The first date after each name is that of the first edition of their works as listed in the preceding chronological book list.

AGRIPPA, H. Cornelius, 1569
ALBERTUS MAGNUS [Pseudo], 1549
ALEXIS OF PIEMONT, 1558
ANDREW, Laurence, 1527
ARISTOTLE, 1528
ARISTOTLE (Pseudo), 1597
ARNALD OF VILLANOVA, 1540
ASCHAM, Anthony, 1550, 1552

B., J., 1598
B., T., 1586
B., W., 1609
BACON, Roger, 1530
BAILEY, Walter, 1586, 1588
BAKER, George, 1574, 1576
BAKER, Humphrey, 1568
BANISTER, John, 1578
BARKER, Christopher, 1575
BARROUGH, Philip, 1583
BARTHOLOMAEUS ANGLICUS, 1582
BATMAN, Stephen, 1582
BATTUS, Charles, 1599
BECON, Thomas, 1563
BELLOT, James, 1589
BERNARD, Saint, 1545
BERTHOLDUS, Andreas, 1587
BEZE, Théodore de, 1580
BILLINGSLEY, H., 1570
BLUNDEVILLE, Thomas, 1599
BOAISTUAU, Pierre, 1569
BOORDE, Andrew, 1540, 1542, 1547

BOSTOCK, Robert, 1585
BOTERO, Giovanni, 1606
BOURNE, William, 1574
BRASBRIDGE, Thomas, 1578
BRIGHT, Timothy, 1580, 1586, 1589
BULLEIN, William, 1558, 1564
BURTON, Robert, 1621
BUTTES, Henry, 1599

C.T., 1579
C.W., 1525.
CAIUS, John, 1552
CALDWELL, Richard, 1585
CAMDEN, William, 1610
CAREW, Richard, 1594
CARYE, Walter, 1583
CAWDRY, Robert, 1604
CHARRON, Pierre, 1606
CHURCHYARD, Thomas, 1593
CICERO, Marcus Tullius, 1569
CLEVER, William, 1590
CLOWES, William, 1579
COGAN, Thomas, 1584
COKE, John, 1550
COOPER, C., 1589
COOPER, T., 1548
COPELAND, Robert, 1528
COX, Leonard, 1524
CROOKE, Helkiah, 1615
CUFFE, Henry, 1607
CULPEPER, Nicholas, 1652
CUNNINGHAM, William, 1564

DAWSON, Thomas 1585, 1596
DEE, John, 1570
DIGBY, Kenelm, 1669
DODOENS, Rembert, 1578, 1606
DRUUMDE, Jonas, 1540
DUBRAVIUS, Janus, 1599
DU LAURENS, André, 1599

E., R., 1580
ELYOT, Thomas, 1531, 1536-1539, 1538, 1548
ENGLAND, Acts of the Privy Council, 1586
ENGLAND, Church of, 1563
ERONDELL, Pierre, 1605
ESTIENNE, Charles, 1600
EUCLID, 1570
EVELYN, John, 1699

F., N., 1608
FENTON, E., 1569
FERNEL, Jean, 1548, 1586
FIORAVANTI, Leonardo, 1579, 1580, 1582
FITZHERBERT, John, 1523
FOURESTIER, James, 1594
FRAMPTON, John, 1577
FUCHS, Leonard, 1562
FULLWOOD, William, 1562

GABELHOUER, Oswaldus, 1599
GALE, Thomas, 1563, 1586
GALEN, 1586
GARDINER, Richard, 1603
GAYTON, Edmund, 1659
GEMINUS, Thomas, 1553
GERARD, John, 1597
GESNER, Conrad, 1559, 1576
GOEUROT, Jehan, 1544
GOOGE, Barnabe, 1577, 1587
GRAHAME, Simion, 1609
GRATAROLUS, Gulielmus, 1562, 1574
GRAUNT, John, 1662
GREENE, Robert, 1591
GROCERS OF LONDON, 1592
GROSSETESTE, Robert, 1510
GUILLIMEAU, James, 1612
GYER, Nicholas, 1592

HAKE, Edward, 1574
HALES, John, 1530
HALL, John, 1565
HARRINGTON, John, 1607
HARRISON, William, 1577
HART, James, 1633
HELMONT, John Baptista van, 1662
HERESBACHIUS, Conradus, 1577
HESTER, John, 1580, 1582, 1594
HIERONYMUS VON BRAUNSCHWEIG, 1527, 1561
HILL, Thomas, 1563, 1568, 1576, 1586
HOLINGSHED, Raphael, 1577
HOLLAND, Philemon, 1610, 1617
HOLLYBUSH, John, 1561
HOLYBAND, Claude, 1576
HOWES, Edmund, 1592
HUARTE NAVARRO, Juan de Dios, 1594

JAMES I, King, 1604
JOHNSON, Christopher, 1577

JONAS, Richard, 1540
JONES, John, 1572, 1574, 1579

K., T., 1588
KELLWAYE, Simon, 1593

LANFRANCUS MEDIOLANESIS, 1565
LANGHAM, William, 1579
LANGTON, Christopher, 1547, 1550
LA PRIMAUDAYE, Pierre de, 1586
LAWSON, William, 1617, 1618
LEMNIUS, Levinus, 1565, 1576
LENNARD, Samson, 1606
LIEBAULT, Jean, 1600
LITURGIES, 1563
LLOYD, Humphry, 1551, 1573
LOWE, Peter, 1596
LUPTON, Thomas, 1579
LYTE, Henry 1578

MALYNES, Gerard de, 1623
MANNING, James, 1604
MASCALL, Leonard, 1572, 1581, 1587, 1590
MOFFATT, Thomas, 1655
MONARDES, Nicholas, 1577
MOORE, Philip, 1565
MORE, Thomas, 1551
MORUS, Horatius, 1585
MORWYNGE, Peter, 1559
MORYSINE, Richard, 1540
MORYSON, Fynes, 1617
MOSAN, Jacob, 1598
MOULTON, Thomas, 1539
MULCASTER, Richard, 1581

NEMESIUS OF EMESA, 1636
NEWTON, Thomas, 1565, 1569, 1574, 1580, 1586

PARTRIDGE, John, 1573
PAYNELL, Thomas, 1528, 1534, 1545
PETERSON, Robert, 1606
PETRUS HISPANUS, 1551
PHAER, Thomas, 1544, 1596
PLATT, Hugh, 1594 (two titles), 1596, 1607, 1608
PLUTARCH, 1530
POWELL, John, 1600
PRUDENS CHOISELAT, 1580

RAM, William, 1606
RECORDE, Robert, 1547
RHODES, Hugh, 1545
RIOLAN, Jean, 1586
ROBINSON, Ralphe, 1551
ROESSLIN, Eucharius, 1540
ROWLANDS, Samuel, 1600

S., W., 1581
SANFORD, James, 1569
SCHOLA SALERNITANA, 1528, 1617
SCHOLARS OF PADUA, 1586
SCOT, Reynolde, 1574
SCOTUS, Michael, 1609
SECURIS, John, 1566
SHUTE, John, 1563
SOUTHERNE, Edmund, 1593
STOCKWOOD, John, 1580
STOW, John, 1592
STUBBES, Philip, 1583
SURPHLET, Richard, 1599, 1600

T., A., 1596
TASSO, Torquato, 1588
TAVERNER, John, 1600
TRAHERON, Bartholomew, 1535, 1543
TURBERVILLE, George, 1575
TURNER, William, 1548, 1551, 1562, 1568
TUSSER, Thomas, 1557
TWYNE, Thomas, 1573, 1576

UDALL, Nicholas, 1553

VAUGHAN, William, 1600
VICARY, Thomas, 1577, 1585
VIGO, Joannes de, 1535, 1543
VIVES, Joannes Ludovicus, 1540

W., A., 1584
WALKINGTON, Thomas, 1607
WALTER OF HENLEY, 1510
WARD, William, 1558
WILKINSON, W., 1580
WINGFIELD, Henry, 1551
WIRTZUNG, Christopher, 1598
WITHER, George, 1636
WRIGHT, Thomas, 1601, 1604

BOOK LIST
SECONDARY SOURCES (18th-20th CENTURY)

ADAMSON, John William. *The Illiterate Anglo-Saxon,* Cambridge, 1946.

ADELMANN, H.P. *The Embryological Treatises of Hieronymous Fabricius of Aquapendente.* Ithaca, N.Y., 1942.

ADELMANN, H.P. *Marcello Malpighi and the Evolution of Embryology,* Ithaca, N.Y., 1966.

AEGINETA, Paulus (Translated by F. Adams). *The Seven Books of Paulus Aegineta,* 3 vols., London, 1884.

ALLISON, A.F. and D. M. ROGERS. *A Catalogue of Catholic Books in English, Printed Abroad or Secretly in England 1558-1640,* Bognor Regis, 1956.

ALLBUTT, T. Clifford. *Science and Medieval Thought,* London, 1901.

ALLBUTT, T. Clifford. *The Historical Relations of Medicine and Surgery to the End of the Sixteenth Century,* London, 1905.

ALLBUTT, T. Clifford. *Greek Medicine in Rome,* London, 1921.

ALSTON, C. (Published from manuscripts by John Hope). *Lectures on Materia Medica,* London, 1770.

ALSTON, R.C. *Bibliography of the English Language,* Vol. V, Leeds, 1966.

AMERINE, M.A., R.M. PANGBORNE and E.B. ROESSLER, *Principles of Sensory Evaluation of Food,* London, 1965.

AMHERST, Alicia. *A History of Gardening in England,* London, 1896. (First edition 1895)

ARBER, A. *Herbals Their Origin and Evolution,* Cambridge, 1938.

ARESTY, E.B. *The Delectable Past,* London, 1965.

ARISTOTLE (Edited by W.D. Ross). *The Works of Aristotle,* Oxford, 1908-1931.

ASHLEY, W. *The Bread of Our Forefathers,* Oxford, 1928.

AUSTEN, T. *Two Fifteenth Century Cookery Books,* London, 1888. (Early English Text Society, reprinted 1964)

AVICENNA (Translated and edited by O. Cameron Gruner). *A Treatise on the Cannon of Medicine of Avicenna,* London, 1930.

AYKROYD, W.R. *Sweet Malefactor,* London, 1967.

AYKROYD, W.R. *Conquest of Deficiency Diseases,* Geneva, 1970. (World Health Organization, Basic Study No. 24)

BABB, Laurence. *The Elizabethan Malady,* East Lansing, Mich., 1951.

BALLANTYNE, J.W. *The "Byrth of Mankynde." Its Author, Editions and Contents,* London, [1907].

BARBER, R. *Cooking and Recipes from Rome to the Renaissance,* London, 1973.

BATHO, G.R. *The Household Papers of the Ninth Earl of Northumberland,* London, 1962.

BEATON, G.H. and E.W. McHENRY, *Nutrition,* New York, 1964.

BEAUJOUAN, Guy. *Médecine Humaine et Vétérinaire à la Fin du Moyen Age,* Geneva, 1966.

BEETON, I. *Beeton's Book of Household Management,* London, 1861.

BEEUWKES, A.M., E. Neige TODHUNTER and E.S. WEIGLEY (Compilers). *Essays on the History of Nutrition and Dietetics,* Chicago, 1967.

BENNETT, H.S. *English Books and Readers 1475-1557,* Cambridge, 1952.

BENNETT, H.S. *English Books and Readers 1558-1603,* Cambridge, 1965.

BERNARD, Claude. *Introduction à l'étude de la médecine expérimentale,* Paris, 1865. Translated by H.C. Greene, *An Introduction to the Study of Experimental Medicine,* New York, 1949. (Life of Science Library Series)

BIBLIOGRAPHIE Gastronomique by G. Vicaire, London, 1954. (First edition 1890)

BICKERDYKE, J. *The Curiosities of Ale and Beer,* London, 1889. (Reprinted 1965)

BINDOFF, S.T. *Tudor England,* London, 1950. (Pelican No. 212)

BINDOFF, S.T., J. HURSTFIELD, and C.H. WILLIAMS. *Elizabethan Government and Society,* London, 1961.

BITTING, Katherine G. *Gastronomic Bibliography,* San Francisco, 1939.

BOHN, H.F. *A Handbook of Proverbs,* London, 1855.

BONSER, Wilfred. *The Medical Background of Anglo-Saxon England,* London, 1963.

BOORDE, A. (Edited F.J. Furnivall). *The Fyrste Boke of the Introduction of Knowledge Made by Andrew Borde,* London, 1870. (E.E.T.S. Extra Series No. 10)

BRIGHT, T. *A Treatise of Melancholie* (Reproduced from the 1586 edition with introduction by Hardin Craig), New York, 1940.

BROOKS, J.E. *Tobacco.* New York, 1937.

BROWNING, D.C. *The Dictionary of Quotations and Proverbs.* London, 1959.

BUNGE, G. (Translated by L.C. Woodridge). *Textbook of Physiological and Pathological Chemistry,* London, 1890.

BURNETT, J. *A History of the Cost of Living,* London, 1969. (Penguin Books)

CANDOLLE, A.P. de. *Origin of Cultivated Plants,* London, 1884.

CANNON, W.B. *The Wisdom of the Human Body,* New York, 1932.

CARPENTER, W.B. *Principles of Human Physiology,* London, 1855. (First edition 1843)

CELSUS (Translated by W.G. Spencer). *Celsus de Medicina,* London, 1935. (Loeb Classical Library)

CHEKE, Val. *The Story of Cheese-making in England,* London, 1959.

CHEYNE, George. *An Essay of Health and Long Life,* London, 1724.

CHITTENDEN, R.H. *Physiological Economy in Nutrition,* New York, 1904.

CHOLMELEY, H.P. *John of Goddesden and Rosa Medicinae,* Oxford, 1912.

CLAGETT, M. *Giovanni Marliani and late Medieval Physics,* New York, 1941.

CLAIR, C. *Of Herbs and Spices,* London, 1961.

CLAIR, C. *Kitchen and Table,* London, 1964.

COCKAYNE, T.O. *Leechdoms, Wortcunning and Starcraft of Early England,* London, 1961. (First edition 1864-66)

COPEMAN, W.S.C. *Doctors and Disease in Tudor Times,* London, 1960.

COPLESTON, F. *A History of Philosophy,* London, 1962.

CREIGHTON, C. *A History of Epidemics,* Cambridge, 1891-1894.

CRIPPS-DAY, F.H. *The Manor Farm,* London, 1931.

CRUICKSHANK, C.G. *Elizabeth's Army.* London, 1968. (second edition in Oxford paperback)

CULE, John. The Wreath on the Crown, Llandysul, 1967.

CULLEN, W. *Institutions of Medicine,* Edinburgh, 1785. (First edition 1772)

CULLEN, W. *First Lines of the Practice of Physic,* Edinburgh, 1786. (First edition 1774-86)

CULLEN, William. *A Treatise of the Materia Medica,* Edinburgh, 1789.

CULPEPPER, N. *The English Physician,* London, 1652.

CURRY, W.C. *Chaucer and the Medieval Sciences,* London, 1960.

DAVIDSON, S. and R. PASSMORE. *Human Nutrition and Dietetics,* Edinburgh, 1966 (3rd edition). (5th edition 1972)

DAWSON, W.L. *A Leech Book or Collection of Medicinal Recipes of the Fifteenth Century,* London, 1934.

DIGBY, Sir Kenelm (Edited by A. MacDonell). *The Closet of Sir Kenelm Digby Knight Opened,* London, 1910.

DEBUS, A.G. *The English Paracelsians,* London, 1965.

DE CANDOLLE, A.P. *Origin of Cultivated Plants,* London, 1884.

DIOSCORIDES (Edited by R.T. Gunther). *The Greek Herbal of Dioscorides,* Oxford, 1934.

DRUMMOND, J.C. and A. WILBRAHAM. *The Englishman's Food,* London, 1939. (2nd revised edition 1957)

DUFFY, P.H. *The Theory and Practice of Medicine in Elizabethan England as Illustrated by Certain Dramatic Texts.* Ph.D. Thesis, Harvard University, 1942.

DU LAURENS, A. *The Preservation of Sight* (facsimile and notes by Sanford V. Larkey), London, 1938.

DUREAU-LAPEYSONNIE, Jeanne Marie. (See under G. BEAUJOUAN)

EDELSTEIN, Ludwig. *Ancient Medicine.* Selected Papers (edited by Oswei and Lilian Temkin), Baltimore, 1967.

EDEN, F.E. *The State of the Poor,* London, 1797.

EDLIN, A. *A Treatise on the Art of Bread-making,* London, 1805.

ELGOOD, C. *A Medical History of Persia,* Cambridge, 1951.

ELYOT, Thomas (Edited by H.S.S. Croft). *The Boke named the Governour (by Thomas Elyot, London, 1531),* London, 1880.

EMMERSON, J.S. *Translations of Medical Classics,* Newcastle-upon-Tyne, 1965.

EMMISON, F.G. *Tudor Secretary,* London, 1961.

EMMISON, F.G. *Tudor Food and Pastimes,* London, 1964.

EMMISON, F.G. *Elizabethan Life: Disorder,* Chelmsford, 1970.

FABRICIUS. *The Embryological Treatises of Hieronymus Fabricius of Aqua-pendente.* (Translated with notes by H. P. Adelmann), Ithaca, N.Y., 1942.

FENN, W.O. and Herman RAHN (editors), *Handbook of Physiology,* Section II, Respiration, Vols. I and II, Washington, D.C. 1964.

FERRIERE-PERCY, H. de la (editor). *Lettres de Catherine de Médicis,* Paris, 1880.

FIGARD, L. *Un Médecin Philosophe au XVIe Siècle,* Paris, 1903.

FOOD and Agriculture Organisation of the United Nations. *Nutritional Studies No. 15.* Rome, 1957.

FOOD and Agriculture Organisation of the United Nations. *Nutrition and Working Efficiency,* Rome, 1962. (Freedom from Hunger Campaign Basic Study No. 5)

FRACASTORIUS, Hieronymous (Translated by W. Cave Wright). *Hieronymous Fracastorius , Contagion, Contagious Diseases and their Treatment,* N.Y., 1930.

FRENCH, R.V. *Nineteen Centuries of Drink in England,* London, c.1891.

FRERE, C.F. *A Proper Newe Booke of Cokerye,* Cambridge, 1913.

FURNIVALL, E.J. (Editor). *Early English Meals and Manners,* London, 1868.

FUSSELL, G.E. *The Old English Farming Books,* London, 1947.

GALDSTON, I. (Editor). *Human Nutrition Historic and Scientific,* New York, 1960.

GALEN (Translated by D.C.G. Kühn). *Opera Omnia*, 22 vols. (numbered as 20), Leipzig, 1821-33.

GALEN (Translated by C.H. Daremberg). *Oeuvres anatomiques physiologiques et médicales de Galien,* 2 vols., Paris, 1854-56.

GALEN (Edited by A.J. Brock). *Galen on the Natural Faculties,* London, 1916. (Loeb Classical Library)

GALEN (Translated by M.T. May). *Galen on the Usefulness of the Parts of the Body,* 2 vols., Ithaca, N.Y., 1968.

GASKINGS, Elizabeth. *Investigations into Generation,* London, 1967.

GAYRE, G.R. *Wassail! in Mazers of Mead,* London, 1948.

GLASSE, H. *The Art of Cookery, Made Plain and Easy,* London, 1760. (7th edition)

GOODFIELD, G.J. *The Growth of Scientific Physiology,* London, 1960.

GOODMAN, L.S. and A. GILMAN (Editors). *The Pharmacological Basis of Therapeutics,* New York, 1967.

GOUBERT, P. *Beauvais et les Bouvaiois de 1600 à 1730,* Paris, 1960.

GRAS, N.S.B. *The Evolution of the English Corn Market,* Cambridge, Mass., 1915.

GREAT BRITAIN, Ministry of Agriculture Fisheries and Food. *Household Food Consumption and Expenditure: 1970 and 1971.* A report of the National Food Survey Committee, London, 1973. (Reports have been made by this Committee since 1940)

GREAT BRITAIN, Dept. of Health and Social Security. *Recommended Intakes of Nutrients for the United Kingdom,* London, 1969.

GREAT BRITAIN, Dept. of Health and Social Security. *First Report by the Sub-Committee on Nutritional Surveillance,* London, 1973.

GREAT BRITAIN, Medical Research Council. *Report on the Present State of Knowledge of Accessory Food Factors (Vitamins),* London, 1924.

GREAT BRITAIN, Medical Research Council. *Vitamins: A Survey of Present Knowledge,* London, 1932.

GREAT BRITAIN, Poor Law Commissioners. *Second Annual Report,* London, 1836.

GREAT BRITAIN. *Fifth Report of the Medical Officer of Health to the Privy Council,* London, 1862.

GREAT BRITAIN. *Sixth Report of the Medical Officer of Health to the Privy Council,* London, 1864.

GRUNER, C.G. and H. HAESER. *Scriptores de Sudore Anglico Superstites,* Jena, 1847.

GUY DE CHAULIAC. *The Middle English Translation of Guy de Chauliac's Anatomy* (translated by B. Wallner), Lund, 1964.

HACKWOOD, F.W. *Good Cheer.* London, 1911.

HALL, Herbert. *Society in the Elizabethan Age,* London, 1886.

HALLIWELL, J.O. *A Dictionary of Archaic and Provincial Words,* London, 1825.

HAMPSON, E.M. *The Treatment of Poverty in Cambridgeshire 1597-1834,* Cambridge, 1949.

HARFORD, G. and M. STEVENSON (Editors). *The Prayer Book Dictionary,* London, 1925.

HARRISON, W. *Harrison's Description of England in Shakespeare's Youth* (ed. F. J. Furnival). London, 1877-1909.

HARTLEY, Dorothy. *Thomas Tusser – 1577,* London, 1931.

HARTLEY, Dorothy. *Food in England,* London, 1954.

HARVEY, William (Translated by Robert Willis). *Circulation of the Blood and Other Writings* London, 1952. (Everyman's Library No. 262)

HAYDN, J. (Revised by B. Vincent). *Haydn's Dictionary of Dates,* London, 1881.

HEATON, Nell. *The Complete Cook,* London, 1947.

HEMARDINQUER, J.-J. (Editor). *Pour une histoire de l'alimentation,* Paris, 1970.

HENDERSON, Alexander. *The History of Ancient and Modern Wines,* London, 1824.

HENTZER, Paul (Translated by R. Bently, Edited by Horace Walpole). *Journey into England in the year 1598,* London, 1757.

HERFORD, C.H. and P. SIMPSON. *Ben Jonson,* 2 vols., London, 1925.

HIPPOCRATES (Translated by E. Littré). *Oeuvres complètes d'Hippocrate,* 10 vols., Paris, 1839-1861.

HIPPOCRATES (Translated by Francis Adams). *The Genuine Works of Hippocrates,* London, 1849.

HIPPOCRATES (Translated by W.H.S. Jones). *Hippocrates,* Vols. I and IV, London, 1923 and 1931. (Loeb Classical Library)

HUNTER, R. and I. MacALPINE. *Three Hundred Years of Psychiatry 1535-1860,* London, 1963.

HUTCHISON, R. *Food and the Principles of Dietetics,* London, 1900. (First edition. The most recent edition - the 12th - has been revised by H.M. Sinclair and D.F. Hollingsworth, 1969)

JACKSON, B.D. *A Catalogue of Plants Cultivated in the Garden of John Gerard 1596-1599,* London, 1876.

JOHNSON, G.W. *History of Gardening,* London, 1829.

JOHNSON, W. *The Anatriptic Art,* London, 1866.

JONES, Paul V.B. *The Household of a Tudor Nobleman,* Urbana, Ill., 1917.

JORDAN, W.K. *Philanthropy in England 1480-1660,* London, 1959.

JORTIN, J. *The Life of Erasmus,* London, 1758-60.

KEEVIL, John Joyce. *Medicine and the Navy,* Edinburgh, 1957-63.

KEYS, Ancel et al. *The Biology of Human Starvation,* Minneapolis, 1950.

KINGSFORD, C.L. *Prejudice and Promise in 15th Century England,* Oxford, 1925.

KLIBANSKY, R., E. PANOFSKY and F. SAXL, *Saturn and Melancholy,* London, 1964.

KOCHER, P.H. *Science and Religion in Elizabethan England,* San Marino, Cal., 1953.

LABARGE, M.W. *A Baronial Household of the Thirteenth Century,* London, 1965.

LAMOND, E. (Editor). *A Discourse on the Common Weal of this Realm of England,* Cambridge, 1893.

LARKEY, Sandford V. *The Versalian Compendium of Geminus and Nicholas Udall's Translation,* ? 1933.

LAVOISIER, Antoine. *Traité élémentaire de Chimie, présenté dans un ordre nouveau et d'après les découvertes modernes,* Paris, 1789. (Translated by R. Kerr, *Elements of Chemistry,* 1790. Facsimile Dover Edition, 1965.)

LAWN, Brian. *The Salernitan Questions,* Oxford, 1963.

LEAGUE OF NATIONS. *The Relation of Nutrition to Health, Agriculture and Economic Policy,* Geneva, 1937.

LEES-MILNE, J. *Tudor Renaissance,* London, 1951.

LEHMBERG, Stanford E. *Sir Thomas Elyot Tudor Humanist,* Austin, Texas, 1960.

LEMERY, L. *Traité des Aliments,* Paris, 1702. (Translated by D. Hay, *A Treatise of All Sorts of Food,* London, 1745.)

LIEBIG, J. von (Translated by W. Gregory). *Animal Chemistry,* London, 1842. (Reprint with an Introduction by F. L. Holmes, New York, 1964)

LIND, J. (Edited by C.P. Stewart and D. Guthrie). *Lind's Treatise on Scurvy,* Edinburgh, 1953. (Reprinted with comments from *A Treatise of the Scurvy,* 1753)

LILLYWHITE, B. *London Coffee Houses,* London, 1963.

LODGE, B. *Palladius on Husbandry,* London, 1873. (Early English Text Society)

LOWTHER-CLARKE, W.K. (Editor). *Liturgy and Worship,* London, 1932.

MACKENZIE, James. *The History of Health and the Art of Preserving It,* Edinburgh, 1759. (2nd edition)

McCANCE, R.A. and E.M. WIDDOWSON. *Breads White and Brown,* London, 1956.

McCANCE, R.A. and E.M. WIDDOWSON. *The Composition of Foods,* London, 1967. (Prepared for the Medical Research Council, first edition 1939)

McDONALD, D. *Agricultural Writers 1200-1800,* London, 1908. (Reprinted New York, 1968)

McGRATH, P.H. *The Marketing of Food and Fodder in the London Area in the Seventeenth Century.* Unpublished M.A. Thesis, London University, 1948.

MEAD, W.E. *The English Medieval Feast,* London, 1931.

MENDELSOHN, Everett. *Heat and Life,* Cambridge, Mass., 1964.

MEYER-STIENER, Th. and Karl SUDHOFF. *Geschichte des Medizin im Uberblick mit Abfildungen,* Jena, 1928.

MOLESCHOTT, J. *Lehre der Nahrungsmittel für das Volk,* Erlangen, 1850. (The place of publication of this book is given as Stuttgart in some bibliographies)

MOLESCHOTT, J. *Physiologie der Nahrungsmittel: ein Handbuch der Diätetik,* Giessen, 1859. (2nd edition)

MONCKTON, H.A. *A History of English Ale and Beer,* London, 1966.

MULLINGER, J.B. *The University of Cambridge from the Earliest Times,* Cambridge, 1888.

MULTHAUF, R.P. *The Origins of Chemistry,* London, 1966.

NAPIER, Mrs. Alexander. *A Noble Boke off Cookry,* London, 1882.

NEEDHAM, J. *A History of Embryology,* Cambridge, 1959.

NICHOLS, John. *A Collection of Ordinances and Regulations for the Government of the Royal Household.....,* London, 1790. (For the Society of Antiquaries)

NICHOLS, John. *Illustration of the Manners and Expences of Antient Times in England,* London, 1797.

O'MALLEY, C.D. *Thomas Geminus Compendiosa totus anatomie delineato,* London, 1959.

O'MALLEY, C.D. *English Medical Humanists,* Lawrence, Kansas, 1965.

OXFORD, A.W. *English Cookery Books to the Year 1850,* London, 1915.

PAGEL, W. *The Religious and Philosophical Aspects of Van Helmont's Science and Medicine,* Baltimore, 1944.

PAGEL, W. *William Harvey's Biological Ideas,* Basle, 1967.

PALMER, H.R. *List of English Editions and Translations of Greek and Latin Classics, Printed before 1641,* London, 1911.

PARIS, J.A. *Elements of Medical Chemistry,* London, 1825.

PARIS, J.A. *A Treatise on Diet,* London, 1826.

PARKINS, "Dr." *The English Physician, an Improvement on Culpeper's Herbal,* London, 1814.

PARTINGTON, J.R. *A History of Chemistry,* London, 1970.

PASTON LETTERS, THE (Edited by J. Gairdner). London, 1904.

PAVEY, F.W. *A Treatise on Food and Dietetics,* London, 1875.

PEARSON, L.E. *Elizabethans at Home,* Stanford, California, 1967.

PEGGE, S. *The Forme of Cury,* London, 1780.

PENKETHMAN, J. *Authentic Accounts of the History and Price of Wheat, Bread, Malt etc.,* London, 1765.

PERCY, Thomas. *The Northumberland Household Book,* London, 1770.

PEREIRA, J. *A Treatise on Food and Diet,* London, 1843.

PEREIRA, J. *The Elements of Materia Medica,* London, 1854 (First edition 1839/40)

PHAIRE, Thomas. *The Boke of Chyldren* (Facsimile and notes by A.V. Neale and Hugh R.E. Wallis), Edinburgh, 1965.

PLATO. *Plato's Timeas* (Translated by F.M. Cornford, edited by Oskar Piest), New York, 1959.

POOLE, H. Edmund. *The Wisdom of Andrew Boorde,* Leicester, 1936.

POWER, E.E. *Peasant Life and Rural Conditions 1100-1500,* London, 1911.

POWER, E.E. *The Goodman of Paris,* London, 1928. (A translation of *Le Ménagier de Paris*)

POYNTER, F.N.L. (Editor). *The Evolution of Pharmacy in Britain,* London, 1965.

POYNTER, F.N.L. *A Bibliography of Gervase Markham, 1568?-1637,* Oxford, 1967.

PROTHERO, Rowland E. *English Farming Past and Present,* London, 1912.

PULLAR, P. *Consuming Passions,* London, 1970.

PUTNAM, G.H. *Books and Their Makers during the Middle Ages,* New York, 1896-97 (Reprint 1962)

QUETELET, A. *Sur l'homme, et le développement de ses facultés,* Paris, 1835. English translation ("under the superintendence of Dr. R. Knox,"), *Treatise on Man,* Edinburgh, 1842

QUINCY, J. *Pharmacopoeia Officinalis and Extemporanea,* London, 1718.

RAMAZZINI, Bernadino (Translated by W.C. Wright). *De Morbis Artificum (1713),* New York, 1940.

RATHER, L.J. *Mind and Body in Eighteenth Century Medicine,* London, 1965.

READ, Conyers. *Bibliography of British History: Tudor Period 1485-1603,* Oxford, 1959.

REGIMEN SANITATIS. Sir John Harrington's, *The School of Salernum* (Edited by F.R. Packard and F.H. Garrison), London, 1920.

REGIMEN SANITATIS. *The Englishman's Doctor or the Schoole of Salerne* (Edited by Alexander Croke), Oxford, 1830.

REGIMEN SANITATIS. *The Code of Health of the School of Salernum* (Edited by John Ordronaux), Philadelphia, 1870.

REGIMEN SANITATIS. *Regimen Sanitatis* (Edited by Cameron Gillies), Glasgow, 1911.

RHODE, E.S. *The Old English Herbals,* London, 1922. (Reprinted 1972)

ROGERS, J.E. Thorold. *A History of Agricultural Prices in England (from 1259-1793),* London, 1866-1903.

ROGERS, J.E. Thorold. *Six Centuries of Work and Wages,* London, 1884.

ROSS, David. *Aristotle,* Oxford, 1964 (University paperback).

ROSSI, Paolo (Translated by Sacha Rabinovitch). *Francis Bacon, From Magic to Science,* London, 1968.

RUBNER, M. *Die Gesetze des Energieverbrauchs bei der Ernährung,* Leipzig, 1902. Translated and reprinted by the United States Army Research Institute of

Environmental Medicine as *The Laws of Energy Consumption in Nutrition,* Natick, Mass., 1968.
RUFFHEAD, O. *Statutes at Large,* London, 1730.

SALAMAN, R.N. *The History and Social Influence of the Potato,* Cambridge, 1949.
SALTER, H.E. *Medieval Archives of the University of Oxford,* Oxford, 1920-21.
SCHOENHEIMER, R. *The Dynamic State of Body Constituents,* Cambridge, Mass., 1942.
SETON-WATSON, R.W. (Editor). *Tudor Studies,* London, 1924.
SHEPARD, O. *The Horn of the Unicorn,* London, 1930.
SHEPPARD, R. and E. NEWTON. *The Story of Bread,* London, 1957.
SHERRINGTON, C. *The Endeavour of Jean Fernel,* Cambridge, 1946.
SHREWSBURY, J.F.D. *A History of Bubonic Plague in the British Isles,* Cambridge, 1970.
SIMON, André L. *The Star Chamber Dinner Accounts,* London, 1959.
SIMON, J.F. (Translated by G.E. Day). *Animal Chemistry with Reference to the Physiology and Pathology of Man,* London, 1846.
SINGER, C., E.J. HOLMYARD, A.R. HALL and T.I. WILLIAMS (Editors). *A History of Technology,* 5 vols., Oxford, 1954-58.
SINGER, C. and E. Ashworth UNDERWOOD. *A Short History of Medicine,* Oxford, 1962 (2nd edition)
SINGER, D.W. and A. ANDERSON. *Catalogue of Latin and Vernacular Alchemical Manuscripts in Great Britain and Ireland Dating from before the XVI Century,* 3 vols., Brussels, 1928-31.
SINGER, D.W. and A. ANDERSON. *Catalogue of Latin and Vernacular Plague Texts in Great Britain and Eire Written before the Sixteenth Century,* Paris, 1950.
SKEAT, W.W. *Introduction to the Book of Husbandry,* London, 1882.
SMITH, Edward. *Foods,* London, 1883.
SMITH, F. *The Early History of Veterinary Literature and its British Development,* London, 1919.
SMITH, W. *Dictionary of Greek and Roman Biography and Mythology by Various Writers,* 2 vols., London, 1880.
SORANUS EPHESIUS. *Soranus' Gynecology* (Translated with an Introduction by O. Temkin), Baltimore, 1956.
STALEY, V. *Hierurgia Anglicana: Or Documents and Extracts Illustrative of the Ritual of the Church of England after the Reformation,* London, 1902-4.
STEELE, Robert. *Medieval Lore from Bartholomew Angelicus,* London, 1924.
STILL, G.F. *The History of Paediatrics,* London, 1965. (First edition 1941)
STONE, Lawrence. *The Crisis of the Aristocracy 1558-1641,* Oxford, 1965.
STONOR PAPERS, THE (Edited by C.L. Kingsford). London, 1919.
STORCK, J. and W.D. TEAGUE. *Flour for Man's Bread,* Minneapolis, 1952.
STRYPE, J. *Annals of the Reformation,* London, 1724-5.
STRYPE, John. *Memorials of Thomas Cranmer,* London, 1848. (First edition in the 16th century)

TALBOT, C.H. *Medicine in Medieval England*, London, 1967.

TAWNEY, R.H. *The Agrarian Problem in the Sixteenth Century*, London, 1912.

TAYLOR, Henry Osborn. *Greek Biology and Medicine*, London, [1922]

TAYLOR, Henry Osborn. *Thought and Expression in the Sixteenth Century*, New York, 1959. (First edition 1920)

TELFER, William (Editor). *Cyril of Jerusalem and Nemesius of Emesa*, London, 1955.

TEMKIN, O. *Galenism*, Ithaca, N.Y., 1973.

THEOPHRASTUS (Translated by A. Hart). *Enquiry into Plants*, London, 1916.

THIRSK, J. (Editor). *The Agrarian History of England and Wales (1500-1640)*, London, 1967, Vol. IV.

THOMPSON, Henry. *Food and Feeding*, London, 1894. (8th edition)

THORNDIKE, L. *A History of Magic and Experimental Science*, New York, 1941.

TILLYARD, E M.W. *The Elizabethan World Picture*, London, 1968.

TOMLINSON, C. *A Natural History of Common Salt*, London, 1968.

TRAILL, H.D. and J.S. Mann. *Social England*, 4 vols., London, 1901-4.

TROW-SMITH, R. *A History of British Livestock Husbandry to 1700*, London. 1957.

TURNER, Thomas Hudson. *Manners and Household Expenses of England in the 13th and 15th Centuries*, London, 1841.

TURNER, W. *A Book of Wines* (facsimile and notes by S.V. Larkey and P.M. Wagner), New York, 1941.

TURNER, W. *William Turner* (Facsimiles by the Ray Society, introductory matter by J. Britten, B. Daydon Jackson and W.T. Stearn), London, 1965.

UNITED STATES, Department of Agriculture. W.O. Atwater, "Chemistry and Economy of Food," *Bulletin No. 21*, Washington, D.C., 1895.

UNITED STATES, Food and Nutrition Board (National Research Council). *Recommended Dietary Allowances*, Washington, D.C., 1943.

VEITH, I. *Hysteria, History of a Disease*, Chicago, 1965.

WALTER OF HENLEY (Transcribed by E. Lamond). *Walter of Henley's Husbandry*, Cambridge, 1890.

WARNER, R. *Antiquitates Culinariae*, London, 1791.

WATT, Robert. *Bibliotheca Britannica: or a General Index to British and Foreign Literature*, Edinburgh, 1824.

WAY, A.S. *The Science of Dining*, London, 1936.

WEBB, Margaret. *Early English Recipes*, Cambridge, 1937.

WELCH, C. *The History of the Worshipful Company of Gardiners. . .*, London, 1900.

WELLCOME, Historical Medical Library. *Catalogue of Western Manuscripts on Medicine and Science*, London, 1962. (Compiled by S.A.J. Moorat.) (Wellcome Institute for the History of Medicine)

WHITNEY *Cookery Collection* (Compiled by Lewis M. Stark), New York Public Library, 1946.

WHYTEHORNE, Thomas (Edited by J.M. Osborn). *The Autobiography of Thomas Whytehorne,* Oxford, 1961.

WIGHTMAN, W.P.D. *Science and the Renaissance,* 2 vols., Edinburgh, 1962.

WILLAN, T.S. *Studies in Elizabethan Foreign Trade,* Manchester, 1959.

WILLAN, T.S. (Editor). *A Tudor Book of Rates,* Manchester, 1962.

WILLIAMS, C. (Translator). *Thomas Platter's Travels in England, 1599,* London, 1937.

WILSON, F.P. *The Plague in Shakespeare's London,* Oxford paperback 1963. (First edition 1927)

WITHINGTON, E.T. *Medical History from the Earliest Times,* London, 1964.

WOODFORDE, James (Edited by John Beresford). *The Diary of a Country Parson,* London, 1967. (World's Classics No. 514; first edition 1924-31).

WRIGHT, L.B. *Middleclass Culture in Elizabethan England,* Ithaca, N.Y., 1935.

WRIGHT, L.B. and Virginia A. LAMAR. *Life and Letters in Tudor and Stuart England,* Ithaca, N.Y., 1962.

WRIGHT, Thomas. *Popular Treatises on Science Written during the Middle Ages,* London, 1841.

WRIGHT, Thomas. *A History of Domestic Manners and Sentiments in England during the Middle Ages,* London, 1862.

INDEX

A

Abstinence, 122, 145

Activity, SEE Exercise

Acts, SEE Statutes

Admixtion, 67

Affections of the mind, SEE Emotions

Age, 40, 46, 57, 72, 108, 138, 143, 158, 174, 175

Agglutination, 67

Agriculture, 21, 39, 41, 193

Agricultural workers, SEE Labourers

Air, 22, 44, 49, 52, 74, 83, 84-87, 98

    Aetological agent, 84, 133

    As food, 86, 87

    Causes of bad, 84, 85

Alchemy, 18

Ale, 110, 119, 130, 131, 161, 176,178, 195, 211, 212, 213, 216-219, 221

    Ale-houses, 130, 131

Aliments, 99, 109

"Alimentary substances," SEE Nutrition

Almonds, 107

Allowances of Foods, SEE Intakes

Alteration, 65, 70, 71

Anadosis, 23

Anger, 80, 95, 96, SEE ALSO Emotions

Antiperistasis, 76, 80

Aphrodisiacs, 248, 268, 273

Appetite, 68, 69, 96, 127, 172, 189, 249, 278, 280

Apples, 110, 114, 143, 165, 195, 219, 220, 249, 252, 255, 257

Aqua vitae, 212, 221

Arteries, 46, 58

Articella, 34, 35, 72,

Assimilation, 66, 67

Assize of Bread, 197-198, 199, 200, 203, 207, SEE ALSO Statutes

Astrology, 18-19

Auction, 64, 65, 81

Authors, in the vernacular, 29-33

B

C

D

(Continues on next page)

F

Foods (Meats and Drinks), 24, 44, 46, 47, 66, 97, 99, 102, 123, 193-196, 288, 297

    CHARACTERISTICS OF: 47, 72
    Fattening, 128, 202, 204, 217
    Fine, 111, 116
    Gross, 111, 116
    "Making lean," 128, 206, 278
    Orders of, 101
    Particular groups and circumstances, SEE Diets
    Sequence to be taken, 183-189
    Valuation, criteria for, 99-116

    TYPES (main references only)
    Ale, 216-219
    Animals, parts of, 228, 230
    Beer, 216-219
    Bread, 197-209
    Cereals, 201-205
    Cheese, 241-243
    Cider (perry), 219-220
    Eggs, 236-238
    Fish, 230-232
    Flesh, 225-230
    Fruits, 248-250
    Herbs, 246-248
    Honey, 281-282
    Metheglyn, 220-221
    Sauces, 275-280
    Spices, 261-275
    Sugar, 280-282
    Water, 211, 212
    Whey, 211, 241
    Wine, 212-216

Formation, 65
Frications (Rubbings), 89, 91, 92
Fruits, 101, 102, 110, 112, 118, 134, 144, 147, 148, 161, 162, 173, 174, 186, 188, 195, 220, 245, 246, 247, 248-250, 253, 255, 258

G

Galenic theories, 21-24, 46-47
Galingale, 269, 271
Gall-bladder, 66
Game, 118
Gardening, 39, 246
Garlic, 100, 112, 113, 116, 128, 144-146, 152, 276, 279
Generation, 59, 64, 65, 81, 150
Ginger, 145, 220, 262, 269-271
Gluttony, 131, 181
Goats, 194, 226, 239
"Grains of Paradise," SEE Cardamon
Growth, 23, 64

H

Habits, SEE Custom
Hare, 104, 112, 227

O

P

(Continues on next page)

ILLUSTRATIONS

All the following (six) illustrations are by courtesy of the Trustees of the Wellcome Institute of the History of Medicine

ℭHereafter folo weth a compendyous Regyment or a dyetary of Helth, made in Mountpyllier, compyled by Andrew Boorde of Physycke doctour, dedycated to the armypotent Prynce, and valyaunt Lorde Thomas Duke of Northfolche.

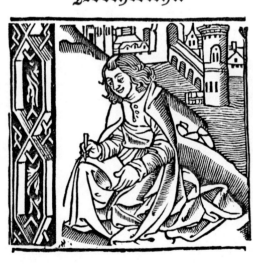

I. THE REGIMEN

From Boorde's *The Regimen or Dyetary of Helth*

Ariſtotle.

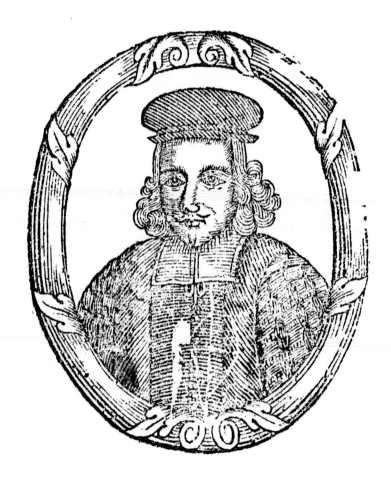

FAm'd *Ariſtotle*, who all Nature knew:

II. ARISTOTLE
From the Pseudo-Aristotelian *Secreta Secretorum*

III. ASSIZE OF BREAD

From the *Assize of Bread* 1600

❡ Here begynneth the Boke

named the Assyse of breade, what it ought to weye
after the pryce of a quarter of Wheete. And also the Assyse of Ale, with all maner of wood
and Cole, Lath, Bowrde, and tymbre, and
the weyght of Butter, and Chese.
❡ Imprynted by me Robert Wyer.

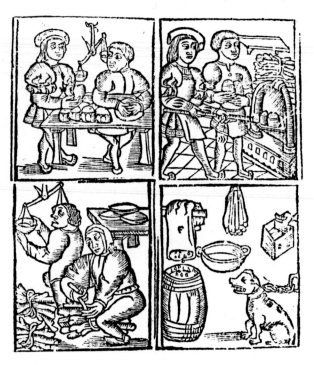

IV. ASSIZE OF BREAD

From the *Assize of Bread 1600*

¶There begynneth a newe tracte or treatyse moost profytable for all husbãde men/and very
frutefull for all other persones to rede newly cor-
recte & amended by the auctour/with dyuerse other
thynges added therunto.

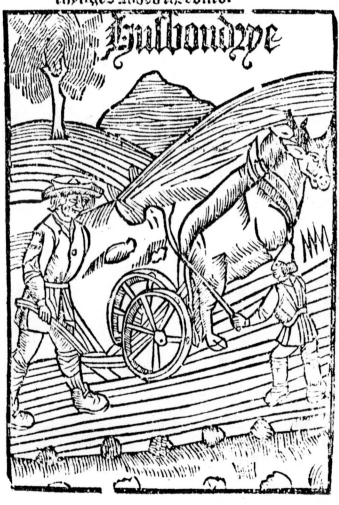

Husbandrye

V. HUSBANDRY
From Fitzherbert's *The Boke of Husbandrye*

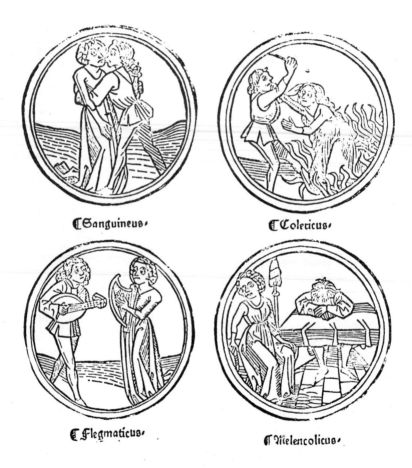

Sanguineus·   Colericus·

Flegmaticus·   Melencolicus·

VI. THE FOUR COMPLEXIONS

Adapted from the Augsburg Calendar